T0327540

# CLINICAL TRIAL DESIGN

# CLINICAL TRIAL DESIGN

## Bayesian and Frequentist Adaptive Methods

**Guosheng Yin**
The University of Hong Kong
The University of Texas M. D. Anderson Cancer Center

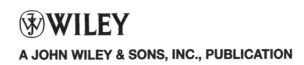

A JOHN WILEY & SONS, INC., PUBLICATION

*Library of Congress Cataloging-in-Publication Data:*

Yin, Guosheng.
  Clinical trial design: Bayesian and frequentist adaptive methods / Guosheng Yin.
     p. ; cm. — (Wiley series in probability and statistics)
  Includes bibliographical references and indexes.
  ISBN 978-0-470-58171-1 (cloth)
  I. Title. II. Series: Wiley series in probability and statistics.
  [DNLM: 1. Clinical Trials as Topic—methods. 2. Bayes Theorem. 3. Statistics as Topic—methods.
QV 771]
  LC-classification not assigned
  610.72'4—dc23                                                                    2011033589

10 9 8 7 6 5 4 3 2 1

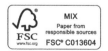

*To my mother and
the memory of my father*

# CONTENTS

# PREFACE

Drug development is a long-term, complex, and expensive process. Each new drug originates from basic biochemical research, moves on to laboratory experiments and animal studies, and eventually reaches clinical trials. Clinical trials are prospective studies of new interventions—such as experimental treatments, combination therapies, or medical devices with human subjects. The entire procedures of clinical trials are rigorously specified and controlled to reduce bias and errors. Clinical trials can generally be classified into four sequential phases: I, II, III, and IV. Phase I trials mainly focus on the safety and toxicity profile of the investigational compound. Once the new agent is considered tolerable, a phase II trial will be undertaken to examine the efficacious activities based on a short-term efficacy endpoint. If the test drug shows promising anti-disease effects, the study will then move forward to a large-scale phase III trial for confirmative evaluation of the drug's efficacy. If the new drug has successfully undergone extensive testing through phase I, II, and III trials, it will be filed to the regulatory authority (e.g., the United States Food and Drug Administration or the European Commission), for approval of widespread use in the general patient population. After the drug becomes available on the market, phase IV trials may be initiated to keep drugs' efficacy, toxicity, and rare side effects under long-term surveillance. New warning labels may be added to the prescription of the drug and, even more seriously, some drugs exhibiting unforeseen excessive toxicities could be withdrawn from the market.

Every clinical trial starts from the design and planning stage, moves to trial conduct and monitoring, and finally to the data analysis and conclusions; each step along the way calls for statistical methods. Without a good design and proper implementation, the trial could be a mess (e.g., leading to inconclusive or false findings), or even a disaster (e.g., causing an undesirably large number of patients to suffer from toxicity or death). Clinical trials should be efficient and ethical; for example, saving resources, benefiting more patients, drawing correct conclusions quicker, and resulting in less unnecessary toxicities. Well-designed and carefully carried-out clinical trials are the most powerful tools for new drugs' discovery. With a focus on the practicality, this book covers a wide range of statistical designs that are commonly used for each phase of clinical trials from both the Bayesian and frequentist perspectives. There has been great interest and extensive development in Bayesian adaptive designs, especially for early-phase clinical trials (i.e., phase I and phase II trials). Nevertheless, frequentist methods still dominate phase III trials by explicitly controlling the type I and type II errors in the hypothesis testing framework. Instead of biasing toward either Bayesian or frequentist methods, this book takes a pragmatic approach and introduces all clinical trial designs that are routinely used.

For beginners in this field, Chapters 1 and 2 provide an overview of the fundamentals of clinical trials and the related terminologies and concepts. For readers without a statistical background, Chapter 3 gives a brief introduction of basic knowledge of statistics including both Bayesian and frequentist estimation and inference procedures, with highlights on the key differences between the two. Chapters 4 through 6 discuss various Bayesian and frequentist designs and their statistical properties and operating characteristics for phase I, II, and III clinical trials, respectively. In particular, phase I and phase II trial designs are mainly based on Bayesian methods, due to small sample sizes in these early-phase studies. Chapters 4 and 5 also cover more advanced methodological development of early-phase trial designs, including Bayesian predictive probability trial monitoring, seamless phase I/II trial designs, and time-to-event toxicity and efficacy trade-offs. Chapter 6, which is dominated by frequentist approaches in the hypothesis testing framework, concentrates on power and sample size calculation for phase III clinical trials with continuous, dichotomous, and survival endpoints, respectively. Sample sizes may be calculated using fixed-sample designs, group sequential methods, or adaptively re-estimated in light of interim data. Noncompliance issues and intent-to-treat analysis are also discussed. In subsequent Chapters 7–10, more specific topics and more up-to-date developments in clinical trials are presented, such as Bayesian adaptive randomization, late-onset toxicity, dose finding in drug-combination studies, and targeted therapy designs.

The impetus of writing this book is to provide comprehensive and systematic coverage of statistical methodologies in clinical trial designs from practical perspectives. It may serve as a textbook for a graduate-level course and also as a reference for statisticians, medical doctors, research nurses, and other clinical trial practitioners, who are interested or involved in designing, conducting, and monitoring clinical trials. My goal is that readers would be able to design clinical trials for each phase on their own and would also understand and evaluate those designed by others. Many clinical trial designs and statistical methods discussed in this book are routinely used at the University of Texas M. D. Anderson Cancer Center and pharmaceutical industries. Most of the software used in this book can be freely downloaded from the website of the Department of Biostatistics at M. D. Anderson Cancer Center:

http://biostatistics.mdanderson.org/SoftwareDownload/

Approximately one-third of the book was written when I was Associate Professor in the Department of Biostatistics at M. D. Anderson Cancer Center, and the rest was finished after I joined the faculty of the Department of Statistics and Actuarial Science at the University of Hong Kong. I would like to express my sincere thanks and gratitude to my colleagues at both institutes for their enormous encouragement and support. In particular, I would like to thank Ying Yuan, J. Jack Lee, Donald Berry, Peter Müller, Peter Thall, Valen Johnson, Yu Shen, Jeffrey Morris, Bradley Carlin, Nan Chen, and Shurong Zheng for many insightful discussions on various issues arising in clinical trials and Bayesian adaptive designs, as well as Jianwen Cai, K. W. Ng, and W. K. Li for their consistent encouragement. Special thanks go to Lee Ann Chastain, Vicki Geall, Robert Golden, Guo-Liang Tian, Yuanshan Wu, and Jiajing Xu for proofreading, Susanne Steitz-Filler, Kristen Parrish, and Amy Hendrickson for editorial help, and all the students and colleagues who took my courses and workshops in this exciting area, which helped me to structure the book from the teaching materials. Finally, I would like to thank my mother, who has always encouraged me but eventually said to me "Son, don't write another book, this is too much work!" and also dedicate this book to the memory of my father; without their guidance, encouragement, and love in my life, this dream would never have come true.

GUOSHENG YIN

*Hong Kong, China; and Houston, USA*
*November, 2011*

# CHAPTER 1

# INTRODUCTION

## 1.1 WHAT ARE CLINICAL TRIALS?

Clinical trials are prospective intervention studies with human subjects to investigate experimental drugs, new treatments, medical devices, or clinical procedures, under rigorously specified conditions. Clinical trials play a critical role in drug development and pharmaceutical research. Conventionally, clinical trials are classified into four sequential phases: I, II, III, and IV. The trial design for each phase is a complicated process, which often requires close collaborations and joint efforts from many stakeholders, such as academic institutions, medical centers/hospitals, pharmaceutical companies, contract research organizations, government organizations (e.g., the National Institute of Health), and regulatory agencies (e.g, the Food and Drug Administration—FDA). From phase I to phase IV trials and from fixed to adaptive designs, all study procedures need to ensure consistency and validity of the findings. Every aspect of the trial design, every stage of the trial conduct, and every interim monitoring and data analysis call upon statistical methods. Therefore, the importance of statistics in the applications of clinical trials can never be overemphasized.

*Clinical Trial Design.* By Guosheng Yin
Copyright © 2012 John Wiley & Sons, Inc.

Before stepping into statistical methods for clinical trial designs, we first provide an overview of clinical trials. If a clinical trial does not involve a comparison treatment or if the patient enrollment and administration of comparison treatments are not concurrent such as use of historical controls, the trial is said to be *uncontrolled*. A *controlled* clinical trial may include an active control (the standard treatment) or a placebo (an inert that mimics the look and the route of administration of the real treatment) for direct comparison so that the difference in the clinical outcome attributable to the experimental therapy can be evaluated objectively.

A clinical trial is said to have internal validity if the observed difference between treatment groups is *real*, not confounded nor due to any bias or chance. Generally speaking, a randomized, double-blind (masking of the identity of treatment to both patients and clinicians), placebo-controlled trial possesses a high level of internal validity. External validity of a clinical trial refers to whether the study conclusions can be generalized to a broader population. The external validity of a trial would not be relevant if its internal validity is questionable. External validity may be enhanced by relaxing patient eligibility criteria.

Clinical trials are the most effective approach to examining and comparing treatment effects of experimental drugs, medical therapies, or any clinical intervention in human beings. A carefully thought-out, well-designed, and appropriately conducted and analyzed clinical trial is a powerful tool for new drug discovery and pharmaceutical development. Most importantly, the findings in clinical trials have a direct and enormous impact on clinical practice.

In a clinical trial, patients are accrued over time and followed prospectively. While participants may not necessarily enter the trial on the same calendar date due to staggered entry, they all progress from a well-defined baseline point by meeting the eligibility criteria of the study. Investigators must take full responsibility to inform the participants of all aspects of the trial—in particular, of the potential benefits and adverse effects of the new intervention.

## 1.2 BRIEF HISTORY AND ADAPTIVE DESIGNS

The *first* controlled clinical trial may be traced back to a study of investigating treatments for scurvy conducted by Lind (1753). In that study, twelve patients aboard the *Salisbury* at sea were divided into six groups, with two in each group. Patients were in similar conditions and had the same diet. Two of the patients were given a quart of cider a day; two took elixir of vitriol three times a day; two took two spoons of vinegar three times a day; the worst two patients were put under a course of seawater; two others had two oranges and one lemon a day; and the remaining two patients took nutmeg three times a day. The most sudden and visible good effects were perceived from the use of oranges and lemons; one of those who had taken them was fit for duty at the end of six days. Obviously, this scurvy study lacks some essential characteristics of modern clinical trials. For one, patients were not properly randomized; for example, the *worst* two patients were treated with seawater. Second, the study was not blinded or masked; that is, both patients and the investigator knew what treatment was used. As a result, there could be selection bias and other confounding effects in the scurvy study.

Early applications of randomization were in agriculture to study which fertilizers affected the great crop yields (Fisher, 1926). The field was divided into plots, and each plot was randomly assigned a specific fertilizer. The goal of randomization here is to obtain a valid test of significance through independent replications, whereas randomization used in clinical trials—for example, the streptomycin trial in pulmonary tuberculosis by Hill (Medical Research Council, 1948)—is to produce comparable groups so that patients in different groups are alike in all aspects except for the treatment. Randomization is essential in clinical trials to control known and unknown biases during patient selection, treatment allocation, outcome evaluation, and so on. Blinding provides another way of reducing the treatment-related bias by intentionally concealing the identity of treatments.

Traditionally, clinical trials are designed with fixed sample sizes and equal randomization (patients are allocated to each treatment with the same probability). This can be illustrated with the following phase III clinical trial of human immunodeficiency virus (HIV) type 1. It is known that maternal-to-infant transmission is the primary means for newborns infected with HIV. To evaluate whether the antiviral therapy zidovudine reduces the risk of maternal-to-infant HIV transmission, the Pediatric AIDS (acquired immune deficiency syndrome) Clinical Trials Group conducted a randomized, double-blind, placebo-controlled, multi-center trial to evaluate the efficacy and safety of the zidovudine regimen (Connor et al., 1994). The primary binary endpoint was whether the newborn infants were HIV-positive (with at least one positive HIV culture of peripheral-blood mononuclear cells). At the first interim analysis, 239 pregnant women received zidovudine and 238 received placebo through equal randomization between zidovudine and placebo, while 12 women withdrew from the study before delivery. Among 363 births with known HIV-infection status, there were 180 newborns in the zidovudine group with 13 infants HIV-positive and 183 in the placebo group with 40 HIV-positive. The interim result was very compelling: Zidovudine reduced the risk of maternal-to-infant HIV transmission by approximately two-thirds. This finding led to early termination of the trial, and the data and safety monitoring board recommended that the patient enrollment be discontinued and that all patients in the trial be offered zidovudine treatment. In a later updated analysis, 20 newborns were HIV-positive in the zidovudine group and 60 were in the placebo group (Zelen and Wei, 1995; Rosenberger, 1996). The results were indeed overwhelming. Had those 60 women with HIV-positive newborns in the placebo group been given zidovudine, many infants would have been saved. This trial reveals a limitation of equal randomization; that is, regardless of the accumulating evidence in the trial, patients are always equally allocated to the experimental treatment and control. By contrast, adaptive randomization, which tends to assign more patients to better treatments based on the accumulating data, may appear to be a more ethical approach.

In fact, adaptive randomization is just one aspect of adaptive designs; adaptations in clinical trials have many other features and meanings (Berry, 2006; Chow and Chang, 2006; Chang, 2008; Berry et al., 2010). In general, adaptive designs may allow trial early stopping for superiority, noninferiority, or futility; adaptive dose escalation/de-escalation or dose insertion in dose-finding studies; dropping or adding treatment arms; adaptive randomization, seamless phase I/II or phase II/III transition; extending accrual or sample size re-estimation; enriching a subpopulation; and so on. No matter how adaptations are undertaken, they all should be completely specified in advance of the trial, so that the type I error rate can be properly controlled. Adaptive clinical trials are much more challenging and demanding than traditional fixed-sample trials. This is true not only in the design stage, but also during the trial conduct. Adaptive designs often require an integrated multidisciplinary research team and the infrastructure to allow for more frequent interim data monitoring. In particular, patients must be examined and treated on the regular basis along with biomarker analysis. We also need to design and oversee the entire trial conduct, implement real-time adaptive randomization, and carry out timely interim analyses.

As an example, adaptation in a phase I dose-finding trial means to escalate or de-escalate the dose based on the accumulating toxicity data. Patients are enrolled sequentially over time and are treated in cohorts. At any time of the trial, a new cohort may be treated at a lower, a higher, or the same dose, depending on whether the current dose is considered overly toxic, safe, or appropriate. Decision making on dose assignment is frequent and spontaneous upon each new cohort's arrival. However, toxicity may be of late onset, such that the outcomes of previous patients are still not available when that information is needed for the next dose assignment. For example, in a dose-finding trial with the combination of oxaliplatin and gemcitabine along with concurrent radiation therapy, toxicity assessment required a nine-week follow-up, while the accrual was one patient every two weeks (Desai et al., 2007). Hence as a new patient entered the trial, some of the patients who had already been treated might have only been partially followed and their toxicity outcomes were missing. Such delayed outcomes inevitably pose great challenges to dose finding. More interestingly, that trial also raises a commonly encountered situation in which multiple therapies are combined for enhancing treatment synergistic effects. Here is another example of a drug-combination study: A seamlessly connected phase I/II trial evaluated both the safety and efficacy of the combination of decitabine and Ara-C in the treatment of acute myelogenous leukemia and myelodysplastic syndrome. Two doses of decitabine, two doses of Ara-C, and two treatment schedules were studied, which led to a total of eight different drug combinations.

## 1.3  MODERN CLINICAL TRIALS

Traditional cancer treatments, such as chemotherapies, take effect by impairing mitosis and act effectively on fast-dividing cancer cells. Unfortunately, these drugs (often known as cytotoxic agents) cannot discriminate fast-dividing normal cells and cancer cells and thus kill both blindly, which often results in substantial toxicity. Nowadays, with enormous expansion of our knowledge on the complex cancer pathways and networks, personalized medicine holds the most promise for the next generation of drug development. Targeted therapies are more specific toward certain disease pathways or inhibiting certain protein profiles. This type of agents utilize pathogenesis at a molecular level to differentiate patients who are more likely to respond from those who are not. Consequently, each patient is treated with individually tailored treatments. For example, imatinib (also called Gleevec) is highly effective in chronic myelogenous leukemia by inhibiting the BCR-ABL fusion protein that promotes cancer cell growth. This "wonder drug" works by seeking out and destroying cancer cells only, while leaving healthy cells virtually untouched. Another example is a monoclonal antibody, called trastuzumab with a trade name of Herceptin, which interferes with the human epidermal growth factor receptor 2 (HER2). Trastuzumab only works effectively in a subset of breast cancer patients with HER2 positive status. As the trend of personalized medicine grows, it is desirable to identify each patient's biomarker profile in order to provide the best available treatment accordingly (Lee, Gu, and Liu, 2010).

Although many new agents are waiting in the pipeline to be tested and a large number of biomarkers (e.g., molecular profiles or protein pathways) have shown promising evidence to be therapeutically useful, efficient diagnosis and treatment as well as biomarker validation have proven to be extremely difficult. To overcome the "biomarker barrier," Bayesian adaptive designs appear to be well-suited because they ideally adapt to information that accrues during the trial. In the modern era of clinical trials, the study design and trial conduct become more sophisticated than ever, which, in turn, demands more advanced and adaptive statistical methods. To appreciate the importance and complexity of the process, we present three recent high-profile clinical trials in the following.

The first trial is known as BATTLE (Biomarkers-Integrated Approaches of Targeted Therapy for Lung Cancer Elimination) at the University of Texas M. D. Anderson Cancer Center (Zhou et al., 2008). This umbrella study consisted of four parallel phase II trials for patients with advanced non-small-cell lung cancer (NSCLC). The trial assessed four targeted agents and four biomarkers simultaneously. Through timely tissue collection and biomarker analysis, BATTLE provided biomarker-based targeted therapies for NSCLC patients.

The statistical design of BATTLE is adaptive, flexible, and ethical. Based on Bayesian hierarchical modeling, the design enhanced borrowing information across different subtypes of biomarker groups. In addition, Bayesian adaptive randomization was used to favor treatments that were more likely to be effective during patient allocation. The trial continued to learn about treatment effects aligning with patients' biomarker profiles. The BATTLE design possesses many desirable operating characteristics, such as

- selecting effective drugs with high probabilities and ineffective drugs with low probabilities;

- treating more patients with more effective drugs according to their tumor biomarker profiles; and

- dropping inefficacious arms with high probabilities based on an early stopping rule.

In conjunction with an early stopping rule, Bayesian adaptive randomization appears to be a rational and smart choice for treating patients and underpinning effective treatments. As a follow-up study, BATTLE 2 is under the way.

Second, we introduce the highly anticipated multi-agent trial, called I-SPY 2 (Investigation of Serial Studies to Predict Your Therapeutic Response with Imaging and Molecular Analysis 2). This is an adaptive neoadjuvant phase II trial for women with newly diagnosed locally advanced breast cancer (Barker et al., 2009). The goal is to examine whether combinations of investigational drugs targeting molecular pathways with standard chemotherapy are better than standard chemotherapy alone. I-SPY 2 evolves from I-SPY 1, which has built an infrastructure to integrate enormous amounts of complex and disparate data from many resources and to facilitate real-time adaptive learning.

The standard biomarkers in I-SPY 2 are hormone receptor, HER2, and MammaPrint, while many other exploratory biomarkers are also involved. Based on practical and clinical relevance, the number of biomarker groups is narrowed down to ten for identifying molecularly tailored treatments. The standard neoadjuvant chemotherapy regimen include weekly paclitaxel (plus trastuzumab for HER2+ patients) followed by doxorubicin and cyclophosphamide. At any time of the trial, up to five novel targeted agents are investigated simultaneously, with the standard therapy added to each.

The primary endpoint in I-SPY 2 is pathologic complete response (pCR) at the six-month follow-up. Patients in each subgroup are adaptively assigned to the treatments that are believed to benefit them the most. However, potentially delayed outcomes may hamper the real-time implementation of adaptive randomization. To overcome this difficulty, the statistical design provides joint modeling of some surrogate endpoints and pCR. For each biomarker signature, the trial continuously updates drugs' predictive probabilities of success in a phase III trial and, consequently, decisions are made on whether an experimental treatment should

- graduate along with the corresponding biomarker signature and move forward to a more informed phase III trial,

- be dropped for futility, or

- continue for further evaluation after accruing more information.

During the trial, new drugs may be added to replace those that have either graduated or been dropped. Unlike the BATTLE trial which considered four fixed therapies, I-SPY 2, being "more" adaptive, allows treatments to "come and go" as the trial progresses.

At last, IPASS (Iressa Pan Asia Study) is a phase III trial to compare oral gefitinib (commonly known as Iressa) monotherapy with intravenous carboplatin and paclitaxel chemotherapy as first-line treatment in chemotherapy-naive Asian patients with advanced NSCLC (Mok et al., 2009). Prior to the IPASS study, there have been several randomized, controlled phase III trials of the epidermal growth factor receptor (EGFR) tyrosine kinase inhibitors for NSCLC treatment, but the results were confusing with some positive and some negative findings (Saijo, Takeuchi, and Kunitoh, 2009).

From a more selective patient population, IPASS enrolled a total of 1,217 patients from Asian countries and equally randomized them to gefitinib or chemotherapy (the combination of carboplatin and paclitaxel). The primary endpoint of IPASS was progression-free survival, and the primary objective of the study was the noninferiority of gefitinib to chemotherapy. Not only the trial concluded the noninferiority of gefitinib, but also demonstrated its superiority over chemotherapy. An interestingly finding was that the survival curves of the two treatment groups crossed at month six, favoring chemotherapy during the first six months and gefitinib thereafter. This suggested that patients could be a mixture of two possible subpopulations that were differentially responsive to the molecular-targeted therapy and cytotoxic agents. Further biomarker analyses showed that patients with EGFR mutations had longer progression-free survival in the gefitinib arm, while patients with wild-type EGFR had longer survival in the chemotherapy arm.

Following the findings of the IPASS study, European Commission granted the marketing authorization for Iressa as treatment of adults with locally advanced or metastatic NSCLC with an EGFR mutation. The endorsement of Iressa's use in a subset of NSCLC patients reflects the growing importance of personalized treatment.

## 1.4  NEW DRUG DEVELOPMENT

Before any further discussion on new drug development, it is important to make a distinction between different types of agents. First of all, most of the oncology drugs are cytotoxic agents, which damage or destroy rapidly growing cancer cells. For example, carboplatin and paclitaxel typically shrink the tumor in a dose-dependent manner: A higher dose would result in more shrinkage of the tumor. The second type of agents are cytostatic; many targeted therapies belong to this family, and they are often directed at molecular targets to inhibit tumor growth or prevent the proliferation of cancer cells (Korn, 2004). Patients may benefit from cytostatic agents even without explicitly shrinking the tumor. For cytostatic agents, lower doses may be as effective as higher doses. For example, a tyrosine kinase inhibitor, lapatinib, specifically targets HER2+ in breast cancer patients. In the treatment of lung cancer, gefitinib prevents cancer cells from growing and multiplying by targeting EGFR through the disruption of EGFR signal transduction for cell division, apoptosis, and angiogenesis. Finally as the third type, biologic agents are substances from a living organism, such as interleukins and vaccines, which are often used in the prevention, diagnosis, or treatment of cancer and other diseases.

For illustration, we describe the intuition behind the four successive phases of clinical trials using cancer drug development as an example. Before initiating a clinical trial for a new chemical compound, extensive preclinical studies must have been carried out. In preclinical settings, *in vitro* (within a controlled environment—e.g., on glass slides or in test tubes) and *in vivo* studies (within a living organism, such as rodents) are performed to test a wide range of doses of the experimental agent. These cell-line and animal experiments mainly provide the preliminary toxicity and efficacy data, along with pharmacokinetics (PK) and pharmacodynamics (PD) information. PK refers to how the body processes the drug, characterizing the relationship between the dosage regimen and the drug concentration in the blood over time; PD studies how the drug works in the body by modeling the relationship between the drug concentration-time profile and therapeutic and adverse effects.

Suppose that laboratory scientists conducted extensive basic research in biochemistry and identified a new chemical compound that appears to be promising to eradicate cancer cells. Every drug comes with certain amount of risk. This chemical compound has never been tested in human subjects; thus the first task is to examine whether the new drug can be tolerated by human beings. We may be willing to accept a certain level of toxicity if the drug's therapeutic benefits outweigh its adverse effects. This is particularly sensible with cancer drugs, because they often induce various levels of toxicity and adverse events.

As the first human study, a phase I clinical trial is launched to investigate the toxicity and side effects of the new agent on a small number of cancer patients. Often these patients are disease-relapsed or refractory to standard treatments, and sometimes there is no other better treatment option for them. In oncology, the goal of a typical phase I trial is to identify the maximum tolerated dose (MTD) and evaluate the drug's dose-limiting toxicities. The MTD is defined as the dose that has a toxicity probability closest to the maximally tolerable level predetermined by the investigator. It is common to assume that both toxicity and efficacy effects of the drug increase as the dose increases. Thus a set of doses of the new drug is explored to find the most toxic dose (presumably also the most therapeutically effective) that can be reasonably tolerated by patients. In a dose-finding study, there is a trade-off between toxicity and efficacy. If the trial design is too conservative, the amount of the dosage may not be sufficient to fully impart the drug's therapeutic effects; however, if the design is too aggressive, the administered dose may be too much to tolerate, and thus the study may result in excessive toxicity, or even death.

After the MTD of the new drug is determined, the next step is to assess whether the drug has sufficient biologic activity in opposition to the disease. For this purpose, a phase II clinical trial is undertaken, in which the drug is often administered at the MTD or the dose immediately lower than the MTD (sometimes called the recommended phase II dose—RP2D). The MTD is the highest dose that can still be tolerated, while use of the RP2D is a more conservative approach. Phase II is a "proof-of-concept" stage, which examines the drug's short-term therapeutic effects and also continues monitoring severe adverse events. Nonworking or unsafe drugs should be "killed" as early as possible. Phase II trials often use a "quick" endpoint to guard the door so that drugs of little therapeutic effects will be blocked out. Once a phase II trial is completed, a decision is made on whether the drug is promising to warrant further investigation. At this stage, compounds found to be ineffective or unsafe should be dropped to avoid wasting more resources.

If a new drug successfully passes through the phase II testing, it will be moved forward to a phase III trial for definitive comparison with the current standard treatment or placebo. Phase III trials are large-scale and long-term randomized studies that may involve hundreds or even thousands of patients. If the drug is proven to be truly effective in such confirmative trials (typically two separate positive phase III trials are required for FDA approval), it will be filed to the regulatory agency for authorization of marketing. If granted approval, the drug prescription will be available to the general patient population in public.

Due to the restrictive eligibility criteria and rigorously specified conditions in phases I–III trials, some rare but serious adverse effects of the drug might not have been surfaced in the previous studies. Hence after the approval, a phase IV trial may be launched with more relaxed eligibility criteria, which will follow a larger number of patients over a much longer period of time. It provides an opportunity to learn more about rare side effects of the approved agent and its interaction with other treatments. Sometimes the findings in a phase IV trial may add a warning label to the drug, or even result in the removal of a drug from the market due to severe adverse events that were unforeseen when the drug was approved.

Conventionally, these four phases of trials are conducted sequentially and separately without any kind of formal borrowing information or strength across them. Each trial, regardless of the phase, requires an independent study design and a completely separate protocol for its own. There is typically a gap between two consecutive phases because it takes time and effort to complete and analyze the previous trial and also to initiate a new trial. Nevertheless, there is an increasing trend of combining phase I and phase II trials—seamless phase I/II trials, and combining phase II and phase III trials—seamless phase II/III trials, in order to expedite the drug development process.

## 1.5   EMERGING CHALLENGES

New drug development, especially in oncology, is becoming a daunting task that requires prohibitive expenditures of time and cost. Although these days much more resources have been devoted to research and development in pharmaceutical industries, fewer drugs make it to the market: Compounds entering phase I trials ultimately approved for sale are about 5% only. Nowadays, on average the number of enrollment criteria has dramatically increased. As a consequence, it becomes more difficult to accrue patients, which, in turn, means that a trial often takes far longer to complete. Moreover, much more medical procedures, such as blood tests or electrocardiograms, are performed on participants for extracting as much information as possible. These changes may be partly due to more complex diseases being tackled in company with the knowledge explosion in genomics. Indeed, clinical trials are becoming more and more complicated and difficult. Every trial has some characteristics unique to itself, albeit the oversimplification of four sequential phases in the conventional setting. There is no shoe that fits all. Therefore, from statistical perspectives, we cannot be more careful, thorough, quantitative, and analytical than ever.

There has been debating about whether clinical trials are being too restrictive to reflect the complexity and diversity of actual clinical practice. It is true that clinical trials must follow strictly specified study conditions and enrollment criteria. By contrast, pragmatic trials are designed and conducted in a more practical way to answer the real questions facing patients and clinicians (Ware and Hamel, 2011). These trials are more relevant to real-world practice and therefore represent less-perfect experiments than the standard randomized controlled trials. The internal validity of pragmatic trials is compromised to achieve higher generalizability. Although randomized controlled trials have limited relevance to clinical practice due to homogeneous patients, carefully defined treatments, double blinding, and rigorous follow-ups and medical exams, they remain as the gold standard approach to examining the benefits and harms of medical interventions.

## 1.6   SUMMARY

In the chapters that follow, we will cover the most commonly used statistical methods for designing clinical trials of each phase. Irrespective of Bayesian or frequentist points of view, we take a practical perspective and introduce various adaptive methods for designing and monitoring clinical trials. Here "adaptive" has a very broad meaning, which includes adaptive dose-finding methods (determining each dose assignment based on the outcomes of previous patients), trial early stopping due to futility or efficacy, dropping or adding an arm if necessary, group sequential methods, sample size re-estimation, adaptive randomization (either covariate-adaptive to balance prognostic factors or response-adaptive to assign more patients to better treatments), enrichment designs to enhance homogeneity of patients, and so on. Adaptation is not exclusively bonded with either Bayesian or frequentist approaches; both can be adaptive.

The remainder of the book is organized as follows. Chapter 2 presents the fundamental concepts and structures of clinical trials. To build the foundation, Chapter 3 introduces both frequentist and Bayesian estimation and inference procedures, and we put an emphasis on the main differences between the two schools of thoughts. Chapters 4 and 5 cover phase I and phase II trial designs, respectively; and most of the statistical methods in these early-phase trials are Bayesian flavored (Biswas et al., 2009; Yin and Yuan, 2010a). This is mainly due to the flexibility of Bayesian adaptive designs and the limited resources and small sample sizes in early-phase trials. Chapter 6 is dominated by frequentist sample size and power calculations in the hypothesis testing framework. Chapter 7 discusses all kinds of randomization procedures and, more importantly, adaptive randomization. Chapter 8 focuses on dose finding with late-onset toxicity (delayed outcomes) and Chapter 9 introduces Bayesian adaptive dose-finding methods for drug-combination trials. With the ground-breaking concept of personalized medicine, prediction and validation of biomarkers for therapeutical use become increasingly important, for which Chapter 10 covers the most updated development in targeted therapy designs. Most of the trial examples in the book were designed at the University of Texas M. D. Anderson Cancer Center. Although we introduce clinical trial design methodologies mainly on the basis of oncology trials, these statistical techniques can also be applied to other disease areas.

**CHAPTER 2**

# FUNDAMENTALS OF CLINICAL TRIALS

## 2.1 KEY COMPONENTS OF CLINICAL TRIALS

For a better understanding of the statistical issues arising from clinical trials, we first introduce necessary concepts and key components that are essential to clinical trial designs in this section. We then give a brief discussion on pharmacokinetics and pharmacodynamics modeling, as well as the intuition behind phase I–IV clinical trials.

## 2.1.1 Protocol

Every clinical trial comes with a study protocol. The protocol is a document that provides a comprehensive description of the entire study. In particular, it includes the general information and background of the disease or condition to be treated, the intervention to be used, the study objectives and rationale, the procedures to assess drugs' efficacy and safety, and the statistical design and methodology (often known as the statistical considerations). The protocol should also describe the known and potential risks and benefits of the treatment to human subjects, the target patient population, the current standard of care, the route of drug administration, and treatment dosages and schedules.

The study protocol may be viewed as a written agreement between the investigators, the trial participants, and the scientific community at large. It is the single document that specifies the detailed research plan and lays out the schematic diagram and organization for the trial. The contents of a protocol are typically confidential, and may contain the following items:

(1)   introduction and rationale;

(2)   study objectives, including primary and secondary aims;

(3)   overall study design and experimental plan;

(4)   patient population and enrollment criteria;

(5)   specific treatment procedures, such as randomization, intervention, outcome measurement, and possible protocol deviations;

(6)   statistical considerations;

(7)   safety data collection and reporting; and

(8)   regulatory, administrative, and legal obligations.

When composing a protocol, all of the issues related to the trial design must be taken into consideration, such as the availability of the drug, the starting time of the trial, the duration of the intervention, needs for special tests or laboratory facilities, and logistics of blinding and randomization. The protocol is a quality control tool for a clinical trial, and the trial conduct should follow the protocol as closely as possible. This is especially important for a multi-center study, in which collaborators from different institutions must all follow a centralized written document.

Statistical considerations in the protocol must ensure the integrity of the trial design. This is the statistical section that specifies the sample size; the probability model; efficacy and toxicity monitoring; stopping rules for superiority, futility, and safety; statistical methods and schedules for analyzing the interim data; the selection of subjects to be included in the analyses; and procedures for assessing any deviations from the original study plan. If any change is made to a protocol, an amendment needs to be added.

Nearly every clinical trial experiences violations of the protocol to some extent. This may be caused by misinterpretation or misunderstanding of some terminologies used in the protocol, or by carelessness or unforeseen circumstances during the trial conduct. Some protocol deviations are inconsequential, but others may have severe effects on the validity of the trial, or even alter the conclusions of the study. Deviations from the protocol should be minimized and their effects on the study findings need to be thoroughly examined.

### 2.1.2 Primary Objective

In general, a clinical trial contains one primary objective and possibly several secondary objectives. All of the objectives must be feasible and clinically meaningful. The primary objective of a clinical trial is the main question that the investigators are most interested in, and the trial should be able to adequately address at its conclusion. The main question needs to be carefully chosen and clearly stated in advance. It is the question on which statistical considerations are centered and sample size computations are based. The secondary objectives are subsidiary questions that are related to the primary one, which may provide additional information on the drug use.

**EXAMPLE 2.1**

In a phase I trial for patients with acute myelogenous leukemia, the primary objective was to determine the maximum tolerated dose (MTD) and the associated dose schedule for a new drug. The secondary objectives included: to characterize the dose-limiting toxicities (DLTs) and the overall safety profile of escalated doses of the drug, to determine the pharmacokinetic parameters and the pharmacodynamic effects, and to assess clinical responses and symptomatic improvement, if any.

The objectives of clinical trials in different phases could be very different, but those in the same phase are more or less similar although still depending on each individual study. As seen in Example 2.1, phase I oncology trials are typically dose-finding studies to identify the MTD of the new agent. On the other hand, phase II trials often aim to evaluate the short-term efficacy of the experimental treatment. In the following example of a phase III clinical trial, the primary goal is to compare patients' survival across different treatment groups.

**EXAMPLE 2.2**

In a phase III trial for patients with HER2 overexpressing advanced or metastatic breast cancer, the primary objective was to evaluate and compare the time to disease progression (i.e., progression-free survival) between an experimental arm and a control arm. Secondary objectives included examining the two treatments with respect to the overall response rate, clinical benefit, time to response, duration of response, and overall survival.

### 2.1.3 Eligibility Criteria and Accrual

Defining the study population is an integral part of posing the primary question in a trial planning stage. The study population is a subset of the general population, which should be defined in advance with unambiguous inclusion or eligibility criteria. We must take into consideration the impact that these criteria will have on the study design, feasibility, and recruitment.

Eligibility criteria are tied with patient safety and the anticipated effects of the intervention. Participants defined in the inclusion criteria of a trial should be those who have the potential to benefit from the intervention and who are likely to adhere to the study protocol. Patients who may be harmed by the intervention must be excluded, and those at a high risk of developing conditions that would prelude the ascertainment of an event of interest should also be excluded.

Due to staggered entry, patients enter the trial at different calendar times. Since all participants must meet the eligibility criteria to enter the trial, they have similar baseline status—that is, the disease and health conditions prior to the initiation of an intervention. All the relevant baseline data should be measured and collected from each subject. Patients in different treatment arms should be comparable with respect to the baseline measurements, including prognostic factors, pertinent demographic and socioeconomic characteristics, and medical history.

Often recruiting a sufficient number of patients in a reasonable period of time is one of the most challenging tasks in a clinical trial. Successful recruitment relies upon devoting extra efforts, maintaining flexibility, and establishing interim goals. Options when the accrual falls short include:

- accepting a smaller number of patients than originally planned,

- relaxing the inclusion criteria,

- extending the time frame for recruitment, and

- adding more recruiting centers in a multi-center study.

A multi-center trial requires collaborative efforts from different institutions to enroll and follow study subjects. Conducting the same trial at multiple centers helps to recruit an adequate number of participants within a reasonable time, and also to assure a more representative sample of the target population. Moreover, investigators with similar research interests and skills can work together on a common problem and share resources.

### 2.1.4 Power and Sample Size

Calculation of the sample size with provision for an appropriate level of significance and power is an essential part of clinical trial planning. The design parameters, such as the effect size including the expected treatment difference and the associated variance, may be obtained from previous studies or expert opinions. Clinical trials should control the type I error to prevent false-positive results and also should have sufficient statistical power to detect the treatment difference considered to be of clinical interest. The primary response variable which characterizes the effectiveness of the intervention must be clearly identified. The endpoint may be dichotomous (whether a patient has responded to treatment or not), continuous (e.g., measuring blood pressures, cholesterol levels, or some biomarker expression), or time-to-event (progression-free survival or overall survival). Different types of endpoints require different statistical methods for sample size calculation.

No matter how thoroughly and rigorously a trial is designed, unexpected events may occur during the trial conduct. For example, the trial may indicate greater-than-expected beneficial effects of the study drug, so that the experimental treatment should be short-tracked to the FDA for approval; or it may become clear in the middle of a trial that it will be impossible to reach a statistically significant difference by the end of the study, and thus the trial should be terminated early for futility. A well-planned clinical trial may allow for appropriate interim decision making for strong positive or negative treatment effects; that is to stop a trial early due to overwhelming efficacious effects, futility, or substantial adverse events of the study drug. Trial designs must preserve the integrity of the study, by controlling the type I and type II errors.

During the planning stage, it may be difficult to obtain reliable estimates of the design parameters due to changes of the study conditions and differences in the patient populations between the current and historical studies. The trial may end up with a sample size that is not adequate to detect a clinically meaningful difference, due to either an overestimation of the treatment difference or an underestimation of the variance. It is thus sensible to adaptively adjust the originally planned sample size using the interim data in order to achieve an adequate power for the study. This additional flexibility in sample size re-estimation calls for more sophisticated statistical methods and trial designs.

## 2.1.5 Blinding

Bias is the systematic error; that is the deviation from the truth caused by any reason other than sampling variability. In a clinical trial, bias can be substantially reduced by blinding the participants and investigators. Bias exists on a conscious and a subconscious level for both patients and investigators. In an open-label (unblinded) study, both patients and investigators know the intervention that each subject is taking. In general, patients tend to believe that they are doing better if these patients know that they are on the new drug, and investigators are more likely to overestimate the response if they know the patient is treated with the experimental drug due to their enthusiasm for the new agent. Due to the conscious and subconscious psychological tendencies of humans, bias may arise in an open-label study, while blinding provides an effective tool to prevent such bias. There are three ways of blinding in clinical trials:

- In a *single-blind* study, patients are not aware of which intervention they receive, but the investigators are.

- In a *double-blind* study, neither the patients nor the investigators who are responsible for patients' follow-up know the identity of the treatment assignment.

- In a *triple-blind* study, not only the patients and investigators are unaware of treatment assignments, the personnel in charge of data analysis (e.g., statisticians) are also not informed of the identity of the treatment groups.

Phase III clinical trials often use double-blind designs to prevent potential bias during data collection and assessment. Triple-blind clinical trials are not common because they are complex and also not regarded as necessary in general.

When conducting a trial under a blinding scheme, great care must be taken to hide the treatment identity from all except those who need to know which medication is active and which is a placebo. Before the trial is finished, this information should be limited only to the drug producers (often the trial sponsors) and possibly the data safety and monitoring board.

### 2.1.6   Randomization

In a comparative study with multiple treatments, each patient is randomly assigned to one of the treatment groups. The use of randomization in a clinical trial helps to remove systematic errors or bias, lay out the foundation for statistical analysis, and also justify the significance level of hypothesis testing. Many factors may affect the primary outcome of a trial, while randomization can reduce the confounding effects that may be incorrectly attributed to the difference between the study groups. For example, if a physician always assigns healthier or younger patients to the experimental therapy and sicker or older patients to the standard treatment, the study may eventually conclude that the experimental therapy is more effective, which, however, could be a false-positive result due to selection bias. To prevent bias in the allocation of patients, randomization helps to produce comparable groups with respect to all the known and unknown risk factors.

The simplest randomization procedure is equal randomization. In a two-arm trial, equal randomization allocates each patient based on a ratio of 1:1, which can be easily achieved by tossing a fair coin. Each participant has the same chance to be assigned to either the intervention or the control group. Randomization probabilities may be fixed throughout the trial, or adaptively changing based on the characteristics or the outcomes of the patients who have already entered the trial. More sophisticated randomization procedures require more advanced statistical modeling. Baseline- or covariate-adaptive randomization adjusts the patient allocation probabilities according to imbalance in the patient baseline characteristics between treatment groups. Response- or outcome-adaptive randomization adjusts the allocation probabilities according to the responses of previously enrolled patients to their assigned treatments, such that a new patient is more likely to receive a better treatment.

### 2.1.7   Parallel and Crossover Designs

The parallel design is the standard approach to comparing several treatments. Patients are randomized to one of the arms and then remain on that treatment throughout the trial. By contrast, a crossover design randomizes patients to a sequence of treatments and allows them to cross over from one treatment to the other instead of fixing the treatment for each subject. There should be a washout period between two consecutive treatments to eliminate the residual effects from the previous treatment. Each patient will be given the new intervention in a crossover design, while a parallel design does not guarantee a patient to be assigned to a certain treatment. In a two-arm crossover trial as shown in Figure 2.1, each participant is evaluated twice, once in the intervention group (treatment A) and once in the control group (treatment B), which lessens the concern over the accuracy of the control data. Moreover, serving as his/her own control, the subject variability is reduced, and investigators can assess whether each participant does better on treatment A or treatment B.

However, crossover designs have some intrinsic limitations. The time interval between using treatments A and B should be sufficiently long to wash out the carryover effects from the previous treatment. Due to the late-onset of certain events, the residual effects of the earlier treatment might affect the subject's response to the later treatment. Moreover, the health status of the patient and the condition of the disease might have already been altered by the previous treatment. Thus only conditions that are likely to be similar in both treatment

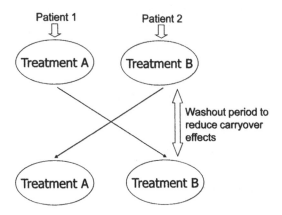

**Figure 2.1**   Crossover design with treatments A and B.

periods are amenable to a crossover design. This restriction greatly limits the applications of crossover designs. For example, surgeries or acute diseases that do not recur are not suitable for a crossover study. Also, in an oncology trial, if a patient has responded to one treatment, it would not be sensible to switch the treatment to something else that is uncertain; or if a patient's disease has progressed, the characteristics of the disease may have changed and will not return back to the original status.

### 2.1.8   Data Collection

Clinical trial data are collected through medical examinations, laboratory tests, interviews, and questionnaires. We need to devote sufficient effort to ensure the key data that are critical to the interpretation and conclusion of the trial of high quality.

Response variables are the outcomes measured in the course of a trial; they must be clinically relevant and also must define and answer the primary and secondary questions. Response variables may be dichotomous, continuous, or time-to-event measurements—for example, the incidence of the DLT, partial or complete response, stable disease, progression-free survival, and overall survival. In general, a single "clean" response variable should be identified to answer the primary question. If there are too many response variables in a trial, the findings may be inconsistent and difficult to interpret and generalize.

In a trial of long duration, intermittent short-term response variables may serve as surrogates for the long-term outcomes. For example, we may measure the percentage of tumor shrinkage instead of mortality, the change in the count of CD-4 (cluster of differentiation 4) lymphocytes for HIV/AIDS patients, or the PSA (prostate-specific antigen) level in prostate cancer as opposed to disease-free survival. The surrogate response variables must be scientifically acceptable such that when the clinical trial is completed, they can be used to speed up the determination of the possible benefits of the new intervention.

After a patient is enrolled in a trial, we should make an effort to monitor and enhance the participant's adherence to the assigned treatment. Patients may not comply with their assigned treatment due to dropping out of the study or switching to a different treatment. Common reasons for noncompliance include that patients experience excessive toxicities and other unexpected side effects, are unwilling to change their behaviors, do not understand instructions given to them, may lack family support, or may change their minds regarding participation.

### 2.1.9   Adverse Events

Drug-related adverse events or side effects are always on the top of the concerns for patients and investigators. Toxicities must be continuously monitored throughout the trial. The potential benefits of the intervention should be maximized, while possible toxicity should be kept to a minimum by appropriately selecting the dose and frequency/schedule of administration of the drug. At any time, a trial should be suspended if excessive toxicities have occurred.

For a thorough evaluation of potential risks of the intervention, we need to pay adequate attention to the assessment, analysis, and reporting of adverse events. When patients are taken off the study medication or have the intervention device removed, the specific reasoning behind such actions should be carefully documented. For example, due to excessive toxicities, patients may be placed on a reduced dosage of the study drug or on a lower intensity of an intervention. Moreover, the type and frequency of participants' complaints are also important for assessing the adverse effects of the intervention.

An external and independent group, known as the data safety monitoring board (DSMB), is often needed to oversee the entire clinical trial, especially for a study involving randomization. The DSMB looks for early evidence of overwhelming benefits or harmful effects related to the experimental intervention. If the treatment is harmful, early termination of the trial should be considered. If the treatment leads to benefits as expected, it would be unethical to continue randomizing patients to other inferior arms. If there appears to be no clear conclusions by the end of the trial, it may be unwise to continue the trial due to the cost and concerns about participants' health.

### 2.1.10  Closeout

The closeout of a clinical trial usually requires careful planning, such as (i) consideration of the date when the last participant is enrolled and (ii) the minimum length of the follow-up that the protocol requires. After completion of the trial, it is important to clean and verify the data to ensure a high quality. Statistical analysis should be thorough and correct. Misspecified models and inappropriate methods may result in misleading findings and impair the credibility of a trial. Questions, as follows, may be asked at the conclusion of the trial:

- Has the trial been carried out as originally planned?

- How do the results of the trial compare with those from other relevant studies?

- What are the clinical implications of the study findings, and how will the trial's conclusion affect clinical practice?

The analysis population should be carefully chosen, because excluding randomized patients from analysis or subgrouping on the basis of response variables may lead to biased results of unknown magnitude and direction. Investigators have an obligation to review their study and the findings critically and to present sufficient information so that others can properly evaluate the trial.

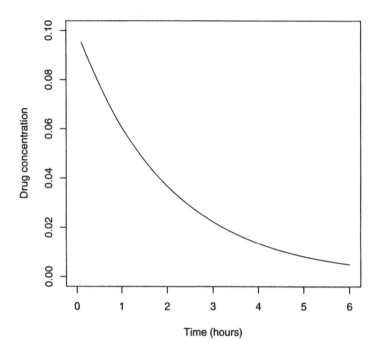

**Figure 2.2**   Drug concentration over time for an intravenous drug.

## 2.2   PHARMACOKINETICS AND PHARMACODYNAMICS

In the preclinical studies and early-phase trials, we need to understand the pharmacokinetics (PK) and pharmacodynamics (PD) of the drug (Hedaya, 2007). PK works on the kinetics of drug absorption, distribution, and elimination; it characterizes the relationship between the dose and the time course of drug concentration in the body.  PD studies the treatment effect once the drug has reached the site of action. Hence intuitively speaking, PK is what the body does to the drug, and PD is what the drug does to the body.

The PK model produces the drug blood concentration-time profile in the body. It describes the motion of the drug in the body over time, in particular, regarding drug absorption, distribution, metabolism, and elimination.  Figure 2.2 shows the plasma concentration-time profile after an intravenous dose administration. Let $C(t)$ denote the drug plasma concentration at time $t$.  The model that characterizes the curve in Figure 2.2 is given by

$$C(t) = \frac{d}{V} \exp(-\beta_e t),$$

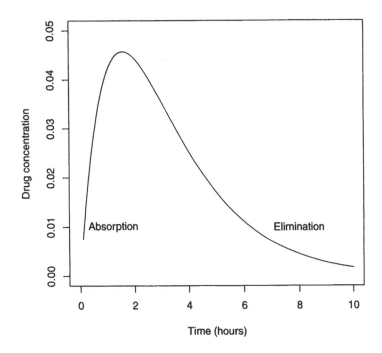

**Figure 2.3**    Drug concentration over time for an orally administered drug.

where $d$ is the dosage of the drug, $V$ is the volume of the distribution, and $\beta_e$ is the elimination rate parameter. If the drug is administered as a single oral dose, the drug blood concentration-time profile is given by

$$C(t) = \frac{\beta_a d}{(\beta_a - \beta_e)V}\{\exp(-\beta_e t) - \exp(-\beta_a t)\},$$

where $\beta_a$ is the absorption rate and other parameters are defined as before. Figure 2.3 displays a typical curve of drug concentration over time for an orally taken agent.

The PD profile of a drug (i.e., a typical dose–response curve) is shown in Figure 2.4. Among various models that characterize the drug concentration-effect profile, the Sigmoid Emax model is particularly popular. The Emax model assumes that the drug effect monotonically increases with respect to the drug concentration until it reaches a plateau corresponding to the maximum drug effect. The Emax model, also known as the Hill (1910) equation, quantifies the

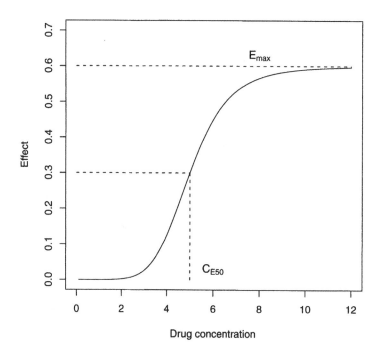

**Figure 2.4**    Drug effect versus drug concentration in an Emax model.

drug's therapeutic effect in the form of

$$E = E_{\max}\frac{C^\alpha}{(C_{E50})^\alpha + C^\alpha},\tag{2.1}$$

where $E_{\max}$ is the maximum effect of the drug, $C_{E50}$ is the drug concentration when the effect is 50% of $E_{\max}$, and $C$ is the drug concentration at the site of action. The parameter $\alpha$ adjusts how quickly this monotonically increasing curve reaches the plateau $E_{\max}$. When $E_{\max} = 1$, (2.1) reduces to a logistic regression model,

$$\log\left(\frac{E}{1 - E}\right) = \alpha\{\log(C) - \log(C_{E50})\} = \beta_0 + \beta_1\log(C),$$

where the intercept and slope are $\beta_0 = -\alpha\log(C_{E50})$ and $\beta_1 = \alpha$, respectively.

## 2.3    PHASES I–IV OF CLINICAL TRIALS

### 2.3.1    Phase I

Following the preclinical studies, the first step of testing a new drug in human beings is to understand how well the agent can be tolerated. The safety of a drug does not mean absolutely harmless, while it is often necessary to accept a certain amount of risk. A drug may be considered "safe" as long as its benefits outweigh the associated risks. Especially in serious and life-threatening diseases, the tolerance for drugs' risks could be higher. For example, chemotherapies are known to potentially induce various severe adverse effects, which, however, may save cancer patients' lives. Exposing human subjects to the risks inherent in experimental research is only justifiable if there is a realistic possibility that the study findings will benefit those participants and future patients, and also lead to substantial scientific progress.

In oncology, phase I trials focus on identifying the MTD, which is the maximum dosage that can be given to patients before they start experiencing an unacceptable level of toxicity. Phase I trials are single-arm studies, and the typical outcome is whether a patient has experienced the DLT, which refers to an unacceptable level of toxicity that prohibits continuing the treatment.

A common assumption in a phase I trial is that toxicity monotonically increases with the dose. Patients are typically grouped according to their enrollment dates and are treated in cohorts. The eligibility criteria in a phase I oncology trial are less restrictive. Most of the participants may have advanced or refractory cancer; that is, the tumor is not responsive to any standard treatment, or the disease has progressed. For safety, the trial starts treating the first cohort of patients at the lowest or the physician-specified dose level. Dose escalation or de-escalation is adaptively determined by the accumulating data from successively accrued patients. Phase I clinical trials are critically important because the identified MTD will be further investigated in the subsequent phase II or phase III trials. If the MTD is misidentified as a dose with higher toxicity, a substantial number of patients would be exposed to over-toxic doses; this may cause a discontinuation of research on an actually working drug due to excessive toxicities. On the other hand, if a dose with lower toxicity is misidentified as the MTD that turns out to be ineffective, it may overlook an otherwise promising drug.

### 2.3.2    Phase II

Phase II trials may be regarded as the "proof-of-principle" stage of drug development. This phase of a trial evaluates whether the drug has any biologic activity or beneficial effect, and it continues monitoring all the possible adverse events. Phase II studies provide critical information for the "go or no-go" decision, that is whether to proceed further to a large confirmatory phase III trial. Nonworking drugs should be dropped from the study or "killed" at this stage to avoid investing more resources and efforts.

Phase II trials may be single-arm assessing one treatment, or multi-arm comparing several treatments. If only one treatment is evaluated, the historical data or the standard response rate will be used for comparison. If the trial examines multiple treatments, patients will be randomized to the experimental and standard arms. Randomized phase II trials may reduce the so-called "trial effect," which often arises due to different patient populations, physician cares, and medical environments between the current and previous studies.

The data collected in a phase II trial characterize the drug's short-term efficacy. The primary endpoint must be ascertainable quickly and be able to establish the treatment benefit convincingly. Examples of such short-term responses include: more than 50% shrinkage of a solid tumor compared with the baseline measurement; partial response (a 30% decrease in the sum of the longest diameter of target lesions) or complete response (disappearance of all target lesions); and partial or complete remission in patients with leukemia as indicated by the levels of platelets, blastic cells, and white blood cells. In principle, a phase II trial is small and can be completed in a relatively short period of time in order to facilitate the "go or no-go" decision to a phase III trial.

### 2.3.3 Phase III

Phase III trials are large-scale in terms of resources, efforts, and costs. This phase collects a large amount of data over a long period of follow-up to examine the ultimate therapeutic effect of a new drug. The standard form of a phase III trial is a double-blind, randomized, and placebo-controlled study. The control arm may be a placebo or the standard of care. The use of a placebo in a randomized trial is only acceptable if there is no other best or standard therapy available. Patients must be informed of the possibility that they may be given a placebo rather than the experimental intervention. The typical endpoint in a phase III trial is a time-to-event measurement, such as progression-free survival. Interim monitoring is often considered for such a long-term confirmatory trial.

### 2.3.4 Phase IV

After a drug successfully passes through phases I, II, and III testing, it will be filed to the FDA for marketing authorization. Upon the drug's approval, a phase IV trial may be initiated as a post-marketing surveillance study. In this phase, the drug-associated adverse events and patients' safety are closely monitored to identify problems that have not be recognized prior to its approval. Rare severe adverse events that arise after the widespread use of the drug in the general patient population may add a warning label to the prescription or even cause the

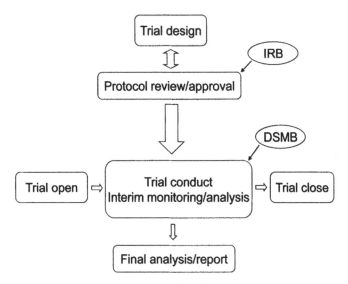

**Figure 2.5**     Diagram of a clinical trial, with Internal Review Board (IRB) and Data Safety Monitoring Board (DSMB).

drug to be withdrawn from the market. A phase IV trial is an integral part of the drug evaluation process, which may lead to new indications or new uses of the approved agent.

## 2.4  SUMMARY

Clinical trials must protect participants' safety in the study and satisfy all ethical constraints. Statistical methods and trial designs should utilize all available resources to detect the treatment effect from confounders, reduce bias, and improve precision (Friedman, Furberg, and DeMets, 1998; Piantadosi, 2005). Properly designed and carefully conducted clinical trials, especially when coupled with blinding and randomization, instill a high level of confidence in the study findings. Figure 2.5 presents the flow chart of a clinical trial from the design, review, approval, and conduct until the final data analysis. As a summary, clinical trial designs aim to

- eliminate bias, quantify and reduce errors,

- produce accurate estimates of treatment effects and the associated precision,

- provide a high degree of credibility, reproducibility, and internal and external validity, and

- most importantly, influence future clinical practice.

## EXERCISES

**2.1**   What are the main objectives and what types of endpoints are typically used in phase I, II, and III clinical trials, respectively?

**2.2**   When can the drug be filed to the FDA for approval? Which phase of the trial is conducted after approval, and for what purposes?

**2.3**   What is the type I error rate and what is power of a statistical test? Describe them in the hypothesis testing framework.

**2.4**   What is the purpose of blinding in a clinical trial, and what is the purpose of randomization?

# CHAPTER 3

# FREQUENTIST VERSUS BAYESIAN STATISTICS

## 3.1 BASIC STATISTICS

### 3.1.1 Probability and Univariate Distributions

A probability space is often denoted by $(\Omega, \mathcal{F}, P)$, where $\Omega$ is the sample space containing all the possible outcomes of an experiment; $\mathcal{F}$, called the $\sigma$-field, is a collection of subsets of $\Omega$; and $P$ is a probability measure. For a set $A \in \mathcal{F}$, its complement $A^c \in \mathcal{F}$; if $A_1, A_2, \ldots \in \mathcal{F}$, then the union $\cup_{i=1}^{\infty} A_i \in \mathcal{F}$; and the empty set $\varnothing \in \mathcal{F}$. For any set $A \in \mathcal{F}$, a probability measure function $P$ with domain $\mathcal{F}$ satisfies

- $P(A) \geq 0$,

- $P(\Omega) = 1$, and

- $P(\cup_{i=1}^{\infty} A_i) = \sum_{i=1}^{\infty} P(A_i)$ for any mutually disjoint sets $A_1, A_2, \ldots \in \mathcal{F}$.

A random variable is a function mapping from the sample space $\Omega$ to the real line $\mathcal{R}$. The cumulative distribution function of random variable $X$ is $F(x) = P(X \leq x)$ for all $x \in \mathcal{R}$. If $X$ is a continuous random variable, the

*Clinical Trial Design.* By Guosheng Yin
Copyright © 2012 John Wiley & Sons, Inc.

probability density function (p.d.f.) of $X$ is defined as

$$f(x) = \frac{\mathrm{d}F(x)}{\mathrm{d}x}.$$

Thus given $f(x)$, the cumulative distribution function of $X$ can be obtained by

$$F(x) = \int_{-\infty}^{x} f(u)\,\mathrm{d}u.$$

If $X$ is a discrete random variable, the probability mass function (p.m.f.) is denoted by $P(X = x)$ or $\Pr(X = x)$. Without loss of generality, we illustrate the expectation and variance for a continuous random variable, while for a discrete random variable the integral is simply replaced by a summation over all of the discrete probability masses. The expectation or the mean of random variable $X$ is

$$\mathrm{E}(X) = \int x f(x)\,\mathrm{d}x,$$

and the variance of $X$ is

$$\mathrm{Var}(X) = \mathrm{E}\{X - \mathrm{E}(X)\}^2 = \mathrm{E}(X^2) - \{\mathrm{E}(X)\}^2.$$

In the following, we list some discrete distribution functions that often arise in clinical trial designs.

- *Discrete uniform distribution*: The p.m.f. of $X$ is

$$P(X = x_k) = \frac{1}{K}, \quad k = 1, \ldots, K,$$

where $x_1, \ldots, x_K$ are different values on the real line and $K$ is a prespecified positive integer. The discrete uniform distribution is often used as a prior distribution in the context of Bayesian model averaging or Bayesian hypothesis testing. For example, a discrete uniform prior distribution may be assigned to the candidate models or hypotheses when there is no preference *a priori* to any specific model/hypothesis.

- *Bernoulli distribution*: $X \sim \mathrm{Bernoulli}(p)$, if $X = 1$ with probability $p$, and $X = 0$ with probability $1 - p$. The p.m.f. of $X$ can be written as

$$P(X = x) = p^x(1 - p)^{1-x}, \quad x = 0, 1,$$

with $\mathrm{E}(X) = p$ and $\mathrm{Var}(X) = p(1 - p)$. The Bernoulli distribution is commonly used in phase I and phase II clinical trials, in which binary endpoints are typically observed, for example, to characterize whether a patient has experienced toxicity or whether a patient has responded to treatment.

- *Binomial distribution*: $Y \sim \text{Bin}(n, p)$, if $Y = X_1 + \cdots + X_n$, where $X_1, \ldots, X_n$ are independent and identically distributed (i.i.d.) random variables from Bernoulli$(p)$. The p.m.f. of $Y$ is given by

$$P(Y = y) = \binom{n}{y} p^y (1 - p)^{n-y}$$

$$= \frac{n!}{y!(n - y)!} p^y (1 - p)^{n-y}, \quad y = 0, 1, \ldots, n,$$

with $\text{E}(Y) = np$ and $\text{Var}(Y) = np(1-p)$. The binomial distribution may be used to model the number of patients who have experienced toxicity or those who have achieved efficacy in a clinical trial.

- *Beta-binomial distribution*: $X \sim \text{Beta-Bin}(n, \alpha, \beta)$, if the p.m.f. of $X$ is

$$P(X = x) = \binom{n}{x} \frac{B(\alpha + x, \beta + n - x)}{B(\alpha, \beta)}, \quad x = 0, 1, \ldots, n,$$

where the beta function is defined as $B(\alpha, \beta) = \Gamma(\alpha)\Gamma(\beta)/\Gamma(\alpha + \beta)$, and the gamma function is given by

$$\Gamma(\alpha) = \int_0^\infty u^{\alpha-1} e^{-u} \, du.$$

The mean and the variance of $X$ are given by

$$\text{E}(X) = \frac{n\alpha}{\alpha + \beta} \quad \text{and} \quad \text{Var}(X) = \frac{n\alpha\beta(\alpha + \beta + n)}{(\alpha + \beta)^2(\alpha + \beta + 1)},$$

respectively. As will be seen in Chapter 5, a beta-binomial distribution often arises as the posterior predictive distribution in a phase II trial with a binary endpoint.

- *Negative binomial distribution*: $X \sim \text{Neg-Bin}(r, p)$, if the p.m.f. of $X$ is

$$P(X = x) = \binom{x + r - 1}{x} p^r (1 - p)^x, \quad x = 0, 1, \ldots,$$

where $r$ is a fixed positive integer, and $\text{E}(X) = rp/(1 - p)$ and $\text{Var}(X) = rp/(1 - p)^2$. Suppose that a sequence of independent Bernoulli experiments are conducted, each with a success probability $p$. Let $X$ be the number of experiments failed until a total of $r$ successes are accumulated, then $X \sim \text{Neg-Bin}(r, p)$. The geometric distribution is a special case of the negative binomial distribution with $r = 1$; that is, the number of experiments failed until the first success is observed.

- *Poisson distribution*: $X \sim \text{Poisson}(\lambda)$, if the p.m.f. of $X$ is

$$P(X = x) = \frac{e^{-\lambda}\lambda^x}{x!}, \quad x = 0, 1, \ldots,$$

where $\lambda > 0$ is the intensity rate parameter, and $E(X) = \text{Var}(X) = \lambda$. For a binomial random variable $Y \sim \text{Bin}(n, p)$, as $n \to \infty$ and $p \to 0$ with $np \to \lambda$ a constant, the distribution of $Y$ converges to a Poisson distribution with intensity parameter $\lambda$.

- *Hypergeometric distribution*: $X \sim \text{Hypergeometric}(N, m, n)$, if the p.m.f. of $X$ is

$$P(X = x) = \frac{\binom{m}{x}\binom{N-m}{n-x}}{\binom{N}{n}},$$

where $x = \max(0, n + m - N), \ldots, \min(m, n)$. If we define $p = m/N$, the expectation and the variance of $X$ are given by

$$E(X) = np \quad \text{and} \quad \text{Var}(X) = \frac{N-n}{N-1}np(1-p),$$

respectively. The hypergeometric distribution can be viewed as the finite population counterpart of a binomial distribution. Consider an urn with a total of $N$ balls, $m$ balls of type A and $(N - m)$ balls of type B. A sample of $n$ balls is randomly drawn without replacement. Let $X$ be the number of balls of type A in the sample, then $X \sim \text{Hypergeometric}(N, m, n)$. However, if each of the $n$ balls is sampled with replacement, this would lead to a binomial distribution, and thus $(N - n)/(N - 1)$ in the variance of $X$ is called the finite population correction factor. The hypergeometric distribution is the fundamental basis to construct the log-rank test when comparing two survival curves.

Besides the discrete random variables, many continuous random variables also play an important role in clinical trials, for which the probability density functions are given as follows.

- *Continuous uniform distribution*: $X \sim \text{Unif}(a, b)$, if the p.d.f. of $X$ is

$$f(x) = \frac{1}{b - a}, \quad a < x < b.$$

The expectation and variance of $X$ are given by

$$E(X) = \frac{a + b}{2} \quad \text{and} \quad \text{Var}(X) = \frac{(b - a)^2}{12},$$

respectively. The simplest continuous uniform distribution is $f(x) = 1$ for $x \in (0, 1)$.

- *Normal distribution*: $X \sim \mathrm{N}(\mu, \sigma^2)$, if the p.d.f. of $X$ is

$$f(x) = \frac{1}{\sqrt{2\pi}\sigma} \exp\left\{-\frac{(x-\mu)^2}{2\sigma^2}\right\},$$

with $\mathrm{E}(X) = \mu$ and $\mathrm{Var}(X) = \sigma^2$. If $\mu = 0$ and $\sigma = 1$, then $\mathrm{N}(0, 1)$ is called the standard normal distribution. If $X \sim \mathrm{N}(\mu, \sigma^2)$ and $Y = \exp(X)$, then random variable $Y$ follows a *log-normal distribution* with the density function

$$f(y) = \frac{1}{\sqrt{2\pi}\sigma y} \exp\left[-\frac{\{\log(y)-\mu\}^2}{2\sigma^2}\right], \quad y > 0,$$

where $\log(\cdot)$ stands for the natural logarithm.

- *Gamma distribution*: $X \sim \mathrm{Ga}(\alpha, \beta)$, if the p.d.f. of $X$ is

$$f(x) = \frac{\beta^\alpha}{\Gamma(\alpha)} x^{\alpha-1} e^{-\beta x}, \quad x > 0,$$

where $\alpha > 0$ is the shape parameter and $\beta > 0$ is the scale parameter. The expectation and the variance of $X$ are given by

$$\mathrm{E}(X) = \frac{\alpha}{\beta} \quad \text{and} \quad \mathrm{Var}(X) = \frac{\alpha}{\beta^2},$$

respectively. When $\alpha = 1$, the gamma distribution reduces to an *Exponential distribution*: $X \sim \mathrm{Exp}(\beta)$ with $\mathrm{E}(X) = 1/\beta$ and $\mathrm{Var}(X) = 1/\beta^2$. The gamma distribution is often used to model the hazard function of failure times in survival analysis.

- *Chi-squared distribution with $\nu$ degrees of freedom*: $X \sim \chi^2_\nu$, if the p.d.f. of $X$ is

$$f(x) = \frac{1}{2^{\nu/2}\Gamma(\nu/2)} x^{\nu/2-1} e^{-x/2}, \quad x > 0,$$

with $\mathrm{E}(X) = \nu$ and $\mathrm{Var}(X) = 2\nu$. The chi-squared distribution $\chi^2_\nu$ is a special case of $\mathrm{Ga}(\alpha, \beta)$ with $\alpha = \nu/2$ and $\beta = 1/2$. If $X \sim \mathrm{N}(0, 1)$, then $X^2 \sim \chi^2_1$. Furthermore, if $X_1, \ldots, X_n$ are independent and each $X_i \sim \chi^2_{\nu_i}$ for $i = 1, \ldots, n$, then

$$X_1 + \cdots + X_n \sim \chi^2_{\nu_1 + \cdots + \nu_n}.$$

If $X_1 \sim \chi^2_{\nu_1}$ and $X_2 \sim \chi^2_{\nu_2}$ are independent, then

$$\frac{X_1/\nu_1}{X_2/\nu_2} \sim F_{\nu_1, \nu_2},$$

which is an $F$ distribution with $\nu_1$ and $\nu_2$ degrees of freedom.

- *Inverse gamma distribution*: If $X \sim \text{Ga}(\alpha, \beta)$ and $Y = X^{-1}$, then $Y \sim \text{IG}(\alpha, \beta)$, and the p.d.f. of $Y$ is given by

$$f(y) = \frac{\beta^\alpha}{\Gamma(\alpha)} y^{-\alpha-1} e^{-\beta/y}, \quad y > 0,$$

with $\text{E}(Y) = \beta/(\alpha-1)$ for $\alpha > 1$, and $\text{Var}(Y) = \beta^2/\{(\alpha-1)^2(\alpha-2)\}$ for $\alpha > 2$. The inverse gamma distribution is often used as a prior distribution for the variance component in Bayesian hierarchical models. For example, let $\sigma^2$ denote the variance of a normal distribution and define $\tau = \sigma^{-2}$, then the prior distribution on $\sigma^2$ can be specified as $\tau \sim \text{Ga}(\alpha, \beta)$, which is equivalent to $\sigma^2 \sim \text{IG}(\alpha, \beta)$.

- *Beta distribution*: $X \sim \text{Beta}(\alpha, \beta)$, if the p.d.f. of $X$ is

$$f(x) = \frac{\Gamma(\alpha + \beta)}{\Gamma(\alpha)\Gamma(\beta)} x^{\alpha-1}(1 - x)^{\beta-1}, \quad 0 < x < 1,$$

where the two shape parameters $\alpha > 0$ and $\beta > 0$, and

$$\text{E}(X) = \frac{\alpha}{\alpha + \beta} \quad \text{and} \quad \text{Var}(X) = \frac{\alpha\beta}{(\alpha + \beta)^2(\alpha + \beta + 1)}.$$

When $\alpha = \beta = 1$, the beta distribution reduces to the uniform distribution on $(0, 1)$. The beta distribution is typically used as a prior distribution for a probability parameter. For example, let $p$ denote the response rate of an experimental drug, and let $Y$ denote the number of patients who have responded among $n$ treated patients. In this case, $Y \sim \text{Bin}(n, p)$ and the prior distribution on $p$ may be given as $p \sim \text{Beta}(\alpha, \beta)$.

- *Student's t distribution with $\nu$ degrees of freedom*: $X \sim t_\nu(\mu, \sigma^2)$, if the p.d.f. of $X$ is

$$f(x) = \frac{\Gamma\{(\nu + 1)/2\}}{\Gamma(\nu/2)\sqrt{\nu\pi}\sigma} \left\{ 1 + \frac{1}{\nu} \left( \frac{x - \mu}{\sigma} \right)^2 \right\}^{-(\nu+1)/2},$$

with $\text{E}(X) = \mu$ for $\nu > 1$, and $\text{Var}(X) = \sigma^2\nu/(\nu - 2)$ for $\nu > 2$. Student's $t$ distribution resembles a normal distribution except with heavier tails. As $\nu \to \infty$, the distribution $t_\nu(\mu, \sigma^2)$ converges to a normal distribution $\text{N}(\mu, \sigma^2)$. When $\nu = 1$, $t_\nu(\mu, \sigma^2)$ becomes *Cauchy distribution* with the density function

$$f(x) = \frac{1}{\pi\sigma\{1 + (x - \mu)^2/\sigma^2\}},$$

whose mean, however, does not exist. In practice, we often encounter a central $t$ distribution with $\mu = 0$ and $\sigma = 1$, simply denoted as $t_\nu$; and we denote a noncentral $t$ distribution with $\mu \neq 0$ and $\sigma = 1$ as $t_\nu(\mu)$. For example, if $X \sim \mathrm{N}(0, 1)$, $Y \sim \chi^2_\nu$, and $X$ and $Y$ are independent, then

$$\frac{X}{\sqrt{Y/\nu}} \sim t_\nu,$$

which is a central $t$ distribution with $\nu$ degrees of freedom.

- *Weibull distribution*: $X \sim \mathrm{Weibull}(\alpha, \beta)$, if the p.d.f. of $X$ is

$$f(x) = \alpha\beta x^{\alpha-1} \exp(-\beta x^\alpha), \quad x > 0,$$

where $\alpha > 0$ is the shape parameter and $\beta > 0$ is the scale parameter. If $\alpha = 1$, the Weibull distribution reduces to an exponential distribution. The Weibull distribution is often used to model the time-to-event data. If the failure time $T \sim \mathrm{Weibull}(\alpha, \beta)$, the survival function of $T$ is

$$S(t) = P(T > t) = \exp(-\beta t^\alpha),$$

and the hazard function is

$$\lambda(t) = \frac{f(t)}{S(t)} = \alpha\beta t^{\alpha-1}.$$

Depending on the value of $\alpha$, the hazard function may be increasing $(\alpha > 1)$, decreasing $(\alpha < 1)$, or constant $(\alpha = 1)$.

As noted, one random variable may be linked with another through a variable transformation. For ease of exposition, denote the density function of $X$ as $f_X(x)$, and let $Y = g(X)$ where $g(\cdot)$ is a monotone function. If the inverse function $g^{-1}(y)$ has a continuous derivative, then the density function of $Y$ is given by

$$f_Y(y) = f_X\{g^{-1}(y)\} \left| \frac{\mathrm{d}g^{-1}(y)}{\mathrm{d}y} \right|.$$

### 3.1.2   Multivariate Distributions

For bivariate random variables $(X, Y)$,

$$P\{(X, Y) \in \mathcal{A}\} = \iint_{(x,y)\in\mathcal{A}} f(x, y)\, \mathrm{d}x\mathrm{d}y,$$

where $\mathcal{A}$ is a subset of $\mathcal{R}^2$ and $f(x, y)$ is the joint p.d.f. of $X$ and $Y$. For a given function $g(\cdot, \cdot)$,

$$\mathrm{E}\{g(X, Y)\} = \iint g(x, y) f(x, y)\, \mathrm{d}x\mathrm{d}y.$$

The marginal density function of $X$ is obtained by integrating out $Y$ from the joint density function,

$$f(x) = \int f(x, y) \, dy,$$

and the conditional density function of $Y$ given $X = x$ is

$$f(y|x) = \frac{f(x, y)}{f(x)}.$$

If $f(x, y) = f(x)f(y)$, then $X$ and $Y$ are said to be independent, which also implies $f(y|x) = f(y)$.

The conditional expectation and the conditional variance of $Y$ given $X = x$ are given by

$$E(Y|X = x) = \int y f(y|x) \, dy$$

and

$$\text{Var}(Y|X = x) = E(Y^2|x) - \{E(Y|x)\}^2,$$

respectively. The covariance between $X$ and $Y$ is defined as

$$\text{Cov}(X, Y) = E[\{X - E(X)\}\{Y - E(Y)\}] = E(XY) - E(X)E(Y),$$

and the correlation coefficient is given by

$$\rho = \frac{\text{Cov}(X, Y)}{\sqrt{\text{Var}(X)\text{Var}(Y)}}.$$

Based on the conditional probability, the expectation and the variance of $X$ can be computed through the following chain rules:

$$E(X) = E\{E(X|Y)\},$$
$$\text{Var}(X) = E\{\text{Var}(X|Y)\} + \text{Var}\{E(X|Y)\}.$$

If $X$ and $Y$ are independent random variables with respective density functions $f_X(x)$ and $f_Y(y)$, the density function of $Z = X + Y$ is

$$f_Z(z) = \int f_X(x) f_Y(z - x) \, dx,$$

which is known as the convolution formula. More importantly, the probability of comparing two independent random variables is given by

$$P(X > Y) = \int_{-\infty}^{\infty} \int_{-\infty}^{x} f_X(x) f_Y(y) \, dy dx,$$

which is useful to ascertain treatment superiority in a randomized trial.

More generally, $f(\mathbf{x})$, which is the joint p.d.f. for a $K$-dimensional random vector $\mathbf{X} = (X_1, \ldots, X_K)^{\mathsf{T}}$, satisfies

$$
\begin{aligned}
P(\mathbf{X} \in \mathcal{A}) &= \int_{\mathcal{A}} f(\mathbf{x}) \, \mathrm{d}\mathbf{x} \\
&= \int \cdots \int_{(x_1, \ldots, x_K) \in \mathcal{A}} f(x_1, \ldots, x_K) \, \mathrm{d}x_1 \cdots \mathrm{d}x_K,
\end{aligned}
$$

where $\mathcal{A}$ is a subset of $\mathcal{R}^K$. For any $k$ between 1 and $K$, the joint density function of $X_1, \ldots, X_k$ can be obtained by integrating out $X_{k+1}, \ldots, X_K$,

$$
f(x_1, \ldots, x_k) = \int \cdots \int f(x_1, \ldots, x_K) \, \mathrm{d}x_{k+1} \cdots \mathrm{d}x_K,
$$

and the conditional density function is given by

$$
f(x_1, \ldots, x_k | x_{k+1}, \ldots, x_K) = \frac{f(x_1, \ldots, x_k, x_{k+1}, \ldots, x_K)}{f(x_{k+1}, \ldots, x_K)}.
$$

Several important discrete and continuous multivariate distributions are given below.

- *Multinomial distribution*: For $i = 1, \ldots, K$, let $p_i$ denote the probability of the occurrence of event $i$, $\sum_{i=1}^{K} p_i = 1$; and let $x_i$ denote the number of occurrences of event $i$ in a total of $n$ experiments, $\sum_{i=1}^{K} x_i = n$. The random vector $\mathbf{X}$ follows a multinomial distribution, if the joint p.m.f. of $\mathbf{X}$ is

$$
f(x_1, \ldots, x_K) = \frac{n!}{x_1! \cdots x_K!} p_1^{x_1} \cdots p_K^{x_K}.
$$

Each $X_i$ marginally follows a binomial distribution, $X_i \sim \mathrm{Bin}(n, p_i)$; and $\mathrm{E}(X_i) = np_i$, $\mathrm{Var}(X_i) = np_i(1 - p_i)$, and $\mathrm{Cov}(X_i, X_j) = -np_i p_j$ for $i \neq j$.

- *Multivariate normal distribution*: The random vector $\mathbf{X}$ follows a $K$-dimensional normal distribution with mean $\boldsymbol{\mu}$ and variance–covariance matrix $\boldsymbol{\Sigma}$; that is, $\mathbf{X} \sim \mathrm{N}_K(\boldsymbol{\mu}, \boldsymbol{\Sigma})$, if the p.d.f. of $\mathbf{X}$ is

$$
f(\mathbf{x}) = \frac{1}{(2\pi)^{K/2} |\boldsymbol{\Sigma}|^{1/2}} \exp \left\{ -\frac{1}{2} (\mathbf{x} - \boldsymbol{\mu})^{\mathsf{T}} \boldsymbol{\Sigma}^{-1} (\mathbf{x} - \boldsymbol{\mu}) \right\}.
$$

- *Dirichlet distribution*: $\mathbf{X} \sim \mathrm{Dir}(\alpha_1, \ldots, \alpha_K)$, if $\mathbf{X}$ has a p.d.f. of

$$
f(\mathbf{x}) = \frac{\Gamma(\alpha)}{\Gamma(\alpha_1) \cdots \Gamma(\alpha_K)} x_1^{\alpha_1 - 1} \cdots x_K^{\alpha_K - 1},
$$

where $\alpha = \sum_{i=1}^{K} \alpha_i$ with $\alpha_i > 0$, and $\sum_{i=1}^{K} x_i = 1$ with $0 < x_i < 1$. Each $X_i$ marginally follows a beta distribution, $X_i \sim \mathrm{Beta}(\alpha_i, \alpha - \alpha_i)$, with $\mathrm{E}(X_i) = \alpha_i/\alpha$,

$$\mathrm{Var}(X_i) = \frac{\alpha_i(\alpha - \alpha_i)}{\alpha^2(\alpha + 1)} \quad \text{and} \quad \mathrm{Cov}(X_i, X_j) = -\frac{\alpha_i \alpha_j}{\alpha^2(\alpha + 1)} \quad (i \neq j).$$

The Dirichlet distribution is a multivariate version of the beta distribution, which reduces to a beta distribution when $K = 2$. In addition, for any $i \neq j$,

$$(X_1, \ldots, X_i + X_j, \ldots, X_K)^\mathsf{T} \sim \mathrm{Dir}(\alpha_1, \ldots, \alpha_i + \alpha_j, \ldots, \alpha_K).$$

- *Wishart distribution*: Suppose that $\mathbf{X}$ is a $\nu \times K$ $(\nu > K)$ random matrix, and the rows of $\mathbf{X}$ are independent zero-mean normal random vectors. Then the $K \times K$ random matrix $\mathbf{W} = \mathbf{X}^\mathsf{T}\mathbf{X}$ follows a Wishart distribution with $\nu$ degrees of freedom; that is, $\mathbf{W} \sim \mathrm{Wishart}(\mathbf{\Sigma}, \nu)$, where $\mathbf{\Sigma}$ is a $K \times K$ symmetric and positive definite parameter matrix. The p.d.f. of $\mathbf{W}$ is given by

$$f(\mathbf{w}) = \frac{|\mathbf{w}|^{(\nu - K - 1)/2}}{c|\mathbf{\Sigma}|^{\nu/2}} \exp\left\{ -\frac{1}{2}\mathrm{trace}(\mathbf{\Sigma}^{-1}\mathbf{w}) \right\},$$

with the normalizing constant

$$c = 2^{\nu K/2} \pi^{K(K-1)/4} \prod_{i=1}^{K} \Gamma\left( \frac{\nu + 1 - i}{2} \right). \tag{3.1}$$

The Wishart distribution is a multivariate version of the gamma distribution.

- *Inverse Wishart distribution*: If $\mathbf{W} \sim \mathrm{Wishart}(\mathbf{\Sigma}, \nu)$ and $\mathbf{U} = \mathbf{W}^{-1}$, then $\mathbf{U}$ follows an inverse Wishart distribution; that is, $\mathbf{U} \sim \mathrm{Inv\text{-}Wishart}(\mathbf{\Sigma}^{-1}, \nu)$ with the density function

$$f(\mathbf{u}) = \frac{|\mathbf{u}|^{-(\nu + K + 1)/2}}{c|\mathbf{\Sigma}|^{\nu/2}} \exp\left\{ -\frac{1}{2}\mathrm{trace}(\mathbf{\Sigma}^{-1}\mathbf{u}^{-1}) \right\},$$

where $c$ is given in (3.1). The inverse Wishart distribution is often used as a prior distribution for the variance–covariance matrix of a multivariate normal distribution in Bayesian hierarchical modeling.

### 3.1.3 Copula

A multivariate distribution can be easily constructed by linking marginal distributions through a copula (Clayton, 1978; Hougaard, 1986; Nelsen, 1999). For the bivariate case, let $H(x, y)$ denote the cumulative distribution function of the bivariate random variables $(X, Y)$, and let $F(x) = H(x, \infty)$ and

$G(y) = H(\infty, y)$ denote the marginal distribution functions of $X$ and $Y$, respectively. Sklar's theorem states that there exists a copula $C_\gamma(\cdot, \cdot)$ such that

$$H(x, y) = C_\gamma\{F(x), G(y)\},$$

where $\gamma$ is the association parameter.

As an illustration, the Gaussian copula is built upon the bivariate normal distribution. Let $\Psi_\rho(\cdot, \cdot)$ denote the cumulative distribution function of the standard bivariate normal distribution with correlation coefficient $\rho$, and let $\Phi(\cdot)$ denote the cumulative distribution function of the standard normal distribution. For $0 \le u, v \le 1$, the Gaussian copula function is given by

$$\Psi_\rho\{\Phi^{-1}(u), \Phi^{-1}(v)\} =$$
$$\int_{-\infty}^{\Phi^{-1}(u)} \int_{-\infty}^{\Phi^{-1}(v)} \frac{1}{2\pi(1-\rho^2)^{1/2}} \exp\left\{-\frac{x^2 - 2\rho xy + y^2}{2(1-\rho^2)}\right\} dy dx.$$

In clinical trials, copulas are particularly useful to model bivariate or multivariate outcomes, such as jointly modeling toxicity and efficacy, or bivariate survival times. The well-known Archimedean copula functions have a special structure of

$$H(x, y) = \eta_\gamma^{-1}[\eta_\gamma\{F(x)\} + \eta_\gamma\{G(y)\}],$$

where the generator function $\eta_\gamma(u)$ satisfies $\eta_\gamma(1) = 0$, $\lim_{u \to 0} \eta_\gamma(u) = \infty$, the first derivative $\eta_\gamma'(u) < 0$, and the second derivative $\eta_\gamma''(u) > 0$. Archimedean copulas encompass the following bivariate distributions:

- The Clayton copula takes the generator function of $\eta_\gamma(u) = u^{-\gamma} - 1$, and thus the bivariate distribution function is given by

$$H(x, y) = \{F(x)^{-\gamma} + G(y)^{-\gamma} - 1\}^{-1/\gamma}.$$

- The Gumbel copula specifies $\eta_\gamma(u) = (-\log u)^{1/\gamma}$, and then

$$H(x, y) = \exp\left[-\{(-\log F(x))^{1/\gamma} + (-\log G(y))^{1/\gamma}\}^\gamma\right].$$

- The Frank copula has $\eta_\gamma(u) = -\log\{(e^{-\alpha u} - 1)/(e^{-\alpha} - 1)\}$, and

$$H(x, y) = -\frac{1}{\gamma} \log\left\{1 + \frac{(e^{-\gamma F(x)} - 1)(e^{-\gamma G(y)} - 1)}{e^{-\gamma} - 1}\right\}.$$

### 3.1.4 Convergence of Sequences of Random Variables

A sequence of random variables, $X_1, X_2, \ldots$, converges in probability to random variable $X$, denoted as $X_n \xrightarrow{\mathcal{P}} X$, if for every $\epsilon > 0$ we have

$$\lim_{n \to \infty} P(|X_n - X| < \epsilon) = 1.$$

*Weak Law of Large Numbers*: Let $X_1, X_2, \ldots$ be i.i.d. random variables with $E(X_i) = \mu$, and define $\bar{X}_n = n^{-1} \sum_{i=1}^{n} X_i$. Then for every $\epsilon > 0$,

$$\lim_{n \to \infty} P(|\bar{X}_n - \mu| < \epsilon) = 1,$$

that is, $\bar{X}_n$ converges to $\mu$ in probability.

*Continuous Mapping Theorem*: Suppose that a sequence of $X_1, X_2, \ldots$ converges in probability to random variable $X$ and $g(\cdot)$ is a continuous function, then the sequence $g(X_1), g(X_2), \ldots$ converges in probability to $g(X)$.

A sequence of random variables, $X_1, X_2, \ldots$, converges almost surely to random variable $X$, denoted as $X_n \xrightarrow{a.s.} X$, if for every $\epsilon > 0$ we have

$$P\left(\lim_{n \to \infty} |X_n - X| < \epsilon\right) = 1.$$

*Strong Law of Large Numbers*: Let $X_1, X_2, \ldots$ be i.i.d. random variables with $E(X_i) = \mu$, then for every $\epsilon > 0$ we have

$$P\left(\lim_{n \to \infty} |\bar{X}_n - \mu| < \epsilon\right) = 1,$$

that is, $\bar{X}_n$ converges to $\mu$ almost surely.

A sequence of random variables, $X_1, X_2, \ldots$, converges in distribution (or weakly converges) to random variable $X$, denoted as $X_n \xrightarrow{D} X$, if the respective cumulative distribution functions of $X_n$ and $X$, $F_{X_n}(x) = P(X_n \leq x)$ and $F_X(x) = P(X \leq x)$, satisfy

$$\lim_{n \to \infty} F_{X_n}(x) = F_X(x)$$

for all $x$ where $F_X(x)$ is continuous. The relationships among the convergence modes are:

- $X_n \xrightarrow{a.s.} X$ implies that $X_n \xrightarrow{P} X$, and

- $X_n \xrightarrow{P} X$ implies that $X_n \xrightarrow{D} X$.

*Slutsky's Theorem*: If $X_n \xrightarrow{D} X$ and $Y_n \xrightarrow{P} a$, where $a$ is a constant, then

$$X_n Y_n \xrightarrow{D} Xa \quad \text{and} \quad X_n + Y_n \xrightarrow{D} X + a.$$

*Central Limit Theorem*: Let $X_1, X_2, \ldots$ be a sequence of i.i.d. random variables and the corresponding moment generating functions exist in a neighborhood of zero. Let $E(X_i) = \mu$ and $\text{Var}(X_i) = \sigma^2$, then

$$\sqrt{n}\left(\frac{\bar{X}_n - \mu}{\sigma}\right) \xrightarrow{D} N(0, 1).$$

*Delta Method*: Let $\bar{X}_n$ be the average of a sequence of i.i.d. random variables as discussed previously, and

$$\sqrt{n}(\bar{X}_n - \mu) \xrightarrow{\mathcal{D}} N(0, \sigma^2).$$

For a given function $g(\cdot)$, suppose that the first derivative $g'(\mu)$ exists and $g'(\mu) \neq 0$. We take the first-order Taylor series expansion of $g(\bar{X}_n)$ around $\mu$,

$$g(\bar{X}_n) = g(\mu) + g'(\mu)(\bar{X}_n - \mu) + o(\bar{X}_n - \mu),$$

where $o(x)$ denotes a quantity such that $o(x)/x \to 0$ as $x \to 0$. Hence, the usual (first-order) Delta method states that

$$\sqrt{n}\{g(\bar{X}_n) - g(\mu)\} \xrightarrow{\mathcal{D}} N(0, \sigma^2\{g'(\mu)\}^2).$$

If $g'(\mu) = 0$, but the second derivative $g''(\mu)$ exists and $g''(\mu) \neq 0$, we take the second-order Taylor series expansion,

$$g(\bar{X}_n) = g(\mu) + \frac{1}{2}g''(\mu)(\bar{X}_n - \mu)^2 + o((\bar{X}_n - \mu)^2),$$

which leads to the second-order Delta method,

$$n\{g(\bar{X}_n) - g(\mu)\} \xrightarrow{\mathcal{D}} \frac{\sigma^2 g''(\mu)}{2}\chi_1^2.$$

## 3.2   FREQUENTIST METHODS

### 3.2.1   Maximum Likelihood Estimation

The maximum likelihood method is the most widely used frequentist approach to estimation and inference. Suppose that the density function of random variable $Y$ is $f(y|\boldsymbol{\theta})$, where $\boldsymbol{\theta}$ is a vector of unknown parameters. Let $\mathbf{y} = \{y_1, \ldots, y_n\}$ denote an i.i.d. sample from $f(y|\boldsymbol{\theta})$, and then the likelihood function is given by

$$L(\boldsymbol{\theta}) = \prod_{i=1}^{n} f(y_i|\boldsymbol{\theta}).$$

The maximum likelihood estimator (MLE) of $\boldsymbol{\theta}$ is obtained by maximizing $L(\boldsymbol{\theta})$ or its logarithm $\log L(\boldsymbol{\theta})$. The first derivative of $\log L(\boldsymbol{\theta})$ with respect to $\boldsymbol{\theta}$ is called the score function,

$$\mathbf{U}_n(\boldsymbol{\theta}) = \frac{\partial \log L(\boldsymbol{\theta})}{\partial \boldsymbol{\theta}} = \sum_{i=1}^{n} \frac{\partial \log f(y_i|\boldsymbol{\theta})}{\partial \boldsymbol{\theta}}, \qquad (3.2)$$

and the MLE $\hat{\boldsymbol{\theta}}$ can be solved from the score equation, $\mathbf{U}_n(\boldsymbol{\theta}) = \mathbf{0}$. Often there is no closed-form solution for the MLE. Hence an iterative procedure, such as the Newton–Raphson algorithm, may be used to solve the score equation. In this iterative procedure, we first specify an initial value $\hat{\theta}_{(0)}$, and then at the $k$th iteration the estimate of $\theta$ is updated as

$$\hat{\theta}_{(k)} = \hat{\theta}_{(k-1)} - \left\{ \frac{\partial \mathbf{U}_n(\theta)}{\partial \theta^{\mathsf{T}}} \right\}^{-1} \Bigg|_{\hat{\theta}_{(k-1)}} \mathbf{U}_n(\hat{\theta}_{(k-1)}), \qquad (3.3)$$

where $\hat{\theta}_{(k-1)}$ is the estimate from the $(k-1)$th iteration. We continue updating the estimate of $\theta$ until some prespecified convergence criteria are met. If we replace $\partial \mathbf{U}_n(\theta)/\partial \theta^{\mathsf{T}}$ by $\mathrm{E}\{\partial \mathbf{U}_n(\theta)/\partial \theta^{\mathsf{T}}\}$ in (3.3), this is called the Fisher-scoring algorithm.

The second derivative of $-\log L(\theta)$ with respect to $\theta$ is the observed information matrix of $\theta$,

$$\mathbf{I}_n(\theta) = -\frac{\partial^2 \log L(\theta)}{\partial \theta \partial \theta^{\mathsf{T}}} = -\sum_{i=1}^{n} \frac{\partial^2 \log f(y_i|\theta)}{\partial \theta \partial \theta^{\mathsf{T}}},$$

and correspondingly, the expected (Fisher) information matrix is given by

$$\begin{aligned} \mathcal{I}(\theta) &= -n\mathrm{E}\left\{ \frac{\partial^2 \log f(Y|\theta)}{\partial \theta \partial \theta^{\mathsf{T}}} \right\} \\ &= n\mathrm{E}\left[ \left\{ \frac{\partial \log f(Y|\theta)}{\partial \theta} \right\} \left\{ \frac{\partial \log f(Y|\theta)}{\partial \theta} \right\}^{\mathsf{T}} \right]. \end{aligned}$$

Under certain regularity conditions, the score function $\mathbf{U}_n(\theta_0)$ evaluated at the true parameter $\theta_0$ asymptotically follows a zero-mean normal distribution with variance–covariance matrix $\mathcal{I}(\theta_0)$. The MLE $\hat{\theta}$ possesses many desirable properties, such as consistency and asymptotic normality; that is, $\hat{\theta} - \theta_0$ converges in distribution to a zero-mean normal distribution with variance–covariance matrix $\mathcal{I}^{-1}(\theta_0)$. Moreover, the MLE is the efficient estimator in the sense that the variance of $\hat{\theta}$ achieves the Cramér–Rao lower bound (Sen and Singer, 1993).

### 3.2.2 Method of Moments

Let $\{y_1, \ldots, y_n\}$ be an i.i.d. sample of random variable $Y$ with a density function $f(y|\theta)$, where $\theta$ is an unknown $\nu$-dimensional parameter vector. The sample moments are given by $n^{-1}\sum_{i=1}^{n} y_i, \ldots, n^{-1}\sum_{i=1}^{n} y_i^{\nu}$, and the corresponding population moments are $\mathrm{E}(Y), \ldots, \mathrm{E}(Y^{\nu})$. By matching respective sample and population moments, a total of $\nu$ estimating equations can be constructed for the

$\nu$ unknown parameters of $\boldsymbol{\theta}$:

$$\frac{1}{n}\sum_{i=1}^{n} y_i = \mathrm{E}(Y),$$

$$\vdots$$

$$\frac{1}{n}\sum_{i=1}^{n} y_i^\nu = \mathrm{E}(Y^\nu),$$

from which we can obtain the estimator for $\boldsymbol{\theta}$.

**EXAMPLE 3.1**

As an illustration, suppose that we observe an i.i.d. sample $\{y_1, \ldots, y_n\}$ from a normal distribution, $\mathrm{N}(\mu, \sigma^2)$ with unknown $\mu$ and $\sigma$. By the method of moments, we have

$$\frac{1}{n}\sum_{i=1}^{n} y_i = \mu \quad \text{and} \quad \frac{1}{n}\sum_{i=1}^{n} y_i^2 = \mu^2 + \sigma^2,$$

which lead to the estimators of $\mu$ and $\sigma^2$ as

$$\hat{\mu} = \bar{y}_n = \frac{1}{n}\sum_{i=1}^{n} y_i,$$

and

$$\hat{\sigma}^2 = \frac{1}{n}\sum_{i=1}^{n} y_i^2 - \bar{y}_n^2 = \frac{1}{n}\sum_{i=1}^{n}(y_i - \bar{y}_n)^2,$$

respectively.

### 3.2.3  Generalized Method of Moments

The generalized method of moments (GMM) is an estimation and inference procedure that has gained much popularity in econometrics (Hansen, 1982; Hall, 2005). The GMM is particularly useful for enhancing efficiency when the likelihood is difficult to derive but the moment conditions are available, and it is also applicable when there are more moment conditions than unknown parameters.

In general, the sample moment can be written as

$$\mathbf{U}_n(\boldsymbol{\theta}) = \frac{1}{n}\sum_{i=1}^{n}\mathbf{u}_i(\boldsymbol{\theta}),$$

which may be the score function in (3.2) or other estimating equations. The GMM estimator $\hat{\boldsymbol{\theta}}$ is obtained by minimizing the quadratic objective function

$$Q_n(\boldsymbol{\theta}) = n\mathbf{U}_n^\mathsf{T}(\boldsymbol{\theta})\boldsymbol{\Sigma}_n^{-1}(\boldsymbol{\theta})\mathbf{U}_n(\boldsymbol{\theta}),$$

where $\Sigma_n(\boldsymbol{\theta})$ is the empirical variance–covariance matrix,

$$\Sigma_n(\boldsymbol{\theta}) = \frac{1}{n} \sum_{i=1}^{n} \mathbf{u}_i(\boldsymbol{\theta})\mathbf{u}_i^{\mathsf{T}}(\boldsymbol{\theta}) - \mathbf{U}_n(\boldsymbol{\theta})\mathbf{U}_n^{\mathsf{T}}(\boldsymbol{\theta}).$$

Via a two-stage iterative procedure, $\hat{\boldsymbol{\theta}}$ is computed as follows:

(1) Insert an initial value $\hat{\boldsymbol{\theta}}_{(0)}$ into $\Sigma_n(\boldsymbol{\theta})$.

(2) At the $k$th iteration, we obtain the estimator $\hat{\boldsymbol{\theta}}_{(k)}$ by minimizing

$$n\mathbf{U}_n^{\mathsf{T}}(\boldsymbol{\theta})\Sigma_n^{-1}(\hat{\boldsymbol{\theta}}_{(k-1)})\mathbf{U}_n(\boldsymbol{\theta})$$

with respect to $\boldsymbol{\theta}$, in which $\Sigma_n(\hat{\boldsymbol{\theta}}_{(k-1)})$ is fixed as known by plugging in the estimate $\hat{\boldsymbol{\theta}}_{(k-1)}$ from the $(k-1)$th iteration.

(3) Continue until some prespecified convergence criteria are met.

The GMM estimator $\hat{\boldsymbol{\theta}}$ may also be obtained by directly minimizing $Q_n(\boldsymbol{\theta})$ (Hansen, Heaton, and Yaron, 1996).

Under certain regularity conditions (Hansen, 1982), the GMM estimator $\hat{\boldsymbol{\theta}}$ exists and converges in probability to the true parameter $\boldsymbol{\theta}_0$, and $\sqrt{n}(\hat{\boldsymbol{\theta}} - \boldsymbol{\theta}_0)$ converges in distribution to a zero-mean normal distribution. Moreover, $Q_n(\boldsymbol{\theta})$ follows a chi-squared distribution when evaluated at $\boldsymbol{\theta}_0$ or $\hat{\boldsymbol{\theta}}$.

### 3.2.4  Confidence Interval

Besides the point estimates for the parameters of interest, the interval estimates are also critically important. For ease of exposition, we consider a scalar parameter $\theta$, whose true value is denoted by $\theta_0$. We are interested in constructing a confidence interval for $\theta$ such that a random interval $[\hat{\theta}_L, \hat{\theta}_U]$ covers $\theta_0$ with a certain probability. Toward this goal, we first derive a pivotal quantity and then construct the interval estimate $[\hat{\theta}_L, \hat{\theta}_U]$ based upon the distribution of the pivot.

For illustration, let $\{y_1, \ldots, y_n\}$ be an i.i.d. sample from $Y \sim \mathrm{N}(\mu, \sigma^2)$, where $\mu$ is unknown and $\sigma$ is known. Denote the sample mean by $\bar{y}_n = n^{-1}\sum_{i=1}^{n} y_i$, and then the pivotal quantity is given by

$$\sqrt{n}\left(\frac{\bar{y}_n - \mu}{\sigma}\right) \sim \mathrm{N}(0, 1).$$

As a result, the $100(1 - \alpha)\%$ confidence interval for $\mu$ is

$$\left[\bar{y}_n - z_{\alpha/2}\frac{\sigma}{\sqrt{n}}, \ \ \bar{y}_n + z_{\alpha/2}\frac{\sigma}{\sqrt{n}}\right],$$

where $z_{\alpha/2}$ is the $100(1 - \alpha/2)$th percentile of the standard normal distribution; that is, $\Pr(Z \leq z_{\alpha/2}) = 1 - \alpha/2$ for $Z \sim \mathrm{N}(0, 1)$. Conventionally, we take

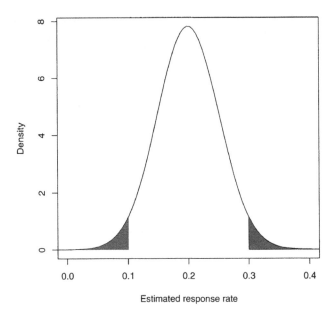

**Figure 3.1**    Estimated 95% confidence interval for the response rate of an experimental drug.

$\alpha = 0.05$ and thus $z_{\alpha/2} \approx 1.96$, which leads to the usual 95% confidence interval of $\mu$. If $\sigma$ is unknown, the $100(1 - \alpha)\%$ confidence interval for $\mu$ is

$$\left[ \bar{y}_n - t_{n-1,\alpha/2} \frac{s_n}{\sqrt{n}}, \quad \bar{y}_n + t_{n-1,\alpha/2} \frac{s_n}{\sqrt{n}} \right],$$

where $t_{n-1,\alpha/2}$ is the $100(1 - \alpha/2)$th percentile of Student's $t$ distribution with $n - 1$ degrees of freedom, and

$$s_n^2 = \frac{1}{n-1} \sum_{i=1}^{n} (y_i - \bar{y}_n)^2.$$

**EXAMPLE 3.2**

Suppose that a clinical trial was conducted to estimate the response rate $p$ of an experimental drug. We observed 13 responses among 65 subjects treated by this drug. Based on the binomial distribution, the estimated response rate is $\hat{p} = 0.2$, and the estimated standard error is $\widehat{\text{SE}} = \sqrt{\hat{p}(1 - \hat{p})/n} \approx 0.05$. We can construct a 95% confidence interval for $p$ using the asymptotic normal approximation; that is, $[\hat{p} - 1.96 \times \widehat{\text{SE}}, \hat{p} + 1.96 \times \widehat{\text{SE}}] \approx [0.1, 0.2]$, which is shown in Figure 3.1.

In practice, confidence intervals may be used to monitor a trial for early stopping. Suppose that for an experimental drug the response rate of $p = 30\%$ is considered clinically relevant. If at any time during the trial the upper bound of the 95% confidence interval of $p$ is smaller than 0.3, we may stop the trial and claim the experimental treatment not promising. As illustrated below, the futility early stopping of a clinical trial may be achieved by the use of the 95% confidence interval $[\hat{p}_L, \hat{p}_U]$.

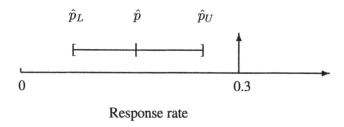

Response rate

### 3.2.5  Hypothesis Testing

Hypothesis testing typically involves a null hypothesis $H_0$ and an alternative hypothesis $H_1$, and each of them poses a statement on the parameter of interest $\theta$. In general, $H_0$ is a hypothesis on $\theta$ that we hope to reject based on the evidence from the data, and $H_1$, which contradicts $H_0$, is expected to hold by rejecting $H_0$.

Depending on how the parameter $\theta$ is specified, we may have

- simple hypotheses

$$H_0\colon \theta = \theta_0 \quad \text{versus} \quad H_1\colon \theta = \theta_1,$$

where $\theta_0$ and $\theta_1$ are the prespecified parameter values and $\theta_0 \neq \theta_1$; or

- composite hypotheses

$$H_0\colon \theta \in \Theta \quad \text{versus} \quad H_1\colon \theta \in \Theta^c,$$

where the parameter value of $\theta$ is not explicitly specified.

Based on the direction of the parameter value, hypothesis testing may also be classified as

- a one-sided test with

$$H_0\colon \theta \leq \theta_0 \quad \text{versus} \quad H_1\colon \theta > \theta_0,$$

if $H_0$ can be rejected when the test statistic exceeds the threshold along one direction only (to the right side in this case); or

- a two-sided test with

$$H_0: \theta = \theta_0 \quad \text{versus} \quad H_1: \theta \neq \theta_0,$$

if $H_0$ can be rejected when the test statistic exceeds the threshold along either direction.

Hypothesis testing is to decide which of the two hypotheses is true or more supported by the observed data. Two different types of error may occur, known as the type I and the type II errors, respectively. The type I error is false positive; that is, it rejects $H_0$ given that $H_0$ is true. The type II error is false negative; that is, it accepts $H_0$ given that $H_1$ is true. Controlling the type I error in clinical trials would prevent a flood of nonworking drugs into the market, while controlling the type II error would prevent overlooking a truly effective treatment. The probability of committing a type I error is the type I error rate, denoted by $\alpha$; the probability of committing a type II error is the type II error rate, denoted by $\beta$. Power is the probability of rejecting $H_0$ given that $H_1$ is true; that is, power $= 1 - \beta$. The type I error rate and power with respect to $H_0$ and $H_1$ are displayed in Figure 3.2.

Hypothesis testing in a clinical trial may formulate the null and the alternative hypotheses as

$H_0$: The experimental treatment is ineffective, and

$H_1$: The experimental treatment is effective.

We can classify $H_0$, $H_1$, and the trial conclusions on whether the drug is effective or not in the following $2 \times 2$ contingency table,

|  | Trial Conclusion: Ineffective | Trial Conclusion: Effective |
|---|---|---|
| $H_0$ | Correct | Type I error rate ($\alpha$) |
| $H_1$ | Type II error rate ($\beta$) | Correct (power) |

Based on a random sample from the population, we first construct a test statistic and then compute the $p$-value which is the probability of obtaining the data as or more extreme than the observed assuming that $H_0$ is true. The $p$-value can be obtained by comparing the test statistic with its associated distribution under the null hypothesis. The smaller the $p$-value, the stronger the evidence contained in the data against $H_0$. The statistical test is said to be *significant* if the resulting $p$-value is smaller than the prespecified significance level. The most widely used significance level is $\alpha = 0.05$. *Statistically significant* means that the observed result is unlikely to have occurred by chance given that the null hypothesis is true. For example, if the null hypothesis states that there is

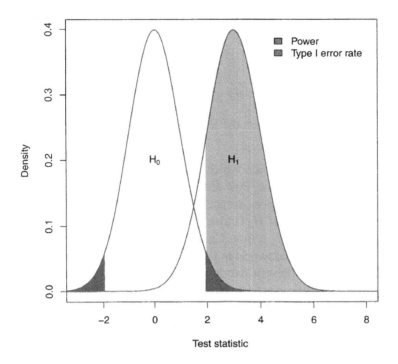

**Figure 3.2**    Type I error rate and power under the null and alternative hypotheses, respectively.

no difference between treatment groups, a $p$-value smaller than 0.05 indicates that the observed difference is so large that this would be very unlikely to occur under the null hypothesis, so we should reject $H_0$. Interestingly, the $p$-value itself under $H_0$ follows a $\mathrm{Unif}(0, 1)$; that is,

$$\Pr(p\text{-value} \leq \alpha | H_0) = \alpha,$$

for every $\alpha \in (0, 1)$.

**EXAMPLE 3.3**

Let $\{y_1, \ldots, y_n\}$ be an i.i.d. sample from the normal distribution $\mathrm{N}(\mu, \sigma^2)$ with unknown mean $\mu$ and variance $\sigma^2$. We are interested in testing

$$H_0\colon \mu = 0 \quad \text{versus} \quad H_1\colon \mu \neq 0.$$

The sample mean

$$\bar{y}_n = \frac{1}{n} \sum_{i=1}^{n} y_i$$

and the sample variance

$$s_n^2 = \frac{1}{n-1} \sum_{i=1}^{n} (y_i - \bar{y}_n)^2$$

are respective unbiased estimators for $\mu$ and $\sigma^2$, since $\mathrm{E}(\bar{y}_n) = \mu$ and $\mathrm{E}(s_n^2) = \sigma^2$. Moreover, $\bar{y}_n \sim \mathrm{N}(\mu, \sigma^2/n)$, $(n-1)s_n^2/\sigma^2 \sim \chi_{n-1}^2$, and $\bar{y}_n$ and $s_n$ are independent. Therefore, a $t$ test statistic can be constructed, $T_n = \sqrt{n}\bar{y}_n/s_n$, which follows Student's $t$ distribution with $n-1$ degrees of freedom under $H_0$.

### EXAMPLE 3.4

Under the MLE framework of Section 3.2.1, suppose that we are interested in testing the $\nu$-dimensional parameter vector $\boldsymbol{\theta}$ with

$$H_0\colon \boldsymbol{\theta} = \boldsymbol{\theta}_0 \quad \text{versus} \quad H_1\colon \boldsymbol{\theta} \neq \boldsymbol{\theta}_0.$$

By the maximum likelihood method, we first compute the MLE $\hat{\boldsymbol{\theta}}$ and the observed information matrix $\mathbf{I}_n(\boldsymbol{\theta})$ and then formulate the following three equivalent statistics,

- Wald's statistic: $(\hat{\boldsymbol{\theta}} - \boldsymbol{\theta}_0)^{\mathsf{T}} \mathbf{I}_n(\hat{\boldsymbol{\theta}})(\hat{\boldsymbol{\theta}} - \boldsymbol{\theta}_0)$,

- Likelihood ratio statistic: $-2\{\log L(\boldsymbol{\theta}_0) - \log L(\hat{\boldsymbol{\theta}})\}$, and

- Rao's score statistic: $\mathbf{U}_n^{\mathsf{T}}(\boldsymbol{\theta}_0)\mathbf{I}_n^{-1}(\boldsymbol{\theta}_0)\mathbf{U}_n(\boldsymbol{\theta}_0)$.

Under the null hypothesis, all three test statistics asymptotically follow the same chi-squared distribution with $\nu$ degrees of freedom.

### 3.2.6  Generalized Linear Model and Quasi-Likelihood

Suppose that we observe the outcome $y_i$ (which may be continuous or discrete) and the associated covariate vector $\mathbf{Z}_i$ for $i = 1, \ldots, n$. To characterize the relationship between $y_i$ and $\mathbf{Z}_i$, generalized linear models are readily applicable to various types of outcomes (McCullagh and Nelder, 1989). For continuous data, we typically assume normality and fit a linear regression model,

$$y_i = \boldsymbol{\beta}^{\mathsf{T}} \mathbf{Z}_i + \epsilon_i,$$

where the error $\epsilon_i \sim \mathrm{N}(0, \sigma^2)$. By taking the first derivative of the log-likelihood, the score function is given by

$$\mathbf{U}_n(\boldsymbol{\beta}) = \sum_{i=1}^{n} \mathbf{Z}_i(y_i - \boldsymbol{\beta}^{\mathsf{T}} \mathbf{Z}_i).$$

The MLE of $\beta$ has a close-form solution,

$$\hat{\beta} = \left( \sum_{i=1}^{n} \mathbf{Z}_i \mathbf{Z}_i^{\mathsf{T}} \right)^{-1} \sum_{i=1}^{n} \mathbf{Z}_i y_i.$$

For dichotomous data, the outcome variable $y_i$ takes a value of 1 with probability $p_i$, and 0 with probability $1 - p_i$. Under the usual logistic regression model,

$$\mathrm{logit}(p_i) \equiv \log\left( \frac{p_i}{1 - p_i} \right) = \beta^{\mathsf{T}} \mathbf{Z}_i,$$

the score function takes the form of

$$\mathbf{U}_n(\beta) = \sum_{i=1}^{n} \mathbf{Z}_i \left\{ y_i - \frac{\exp(\beta^{\mathsf{T}} \mathbf{Z}_i)}{1 + \exp(\beta^{\mathsf{T}} \mathbf{Z}_i)} \right\}.$$

The MLE of $\beta$ does not have an explicit form and may be obtained by the Newton–Raphson algorithm. If $y_i$ is an integer representing a count outcome, the Poisson (log-linear) model is readily applicable,

$$\log(\mu_i) = \beta^{\mathsf{T}} \mathbf{Z}_i,$$

where $\mu_i$ is the Poisson mean; and correspondingly, the score function is

$$\mathbf{U}_n(\beta) = \sum_{i=1}^{n} \mathbf{Z}_i \{ y_i - \exp(\beta^{\mathsf{T}} \mathbf{Z}_i) \}.$$

Besides the identity, logit-, and log-link functions, other commonly used link functions include the complementary log–log transformation $\log\{-\log(\cdot)\}$ and the probit function $\Phi^{-1}(\cdot)$.

The aforementioned score functions are special cases of the more general quasi-likelihood approach (Wedderburn, 1974; McCullagh, 1983). If we denote $\mu_i$ and $V_i$ as the respective mean and variance of the outcome variable $y_i$, the quasi-likelihood estimator can be solved from

$$\sum_{i=1}^{n} \frac{\partial \mu_i}{\partial \beta} V_i^{-1} (y_i - \mu_i) = \mathbf{0}.$$

So far, the observed data are assumed to be i.i.d., which, however, may not be true in many cases, such longitudinal measurements or clustered/grouped data. In this regard, statistical methods need to account for the underlying correlations for valid inference (Diggle et al., 2002). Liang and Zeger (1986) propose the generalized estimating equation (GEE) for such data, which provides a population-average approach to modeling the marginal mean while treating the correlation as nuisance.

For $i = 1, \ldots, n$, let $\mathbf{y}_i = (y_{i1}, \ldots, y_{iK})^\mathsf{T}$ denote a $K$-vector of outcome variables for cluster $i$, and let $\boldsymbol{\mu}_i = (\mu_{i1}, \ldots, \mu_{iK})^\mathsf{T}$ denote the marginal mean of $\mathbf{y}_i$. Via a link function $\eta(\cdot)$, the generalized linear model specifies

$$\eta(\mu_{ik}) = \boldsymbol{\beta}^\mathsf{T}\mathbf{Z}_{ik},$$

for $i = 1, \ldots, n$ and $k = 1, \ldots, K$. If we denote $\mathbf{C}_i$ as the working correlation matrix, which may not be identical to the true correlation matrix, the GEE is given by

$$\sum_{i=1}^{n} \left(\frac{\partial \boldsymbol{\mu}_i}{\partial \boldsymbol{\beta}}\right)^\mathsf{T} \mathbf{V}_i^{-1}(\mathbf{y}_i - \boldsymbol{\mu}_i) = \mathbf{0}, \tag{3.4}$$

where $\mathbf{V}_i = \boldsymbol{\Gamma}_i^{1/2}\mathbf{C}_i\boldsymbol{\Gamma}_i^{1/2}$ and $\boldsymbol{\Gamma}_i$ is the diagonal matrix of the marginal variances for cluster $i$. Under certain regularity conditions, the GEE estimator $\hat{\boldsymbol{\beta}}$ solved from (3.4) is consistent and asymptotically normal with a sandwich (robust) variance–covariance matrix.

### 3.2.7  Random Effects Model

In contrast to the marginal approach such as the GEE, the random effects model is a subject-specific approach by explicitly formulating the dependence structure through random effects. The observed data are assumed to be conditionally independent, given the unobservable random effects. For illustration, let $y_{ik}$ denote the outcome of measurement $k$ on subject $i$ in a longitudinal study, for $i = 1, \ldots, n$ and $k = 1, \ldots, K$. The linear random effects (or mixed) model is given by

$$y_{ik} = \boldsymbol{\beta}^\mathsf{T}\mathbf{Z}_{ik} + \mathbf{b}_i^\mathsf{T}\mathbf{X}_{ik} + \epsilon_{ik}, \tag{3.5}$$

where $\boldsymbol{\beta}$ is a vector of fixed effects, $\mathbf{b}_i$ is a vector of random effects, and $\mathbf{Z}_{ik}$ and $\mathbf{X}_{ik}$ are covariates. Let $\mathbf{y}_i = (y_{i1}, \ldots, y_{iK})^\mathsf{T}$, $\mathbf{Z}_i = (\mathbf{Z}_{i1}, \ldots, \mathbf{Z}_{iK})^\mathsf{T}$, and $\mathbf{X}_i$ and $\epsilon_i$ are defined similarly. In a more compact form, model (3.5) can be rewritten as

$$\mathbf{y}_i = \mathbf{Z}_i\boldsymbol{\beta} + \mathbf{X}_i\mathbf{b}_i + \epsilon_i.$$

We assume that $\mathbf{b}_i$ and $\epsilon_i$ are independent and normally distributed with mean zero and variance–covariance matrices $\mathbf{G}$ and $\mathbf{R}$, respectively.

Model parameters in (3.5) can be estimated by iterating between the generalized least squares estimation of $\boldsymbol{\beta}$ and the restricted maximum likelihood estimation of the variance components (Harville, 1977). Let $\boldsymbol{\Sigma}_i$ denote the variance of $\mathbf{y}_i$; that is, $\boldsymbol{\Sigma}_i = \mathbf{X}_i\mathbf{G}\mathbf{X}_i^\mathsf{T} + \mathbf{R}$. For a fixed $\boldsymbol{\Sigma}_i$, the MLE of $\boldsymbol{\beta}$ can be obtained by minimizing

$$\sum_{i=1}^{n}(\mathbf{y}_i - \mathbf{Z}_i\boldsymbol{\beta})^\mathsf{T}\boldsymbol{\Sigma}_i^{-1}(\mathbf{y}_i - \mathbf{Z}_i\boldsymbol{\beta}),$$

which leads to an explicit solution of

$$\hat{\boldsymbol{\beta}} = \sum_{i=1}^{n} (\mathbf{Z}_i^{\mathsf{T}} \boldsymbol{\Sigma}_i^{-1} \mathbf{Z}_i)^{-1} \mathbf{Z}_i^{\mathsf{T}} \boldsymbol{\Sigma}_i^{-1} \mathbf{y}_i.$$

The restricted MLE is often preferred over the usual MLE, as the latter may yield biased estimates for the variance components.

## 3.3 SURVIVAL ANALYSIS

Often, the primary endpoint in a phase III clinical trial is concerned with patient survival. For example, progression-free survival measures the length of the time after treatment during which the disease remains stable without any sign of progression; overall survival is the time from the initiation of treatment to death due to any cause. Survival data are subject to random censoring, which may be caused by loss of follow-up, interim analysis, or the termination of the study. The most common case, right censoring, occurs if a patient is only known to have survived up to a (censoring) time point, but not exactly when the event occurred afterwards (Kalbfleisch and Prentice, 2002). Interval censored data arise if a patient is known to experience the event between two time points, but the exact failure time is unknown (Sun, 2006).

Let $f(t)$ denote the probability density function of failure time $T$, and let $S(t) = P(T > t)$ denote the survival function. The hazard function

$$\lambda(t) = \lim_{\delta \to 0} \frac{P(t \leq T < t + \delta | T \geq t)}{\delta}$$

specifies the instantaneous failure rate, given that a subject has survived up to time $t$; and the cumulative hazard function is defined as

$$\Lambda(t) = \int_0^t \lambda(u) \, du.$$

It is easy to show that $S(t) = \exp\{-\Lambda(t)\}$ and $\lambda(t) = f(t)/S(t)$. Therefore, $f(t)$, $S(t)$, $\lambda(t)$, and $\Lambda(t)$ are one-to-one related; that is, any one of these functions uniquely determines the others.

### 3.3.1 Kaplan–Meier Estimator

As shown in Figure 3.3, the calendar time in a clinical trial can be divided into the accrual period and the follow-up period. Although patients are enrolled into a trial at different calendar times due to staggered entry, they can all be aligned at the same baseline condition for the purpose of analysis.

For $i = 1, \ldots, n$, let $T_i$ be the failure time, let $C_i$ be the censoring time, and we observe $X_i = \min(T_i, C_i)$ and the censoring indicator $\Delta_i = I(T_i \leq C_i)$,

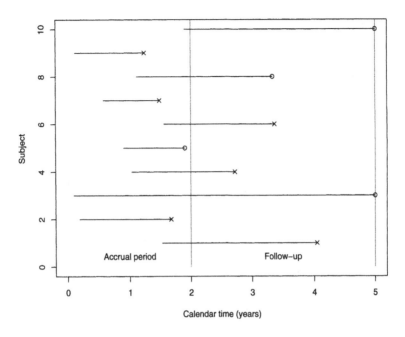

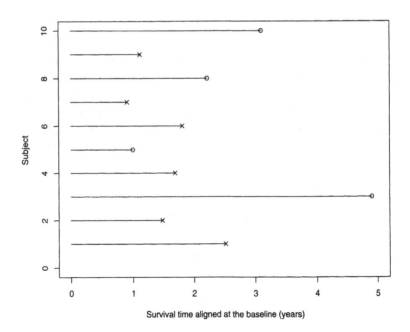

**Figure 3.3**  Patients' accrual period and follow-up period, with crosses denoting events and circles denoting censoring.

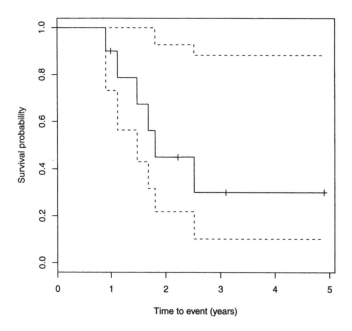

**Figure 3.4**   Kaplan–Meier estimator of the survival function with its pointwise 95% confidence interval, with "+" indicating censored observations.

where $I(\cdot)$ is the indicator function. We assume that $T_i$ and $C_i$ are independent; that is, censoring times do not carry any information about failure times. Let $D_i$ denote the number of events occurred at time $X_i$, and let $R_i$ denote the number of subjects at risk just prior to $X_i$, so $R_i$ includes those who have not experienced the event or been censored yet. Under the independent censoring assumption, the Kaplan–Meier (or product-limit) estimator (Kaplan and Meier, 1958) for the survival function $S(t)$ is given by

$$\hat{S}(t) = \prod_{i:X_i \leq t} \left( 1 - \frac{D_i}{R_i} \right), \qquad (3.6)$$

and the variance of $\hat{S}(t)$ can be estimated by the Greenwood (1926) formula,

$$\widehat{\mathrm{Var}}\{\hat{S}(t)\} = \hat{S}^2(t) \sum_{i:X_i \leq t} \frac{D_i}{R_i(R_i - D_i)}.$$

For the data presented in Figure 3.3, the Kaplan–Meier estimator of the survival function and its pointwise 95% confidence intervals are displayed in Figure 3.4.

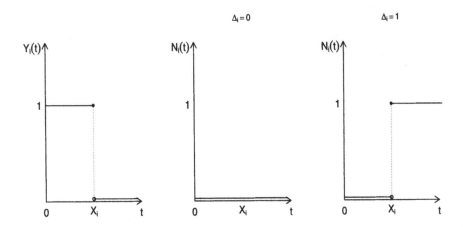

**Figure 3.5** At-risk process $Y_i(t) = I(X_i \geq t)$ and counting process $N_i(t) = I(X_i \leq t, \Delta_i = 1)$.

Starting from 1 toward 0, the Kaplan–Meier estimator is a nonincreasing step function with jumps at failure times only.

In survival analysis, it is easier to develop asymptotic theories based on the counting process and martingale (Andersen and Gill, 1982; Fleming and Harrington, 1991). As shown in Figure 3.5, the at-risk process $Y_i(t) = I(X_i \geq t)$ indicates whether subject $i$ is still at risk at time $t$; and the counting process $N_i(t) = I(X_i \leq t, \Delta_i = 1)$ indicates whether subject $i$ has experienced the event by time $t$. Let $Y(t) = \sum_{i=1}^{n} Y_i(t)$ and $N(t) = \sum_{i=1}^{n} N_i(t)$. The Kaplan–Meier estimator in (3.6) can be rewritten as

$$\hat{S}(t) = \prod_{i:X_i \leq t} \left\{ 1 - \frac{\Delta N(X_i)}{Y(X_i)} \right\},$$

where $\Delta N(t) = N(t) - N(t-)$. The cumulative hazard function $\Lambda(t)$ can be estimated by the Nelson–Aalen estimator,

$$\hat{\Lambda}(t) = \sum_{i:X_i \leq t} \frac{\Delta N(X_i)}{Y(X_i)},$$

which is a nondecreasing step function taking jumps at failure times only. The estimate for the variance of $\hat{\Lambda}(t)$ is given by

$$\widehat{\mathrm{Var}}\{\hat{\Lambda}(t)\} = \sum_{i:X_i \leq t} \frac{\Delta N(X_i)}{Y^2(X_i)}.$$

### 3.3.2 Log-Rank Test

In a two-sample comparison with time-to-event data, the log-rank test is the most commonly used approach to testing whether the two survival curves are the same. Let $S_1(t)$ and $S_2(t)$ denote the survival functions for treatment groups 1 and 2, respectively. The null hypothesis is

$$H_0\colon S_1(t) = S_2(t) \ \text{ for all } t,$$

and the alternative hypothesis is

$$H_1\colon S_1(t) \neq S_2(t) \ \text{ for some } t.$$

To construct the log-rank test, we first sort the distinct failure times in the pooled sample, $t_1 < \cdots < t_m$, where $m$ is the total number of unique failure times. Then at each distinct failure time $t_i$, we create a $2 \times 2$ contingency table as follows:

|  | Group 1 | Group 2 |  |
|---|---|---|---|
| Number of failures | $D_{1i}$ | $D_{2i}$ | $D_i$ |
| Number of survivors | $R_{1i} - D_{1i}$ | $R_{2i} - D_{2i}$ | $R_i - D_i$ |
| Number of subjects at risk | $R_{1i}$ | $R_{2i}$ | $R_i$ |

Under $H_0$, the number of events in group 1 follows a hypergeometric distribution conditional on all the marginal counts, i.e., $D_{1i} \sim \text{Hypergeometric}(R_i, R_{1i}, D_i)$. Under the hypergeometric distribution, the expected number of failures in group 1 is $R_{1i}D_i/R_i$, and the variance of $D_{1i}$ is

$$V_i = \frac{R_{1i}R_{2i}D_i(R_i - D_i)}{R_i^2(R_i - 1)}.$$

Hence, by comparing the observed number of events with the expected count, the standardized log-rank test statistic is given by

$$T_n = \frac{\sum_{i=1}^{m}(D_{1i} - R_{1i}D_i/R_i)}{(\sum_{i=1}^{m} V_i)^{1/2}},$$

which asymptotically follows the standard normal distribution under $H_0$.

### 3.3.3 Proportional Hazards Model

When covariates are involved in survival analysis, it is often assumed that the failure time $T_i$ and the censoring time $C_i$ are conditionally independent given covariates $\mathbf{Z}_i$. The observed data $\{X_i = \min(T_i, C_i), \Delta_i = I(T_i \leq C_i), \mathbf{Z}_i\}$ are i.i.d. replicates of $(X, \Delta, \mathbf{Z})$ for $i = 1, \ldots, n$. If we denote $\lambda(t|\mathbf{Z}_i)$ as the hazard function for subject $i$ with covariates $\mathbf{Z}_i$, the Cox (1972) proportional hazards model takes the form of

$$\lambda(t|\mathbf{Z}_i) = \lambda_0(t)\exp(\boldsymbol{\beta}^{\mathsf{T}}\mathbf{Z}_i), \tag{3.7}$$

where $\beta$ is the parameter of interest and $\lambda_0(t)$ is the unknown baseline hazard function. If $\lambda_0(t)$ is not specified, (3.7) becomes a semiparametric regression model.

For subjects who have experienced the event of interest, their contributions to the likelihood are the density functions evaluated at their failure times; and for those who have been censored, their contributions to the likelihood are their survival functions (i.e., all the information we know are that these subjects have survived up to their respective censoring time points). As a result, the likelihood function is given by

$$ L(\beta) = \prod_{i=1}^{n} f(X_i|\mathbf{Z}_i)^{\Delta_i} S(X_i|\mathbf{Z}_i)^{1-\Delta_i} = \prod_{i=1}^{n} \lambda(X_i|\mathbf{Z}_i)^{\Delta_i} S(X_i|\mathbf{Z}_i), $$

where $f(X_i|\mathbf{Z}_i)$ is the density function and $S(X_i|\mathbf{Z}_i)$ is the survival function of subject $i$. Let $\mathcal{R}(t) = \{j: X_j \geq t\}$ denote the risk set prior to time $t$. The partial likelihood (Cox, 1975) takes the form of

$$ L_p(\beta) = \prod_{i=1}^{n} \left\{ \frac{\exp(\beta^\mathsf{T} \mathbf{Z}_i)}{\sum_{j \in \mathcal{R}(X_i)} \exp(\beta^\mathsf{T} \mathbf{Z}_j)} \right\}^{\Delta_i}, $$

in which the infinite-dimensional parameter $\lambda_0(t)$ is eliminated so that the only remaining parameter is $\beta$. By taking the first derivative of $\log L_p(\beta)$ with respect to $\beta$, we have the score function,

$$ \mathbf{U}_n(\beta) = \sum_{i=1}^{n} \Delta_i \left\{ \mathbf{Z}_i - \frac{\sum_{j \in \mathcal{R}(X_i)} \mathbf{Z}_j \exp(\beta^\mathsf{T} \mathbf{Z}_j)}{\sum_{j \in \mathcal{R}(X_i)} \exp(\beta^\mathsf{T} \mathbf{Z}_j)} \right\}. \tag{3.8} $$

The maximum likelihood estimator of $\beta$ can be solved from $\mathbf{U}_n(\beta) = \mathbf{0}$.

Let $\Lambda_0(t)$ denote the baseline cumulative hazard function, $\Lambda_0(t) = \int_0^t \lambda_0(u)du$. As defined before, let $N_i(t) = I(X_i \leq t, \Delta_i = 1)$ and $Y_i(t) = I(X_i \geq t)$, and then the martingale under the Cox proportional hazards model is given by

$$ M_i(t) = N_i(t) - \int_0^t Y_i(u) \exp(\beta^\mathsf{T} \mathbf{Z}_i) \, d\Lambda_0(u). $$

The score process is written as

$$ \mathbf{U}_n(\beta, t) = \sum_{i=1}^{n} \int_0^t \left\{ \mathbf{Z}_i - \frac{\sum_{j=1}^{n} Y_j(u) \exp(\beta^\mathsf{T} \mathbf{Z}_j) \mathbf{Z}_j}{\sum_{j=1}^{n} Y_j(u) \exp(\beta^\mathsf{T} \mathbf{Z}_j)} \right\} dM_i(u), $$

which reduces to (3.8) by taking $t = \infty$. The Aalen–Breslow estimator (Breslow, 1974) of $\Lambda_0(t)$ is given by

$$ \hat{\Lambda}_0(t, \beta) = \int_0^t \frac{\sum_{i=1}^{n} dN_i(u)}{\sum_{i=1}^{n} Y_i(u) \exp(\beta^\mathsf{T} \mathbf{Z}_i)}, $$

where $dN_i(u) = N_i((u + du)-) - N_i(u-)$.

### 3.3.4 Cure Rate Model

The entire population may be a mixture of patients who would eventually experience the event of interest if a sufficient follow-up is taken, and those who would never experience the event. For example, cancer patients after intensive chemotherapy treatment, may develop drug resistance and will not achieve partial or complete response under another treatment no matter how long they are followed. To incorporate a cure/insusceptible fraction in the population, cure rate models are developed for such time-to-event data.

Let $S_{\text{pop}}(t|\mathbf{Z}_i)$ denote an improper survival function for the population; that is, $\lim_{t\to\infty} S_{\text{pop}}(t|\mathbf{Z}_i) > 0$, where $\mathbf{Z}_i$ is a vector of covariates for subject $i$. The mixture cure model (Berkson and Gage, 1952) takes the form of

$$S_{\text{pop}}(t|\mathbf{Z}_i) = 1 - \theta(\mathbf{Z}_i) + \theta(\mathbf{Z}_i)S(t),$$

where $S(t)$ is a usual proper survival function and $1 - \theta(\mathbf{Z}_i)$ represents the proportion of the population that is cured or insusceptible to the event. Often, $\theta(\mathbf{Z}_i)$ is modeled by the logistic regression,

$$\theta(\mathbf{Z}_i) = \frac{\exp(\boldsymbol{\beta}^\mathsf{T}\mathbf{Z}_i)}{1 + \exp(\boldsymbol{\beta}^\mathsf{T}\mathbf{Z}_i)}.$$

In an alternative formulation (Yakovlev et al., 1993; Yin and Ibrahim, 2005), the cure rate model takes the form of

$$S_{\text{pop}}(t|\mathbf{Z}_i) = \exp\{-\theta(\mathbf{Z}_i)F(t)\}, \tag{3.9}$$

where $\theta(\mathbf{Z}_i) = \exp(\boldsymbol{\beta}^\mathsf{T}\mathbf{Z}_i)$ and $F(t)$ is the baseline cumulative distribution function. The cure rate under model (3.9) is $\lim_{t\to\infty} S_{\text{pop}}(t|\mathbf{Z}_i) = \exp\{-\theta(\mathbf{Z}_i)\}$, and the population hazard function is $\lambda_{\text{pop}}(t|\mathbf{Z}_i) = \theta(\mathbf{Z}_i)f(t)$, where $f(t) = dF(t)/dt$. For more detailed discussions on cure rate models, see Kuk and Chen (1992), Maller and Zhou (1996), Tsodikov (1998), and Ibrahim, Chen, and Sinha (2001).

## 3.4 BAYESIAN METHODS

### 3.4.1 Bayes' Theorem

According to Bayes' rule, if $A$ and $B$ are two events in the sample space $\Omega$, then the conditional probability of $A$ given $B$ is

$$P(A|B) = \frac{P(A\cap B)}{P(B)} = \frac{P(B|A)P(A)}{P(B)},$$

where $P(B) \neq 0$. If $P(A\cap B) = P(A)P(B)$, $A$ and $B$ are said to be statistically independent. More generally, if $\{A_1, \ldots, A_m\}$ is a partition of $\Omega$, then for each

$i = 1, \ldots, m,$

$$P(A_i|B) = \frac{P(B|A_i)P(A_i)}{\sum_{j=1}^{m} P(B|A_j)P(A_j)}.$$

Bayesian methods adhere to the likelihood principle: All that we know about the data/sample is contained in the likelihood function. If the likelihood functions under two different sampling plans/distributions are proportional with respect to the parameter of interest $\theta$, statistical inferences on $\theta$ should be identical based on these two sampling distributions.

**EXAMPLE 3.5**

We consider an experiment in which a coin was tossed 12 times, with 9 heads and 3 tails observed (Lindley and Phillips, 1976). Let $\theta$ be the probability of observing a head for a toss of the coin, and we are interested in testing the hypotheses,

$$H_0: \theta = 0.5 \quad \text{versus} \quad H_1: \theta > 0.5.$$

There is no further information on the sampling plan.

Based on the observed data, there may be two choices for the likelihood function. First, let $Y$ denote the number of heads after a fixed number of $n$ tosses; that is, $Y \sim \text{Bin}(n, \theta)$. Under the binomial distribution with $n = 12$ tosses and $y = 9$ heads observed, the likelihood function is given by

$$L_1(\theta) = \binom{n}{y} \theta^y (1 - \theta)^{n-y} = \binom{12}{9} \theta^9 (1 - \theta)^3.$$

Second, let $Y$ be the number of heads for the tosses of the coin until the third tail ($r = 3$) is observed; that is, $Y \sim \text{Neg-Bin}(r, \theta)$. Under the negative binomial distribution, the likelihood function is given by

$$L_2(\theta) = \binom{y + r - 1}{y} \theta^y (1 - \theta)^r = \binom{11}{9} \theta^9 (1 - \theta)^3.$$

Clearly, $L_1(\theta) \propto L_2(\theta)$ except for a normalizing constant, and the posterior distributions of $\theta$ under these two sampling distributions are identical in the Bayesian framework. However, frequentist inferences about $\theta$ are very different, which depends on the sampling distribution. Based on the binomial likelihood, the $p$-value is

$$p_1\text{-value} = \Pr(y \geq 9|H_0) = \sum_{y=9}^{12} \binom{12}{y} 0.5^{12} \approx 0.073,$$

while under the negative binomial distribution,

$$p_2\text{-value} = \Pr(y \geq 9|H_0) = \sum_{y=9}^{\infty} \binom{y+2}{y} 0.5^{3+y} \approx 0.033.$$

If we set the significance level at $\alpha = 0.05$, the frequentist hypothesis test yields conflicting results: The null hypothesis is accepted under the binomial distribution, but it is rejected under the negative binomial distribution.

Let $\mathbf{y} = \{y_1, \dots, y_n\}$ be an i.i.d. sample from a density function $f(y|\theta)$ which is characterized by a vector of unknown parameters $\theta$. The likelihood function is

$$L(\mathbf{y}|\theta) = \prod_{i=1}^{n} f(y_i|\theta),$$

for which we use the notion of the data conditioning on the parameters to highlight one of the major differences between the Bayesian and frequentist methods. That is, the data are observed (fixed) and the parameters are random in the Bayesian paradigm, while the data are random and the parameters are fixed from the frequentist perspective. Given a prior distribution $p(\theta)$, the posterior distribution of $\theta$ is given by

$$p(\theta|\mathbf{y}) \propto L(\mathbf{y}|\theta)p(\theta).$$

We may incorporate the normalizing constant to make $p(\theta|\mathbf{y})$ a valid density function; that is,

$$p(\theta|\mathbf{y}) = \frac{L(\mathbf{y}|\theta)p(\theta)}{\int L(\mathbf{y}|\theta)p(\theta)\,d\theta}.$$

The usual Markov chain Monte Carlo (MCMC) algorithms can then be used to draw posterior samples of $\theta$ from $p(\theta|\mathbf{y})$ for statistical inference.

As one step further, the Bayesian posterior predictive distribution is concerned with a future observation $\tilde{y}$ conditional on the current data $\mathbf{y}$. If $\tilde{y}$ and $\mathbf{y}$ are conditionally independent given $\theta$, which is often the case, then

$$f(\tilde{y}, \theta|\mathbf{y}) = f(\tilde{y}|\theta, \mathbf{y})p(\theta|\mathbf{y}) = f(\tilde{y}|\theta)p(\theta|\mathbf{y}).$$

By integrating out $\theta$ from $f(\tilde{y}, \theta|\mathbf{y})$, we obtain the posterior predictive distribution,

$$f(\tilde{y}|\mathbf{y}) = \int f(\tilde{y}|\theta)p(\theta|\mathbf{y})\,d\theta.$$

Bayesian clinical trial designs can naturally incorporate prior information through the prior distributions on the model parameters. The prior distribution characterizes all the information available before the trial is conducted, which, if properly calibrated, may improve the design properties. However, the prior specification is also the most criticized part of Bayesian methods due to the subjectivity involved in the prior distribution. During the trial, the Bayesian machinery updates the prior to the posterior distribution coherently based on the accumulating data. Decisions are adaptively made based upon the posterior probabilities, credible intervals, Bayes factors, and so on.

### 3.4.2 Prior Elicitation

Prior distributions may be elicited from clinical investigators (expert opinions) or from previous studies (historical data). Before a trial is carried out, clinicians often have more or less knowledge on the effectiveness of the treatment, such as the drug's response and toxicity probabilities at certain dose levels, or the patients' median survival times in certain groups. Through communication with physicians, we should extract as much information as possible about the trial. For example, questions as follows may be asked:

- What are the typical responses and toxicities for this patient population under treatment?

- What percentage of patients will experience each of the clinically meaningful events?

- What is the highest dose that has negligible toxicity, and what is the lowest dose that induces a positive response?

- What are the prediction intervals for patients' responses treated at certain dose levels?

- What are the median survival times for certain prognostic groups?

Based on the knowledge acquired from medical experts, we match the elicited information with the prior distributions by choosing appropriate hyperparameters.

On the other hand, historical data offer another route for prior elicitation. Due to patients' heterogeneity and differences in eligibility criteria, and treatment and assessment procedures, patients in the previous studies may not be exchangeable with those in the current trial. Hence, we need to discount the historical data by inflating the variance in the prior distribution or only using partial data.

In general, the prior distribution may be classified into four categories as follows:

- *Noninformative prior* refers to a flat or vague prior distribution, under which the posterior distribution is approximately proportional to the likelihood, so that the data fully dominate the posterior distribution and statistical inference.

- *Skeptical prior* is a more conservative prior distribution, which often represents the standing point of the regulatory agency with a doubting view about the new therapy.

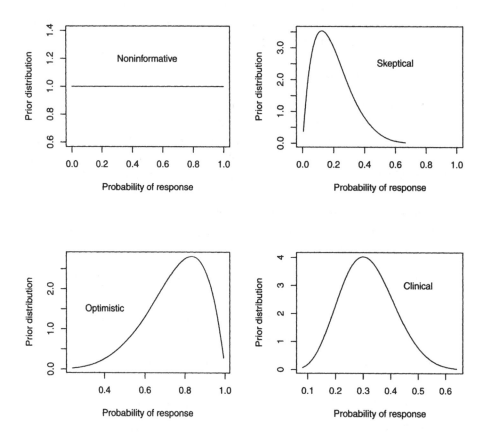

**Figure 3.6**   Four different prior distributions for the probability of response of an experimental drug in a clinical trial.

- *Optimistic prior* is a more enthusiastic prior distribution, which is often dominated by the investigator's optimism about the new drug and thus puts most of the prior probability mass at favorable values of the treatment effect.

- *Clinical prior* is a relatively objective prior distribution, which tries to eliminate the potential subjectivity by taking an average of several prior distributions elicited from different clinical experts.

Figure 3.6 illustrates the aforementioned four types of prior distributions for the probability of response of a new drug. In order to be comparable with frequentist approaches, Bayesian clinical trial designs may simply use noninformative (improper or flat) prior distributions.

### 3.4.3  Conjugate Prior Distribution

Let $\theta$ be the response rate of an experimental drug, and let $p(\theta)$ be the prior distribution of $\theta$, which represents uncertainty on $\theta$ before observing any data. We take $\theta \sim \text{Beta}(\alpha, \beta)$; that is, a beta prior distribution for $\theta$ with the density function of

$$p(\theta) = \frac{\Gamma(\alpha + \beta)}{\Gamma(\alpha)\Gamma(\beta)} \theta^{\alpha - 1} (1 - \theta)^{\beta - 1}.$$

The parameters $\alpha$ and $\beta$ in the beta prior distribution can be viewed as the numbers of prior successes (responders) and failures (nonresponders), respectively; $\alpha + \beta$ can be regarded as the number of prior observations measuring how informative the prior distribution is. For example, $\text{Beta}(0.5, 1.5)$ is a vague prior distribution, which contains information as much as two observations only, while $\text{Beta}(5, 15)$ is a more informative prior distribution, which contains the amount of information corresponding to 20 subjects.

If we observe $y$ responders among $n$ subjects treated by the investigational drug, the posterior distribution for the response rate $\theta$ is given by

$$p(\theta|y) \propto L(y|\theta)p(\theta),$$

where the likelihood under the binomial distribution is

$$L(y|\theta) = \binom{n}{y} \theta^y (1 - \theta)^{n-y}.$$

The posterior distribution of $\theta$ is also a beta distribution,

$$\theta|y \sim \text{Beta}(\alpha + y, \beta + n - y). \qquad (3.10)$$

If we take a uniform prior distribution, $\theta \sim \text{Beta}(1, 1)$, this is equivalent to adding two observations to the data, one success and one failure; so the posterior mean of $\theta$ in (3.10) is

$$\frac{\alpha + y}{\alpha + \beta + n} = \frac{1 + y}{2 + n}.$$

If the posterior and the prior distributions are from the same distributional family as in the beta-binomial case, the prior distribution is called a conjugate prior. For example, a Dirichlet prior distribution is conjugate with the likelihood function under a multinomial distribution; and a gamma prior distribution is conjugate with the likelihood function under an exponential distribution. Multiplying the likelihood with a conjugate prior distribution is equivalent to increasing the sample size; thus it is easier to assess the influence of different values of the hyperparameters in a conjugate prior distribution.

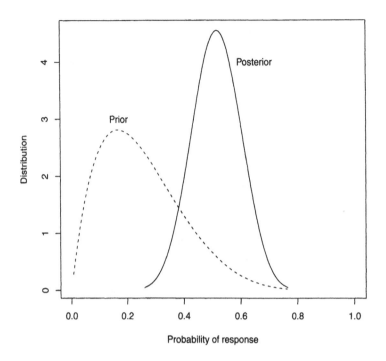

**Figure 3.7**    Update the probability of response from the prior to the posterior distribution using a beta prior distribution.

**EXAMPLE 3.6**

As an illustration, we specify a beta prior distribution for the response rate of an experimental drug, $\theta \sim \text{Beta}(2, 6)$. If we observe $y = 15$ responders among $n = 25$ patients treated in the trial, the posterior distribution of $\theta$ is updated as $\theta|y \sim \text{Beta}(17, 16)$. Figure 3.7 shows that from the prior to the posterior distribution of $\theta$, the distribution is shifted to the right in light of the observed data.

The multinomial distribution is a generalization of the binomial distribution, which is particularly useful for monitoring multivariate outcomes in a clinical trial. Correspondingly, the Dirichlet distribution is the multivariate version of the beta distribution. For $k = 1, \ldots, K$, let $\theta_k$ denote the probability of the occurrence of the $k$th event, satisfying $\sum_{k=1}^{K} \theta_k = 1$. Define $\boldsymbol{\theta} = (\theta_1, \ldots, \theta_K)^\mathsf{T}$; then we can specify a Dirichlet prior distribution for $\boldsymbol{\theta}$,

$$p(\boldsymbol{\theta}) = \frac{\Gamma(\alpha_1 + \cdots + \alpha_K)}{\Gamma(\alpha_1) \cdots \Gamma(\alpha_K)} \theta_1^{\alpha_1 - 1} \cdots \theta_K^{\alpha_K - 1}.$$

If the observed data $\mathbf{y} = \{y_1, \ldots, y_K\}$ follow a multinomial distribution with $\sum_{k=1}^{K} y_k = n$, the likelihood function is

$$L(\mathbf{y}|\boldsymbol{\theta}) = \frac{n!}{y_1! \cdots y_K!} \theta_1^{y_1} \cdots \theta_K^{y_K}.$$

Given the prior distribution $\boldsymbol{\theta} \sim \text{Dir}(\alpha_1, \ldots, \alpha_K)$, the posterior distribution of $\boldsymbol{\theta}$ is also a Dirichlet distribution,

$$\boldsymbol{\theta}|\mathbf{y} \sim \text{Dir}(\alpha_1 + y_1, \ldots, \alpha_K + y_K),$$

due to the conjugate property.

### 3.4.4  Bayesian Generalized Method of Moments

Bayesian inference for a vector of unknown parameters $\boldsymbol{\theta}$ depends on the posterior distribution of $\boldsymbol{\theta}$,

$$p(\boldsymbol{\theta}|\mathbf{y}) \propto L(\mathbf{y}|\boldsymbol{\theta})p(\boldsymbol{\theta}),$$

where $L(\mathbf{y}|\boldsymbol{\theta})$ is the likelihood function and $p(\boldsymbol{\theta})$ is the prior distribution. However, if there is not enough information to construct the likelihood, the Bayesian posterior estimation and inference can be difficult (Zellner, Tobias, and Ryu, 1997). In this regard, Zellner (1997) proposes the Bayesian method of moments by computing the maximum entropy density that is consistent with the moment conditions. Kim (2002) develops the limited information likelihood by minimizing the distance of the Kullback–Leibler information criterion. Chernozhukov and Hong (2003) study MCMC approaches to Laplace-type estimators, and Yin (2009) propose the Bayesian generalized method of moments to circumvent the difficulty of constructing the likelihood function.

As discussed in Section 3.2.3, the GMM is based on the sample moment condition,

$$\mathbf{U}_n(\boldsymbol{\theta}) = \frac{1}{n} \sum_{i=1}^{n} \mathbf{u}_i(\boldsymbol{\theta}),$$

which has a mean zero. The frequentist GMM estimator is obtained by minimizing

$$Q_n(\boldsymbol{\theta}) = n\mathbf{U}_n^{\mathsf{T}}(\boldsymbol{\theta})\boldsymbol{\Sigma}_n^{-1}(\boldsymbol{\theta})\mathbf{U}_n(\boldsymbol{\theta}),$$

where $\boldsymbol{\Sigma}_n(\boldsymbol{\theta})$ is the empirical variance–covariance matrix in the form of

$$\boldsymbol{\Sigma}_n(\boldsymbol{\theta}) = \frac{1}{n} \sum_{i=1}^{n} \mathbf{u}_i(\boldsymbol{\theta})\mathbf{u}_i^{\mathsf{T}}(\boldsymbol{\theta}) - \mathbf{U}_n(\boldsymbol{\theta})\mathbf{U}_n^{\mathsf{T}}(\boldsymbol{\theta}).$$

Observing that $Q_n(\boldsymbol{\theta})$ behaves exactly like $-2 \log L(\mathbf{y}|\boldsymbol{\theta})$, we can build a pseudo-likelihood function

$$\widetilde{L}(\mathbf{y}|\boldsymbol{\theta}) \propto \exp\left\{-\frac{1}{2}Q_n(\boldsymbol{\theta})\right\},$$

which may be used to substitute the original likelihood $L(\mathbf{y}|\boldsymbol{\theta})$.

Following the usual MCMC procedure, if we specify a prior distribution $p(\boldsymbol{\theta})$, the pseudo-posterior distribution of $\boldsymbol{\theta}$ is given by

$$\widetilde{p}(\boldsymbol{\theta}|\mathbf{y}) \propto \widetilde{L}(\mathbf{y}|\boldsymbol{\theta})p(\boldsymbol{\theta}),$$

from which we draw samples to obtain the posterior inference for $\boldsymbol{\theta}$. The Bayesian GMM is a moment-based approach, so that it can be generally constructed whenever moments or estimating equations are available. The likelihood may be vulnerable to model misspecification, while the Bayesian GMM only depends on moments and thus is more robust. Nevertheless, the pseudo-posterior distribution in the Bayesian GMM is complicated and nonstandard, which makes posterior sampling very challenging (Yin et al., 2011).

### 3.4.5   Credible Interval

In the frequentist paradigm, the parameter is fixed, but the confidence interval is random. The usual 95% confidence interval has an interpretation that by replicating the same experiment for a large number of times, the probability that these intervals contain the true parameter is 0.95. By contrast, the Bayesian credible interval given the data is fixed, while the parameter is considered to be random. Hence, the probability that the parameter is covered by (or falls inside) the 95% credible interval is 0.95.

Let $f(\theta|\mathbf{y})$ be the posterior distribution of $\theta$, and let $\Theta$ be the support of $\theta$. For a subset of $\Theta$, say $\mathcal{A}$, the posterior probability of the credible set $\mathcal{A}$ is

$$\Pr(\theta \in \mathcal{A}|\mathbf{y}) = \int_{\mathcal{A}} f(\theta|\mathbf{y}) \, \mathrm{d}\theta.$$

Let $F(\theta|\mathbf{y})$ denote the posterior cumulative distribution function of $\theta$, and let $F^{-1}(\alpha|\mathbf{y})$ denote the $\alpha$th quantile of $\theta$, where $F^{-1}(\cdot|\mathbf{y})$ is the inverse function. Then, the usual $100(1-\alpha)\%$ credible interval for $\theta$ is given by

$$\left[F^{-1}(\alpha/2|\mathbf{y}), \; F^{-1}(1-\alpha/2|\mathbf{y})\right].$$

A more meaningful Bayesian interval estimate is called the highest posterior density (HPD) interval (Chen, Shao, and Ibrahim, 2000). As shown in Figure 3.8, if $f(\theta|\mathbf{y})$ is unimodal, the $100(1-\alpha)\%$ HPD interval for $\theta$ is given by

$$\mathcal{A}(\pi_\alpha) = \{\theta\colon f(\theta|\mathbf{y}) \geq \pi_\alpha\},$$

where $\pi_\alpha$ is the largest constant such that

$$\int_{\mathcal{A}(\pi_\alpha)} f(\theta|\mathbf{y})\mathrm{d}\theta = 1 - \alpha.$$

If $f(\theta|\mathbf{y})$ is symmetric and unimodal, the credible interval and the HPD interval coincide.

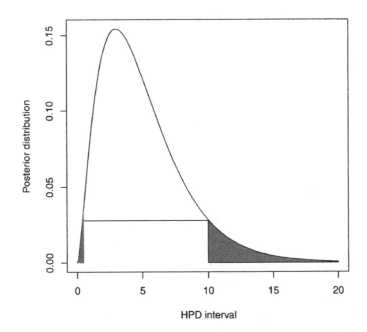

**Figure 3.8**    Illustration of the highest posterior density (HPD) interval.

### 3.4.6  Bayes Factor

Given the observed data $D$, we consider two candidate models, $M_0$ and $M_1$, characterized by parameters $\theta_0$ and $\theta_1$, respectively. Let $L(D|\theta_k, M_k)$ denote the likelihood function under model $M_k$ for $k = 0, 1$. We specify the prior distributions for $\theta_0$ and $\theta_1$ as $f(\theta_0|M_0)$ and $f(\theta_1|M_1)$, and the prior model probabilities for $M_0$ and $M_1$ as $P(M_0)$ and $P(M_1)$, respectively. The marginal likelihood for model $M_k$ is obtained by integrating out the model parameter in the likelihood function with respect to the prior distribution,

$$P(D|M_k) = \int L(D|\theta_k, M_k) f(\theta_k|M_k) \, d\theta_k. \tag{3.11}$$

The posterior model probability for $M_k$ is given by

$$P(M_k|D) = \frac{P(D|M_k)P(M_k)}{P(D|M_0)P(M_0) + P(D|M_1)P(M_1)}.$$

Noting that $P(M_1)/P(M_0)$ is the prior odds in favor of model $M_1$ over $M_0$, the posterior odds is given by

$$\frac{P(M_1|D)}{P(M_0|D)} = \frac{P(M_1)}{P(M_0)} \times \frac{P(D|M_1)}{P(D|M_0)}.$$

The Bayes factor (BF) is defined as the ratio of the posterior odds to the prior odds in favor of model $M_1$ over $M_0$,

$$\mathrm{BF}_{1,0} = \frac{P(M_1|D)/P(M_0|D)}{P(M_1)/P(M_0)} = \frac{P(D|M_1)}{P(D|M_0)}.$$

Similarly in the Bayesian hypothesis testing, let $P(H_0)$ and $P(H_1)$ denote the prior probabilities assigned to the null and alternative hypotheses, respectively. The posterior odds of favoring $H_1$ over $H_0$ is

$$\frac{P(H_1|D)}{P(H_0|D)} = \frac{P(H_1)}{P(H_0)} \times \frac{P(D|H_1)}{P(D|H_0)} = \frac{P(H_1)}{P(H_0)} \times \mathrm{BF}_{1,0}.$$

Therefore, the Bayes factor $\mathrm{BF}_{1,0}$ can be interpreted as the weight or strength of evidence contained in the data to support $H_1$ against $H_0$ (Jeffreys, 1961; Kass and Raftery, 1995). In the case of testing two simple hypotheses, $H_0$: $\theta = \theta_0$ versus $H_1$: $\theta = \theta_1$, the Bayes factor reduces to the likelihood ratio. To quantify the strength of the data information in favor of $H_1$ against $H_0$, the Bayes factor may be categorized in the unit of $1/2$ on the $\log_{10}(\cdot)$ scale as follows:

- If $0 < \log_{10}(\mathrm{BF}_{1,0}) \leq 1/2$, the evidence in the data favoring $H_1$ over $H_0$ is not worth more than a bare mention.

- If $1/2 < \log_{10}(\mathrm{BF}_{1,0}) \leq 1$, the data contain substantial evidence against $H_0$.

- If $1 < \log_{10}(\mathrm{BF}_{1,0}) \leq 2$, the data contain strong such evidence.

- If $\log_{10}(\mathrm{BF}_{1,0}) > 2$, the evidence in favor of $H_1$ against $H_0$ appears to be decisive.

### 3.4.7  Bayesian Model Averaging

Suppose that there are $K$ candidate models, $M_1, \ldots, M_K$, to fit the observed data $D$. Let $P(M_k)$ be the prior probability that $M_k$ is the true model, $k = 1, \ldots, K$. If there is no preference *a priori* to any single model, an equal probability mass is assigned to each model by simply setting $P(M_k) = 1/K$, which represents a discrete uniform prior distribution. When there is a preference to a certain model, we can incorporate such prior information into $P(M_k)$. Let $\theta_k$ be the parameter associated with model $M_k$, and let $f(\theta_k|M_k)$ be the prior distribution of $\theta_k$.

For $k = 1, \ldots, K$, the posterior model probability for $M_k$ is given by

$$P(M_k|D) = \frac{P(D|M_k)P(M_k)}{\sum_{j=1}^{K} P(D|M_j)P(M_j)},$$

where $P(D|M_k)$ is the marginal likelihood under model $M_k$ as given in (3.11). The Bayes factor $\mathrm{BF}_{k,0}$ for model $M_k$ against the reference model $M_0$ is the ratio of the marginal likelihoods,

$$\mathrm{BF}_{k,0} = \frac{P(M_k|D)/P(M_0|D)}{P(M_k)/P(M_0)} = \frac{P(D|M_k)}{P(D|M_0)}.$$

We can construct such a Bayes factor for each of the $K$ models versus model $M_0$, and denote them by $\mathrm{BF}_{1,0}, \ldots, \mathrm{BF}_{K,0}$, respectively. Then, the posterior model probability of $M_k$ can be naturally linked to the Bayes factors,

$$P(M_k|D) = \frac{\mathrm{BF}_{k,0}P(M_k)}{\sum_{j=1}^{K} \mathrm{BF}_{j,0}P(M_j)} = \frac{\mathrm{BF}_{k,0}}{\sum_{j=1}^{K} \mathrm{BF}_{j,0}},$$

if all the models are equally probable *a priori*.

The Bayesian model averaging (BMA) procedure provides a coherent mechanism to account for the uncertainty associated with each candidate model (Raftery, Madigan, and Hoeting, 1997). For the model parameter $\theta$, the BMA estimator is given by

$$\bar{\theta} = \sum_{k=1}^{K} \hat{\theta}_k P(M_k|D),$$

where $\hat{\theta}_k$ is the posterior mean of $\theta$ under model $M_k$,

$$\hat{\theta}_k = \int \theta_k \frac{L(D|\theta_k, M_k)f(\theta_k|M_k)}{\int L(D|\theta_k, M_k)f(\theta_k|M_k)\,\mathrm{d}\theta_k}\,\mathrm{d}\theta_k.$$

By assigning the posterior mean $\hat{\theta}_k$ a weight of $P(M_k|D)$, BMA automatically lean toward the best fitting model, and thus $\bar{\theta}$ will be close to the best parameter estimate (Madigan and Raftery, 1994; Hoeting et al., 1999).

### 3.4.8 Bayesian Hierarchical Model

Bayesian hierarchical modeling often contains several layers of hierarchies, which is typically used to model dependent data, borrow information or strength across different subgroups, or pool separate studies together for joint inference. For illustration, we consider a longitudinal study, in which each subject is repeatedly measured over time. For $i = 1, \ldots, n$ and $k = 1, \ldots, K$, the linear random effects model, as discussed in Section (3.2.7), may be used to account for the intra-patient correlation,

$$y_{ik} = \boldsymbol{\beta}^{\mathsf{T}}\mathbf{Z}_{ik} + \mathbf{b}_i^{\mathsf{T}}\mathbf{X}_{ik} + \epsilon_{ik}, \tag{3.12}$$

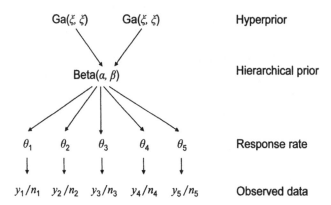

**Figure 3.9**   Illustration of Bayesian hierarchical modeling.

where $\beta$ is the $p$-dimensional fixed effects, $\mathbf{b}_i$ is the $q$-dimensional random effects, $\mathbf{b}_i \sim N_q(\mathbf{0}, \mathbf{G})$, and the error $\epsilon_{ik} \sim N(0, \sigma^2)$. The Bayesian hierarchical model for (3.12) can be formulated as

$$y_{ik}|(\mathbf{b}_i, \sigma^2) \sim N(\boldsymbol{\beta}^\mathsf{T} \mathbf{Z}_{ik} + \mathbf{b}_i^\mathsf{T} \mathbf{X}_{ik}, \sigma^2),$$
$$\mathbf{b}_i|\mathbf{G} \sim N_q(\mathbf{0}, \mathbf{G}),$$
$$\mathbf{G} \sim \text{Inv-Wishart}((\eta\boldsymbol{\Omega})^{-1}, \eta),$$
$$\sigma^2 \sim \text{IG}(\xi, \xi),$$

where $\boldsymbol{\Omega}$ is a $q \times q$ symmetric and positive definite matrix, $\eta$ is a scalar parameter, and $\xi$ is a hyperparameter.

**EXAMPLE 3.7**

In a multi-arm randomized trial, it is desirable to borrow information across different subgroups. As shown in Figure 3.9, let $\theta_1, \ldots, \theta_5$ denote the response rates for the five treatments, respectively. Suppose that we observe $y_k$ responses among $n_k$ patients treated in arm $k$, $k = 1, \ldots, 5$. The Bayesian hierarchical model can be formulated as follows,

$$y_k|\theta_k \sim \text{Bin}(n_k, \theta_k),$$
$$\theta_k|(\alpha, \beta) \sim \text{Beta}(\alpha, \beta),$$
$$\alpha \sim \text{Ga}(\xi, \xi),$$
$$\beta \sim \text{Ga}(\xi, \xi),$$

where the hyperparameter $\xi$ in the gamma distribution may take a small value (e.g., $\xi = 0.001$) to induce noninformative prior distributions.

Let $\mathbf{y} = (y_1, \ldots, y_5)$ denote the observed data. The joint posterior distribution is given by

$$f(\theta_1, \ldots, \theta_5, \alpha, \beta | \mathbf{y}) \propto \left\{ \prod_{k=1}^{5} L_k(y_k | \theta_k) f(\theta_k | \alpha, \beta) \right\} f(\alpha) f(\beta),$$

where the binomial likelihood function is

$$L_k(y_k | \theta_k) = \binom{n_k}{y_k} \theta_k^{y_k} (1 - \theta_k)^{n_k - y_k},$$

$f(\theta_k | \alpha, \beta)$ denotes the beta distribution, and $f(\alpha)$ and $f(\beta)$ denote the gamma prior distributions. The full conditional distribution of $\theta_k$ is

$$\theta_k | (\alpha, \beta, \mathbf{y}) \sim \text{Beta}(\alpha + y_k, \beta + n_k - y_k),$$

while those of $\alpha$ and $\beta$ do not have closed forms.

### 3.4.9  Decision Theory

Bayesian decision theory provides a statistical foundation for quantifying the trade-offs between decisions and the associated rewards/costs (Berger, 1985). Let $r$ denote a reward, and let $\mathcal{U}(r)$ denote a utility function. The expected utility under a probability distribution $P$ is written as $\mathrm{E}_P\{\mathcal{U}(r)\}$. The probability distribution $P_2$ is preferred to $P_1$ if and only if $\mathrm{E}_{P_1}\{\mathcal{U}(r)\} < \mathrm{E}_{P_2}\{\mathcal{U}(r)\}$. Let the parameter $\theta$ denote the state of nature, which has an influence on the decision process. The loss function is the opposite of an utility function, which is associated with the cost for a decision. If an action $a$ is taken, a loss $\mathcal{L}(\theta, a)$ may be incurred. Three standard loss functions are given below.

- The squared-error loss function takes the form of

$$\mathcal{L}(\theta, a) = (\theta - a)^2,$$

which has an analogy to the least-squares estimation.

- The linear loss function specifies

$$\mathcal{L}(\theta, a) = \begin{cases} c_0(\theta - a), & \text{if } \theta - a \geq 0, \\ c_1(a - \theta), & \text{if } \theta - a < 0, \end{cases}$$

which reduces to the absolute-error loss function $\mathcal{L}(\theta, a) = |\theta - a|$, if the constants $c_0$ and $c_1$ are the same; for example, $c_0 = c_1 = 1$.

- The zero-one loss function is given by

$$\mathcal{L}(\theta, a_j) = \begin{cases} 0, & \text{if } \theta \in \Theta_j, \\ 1, & \text{if } \theta \in \Theta_k \ (k \neq j). \end{cases}$$

In a two-action decision problem, if $\theta \in \Theta_0$, action $a_0$ is correct with no loss and action $a_1$ is incorrect with a loss of 1.

Based on the likelihood $L(\mathbf{y}|\theta)$ and the prior distribution $f(\theta)$, the posterior distribution of $\theta$ is given by

$$f(\theta|\mathbf{y}) \propto L(\mathbf{y}|\theta)f(\theta).$$

In the posterior decision analysis, we can compute the posterior expected loss for an action $a$,

$$\mathrm{E}\{\mathcal{L}(\theta, a)|\mathbf{y}\} = \int_{\Theta} \mathcal{L}(\theta, a)f(\theta|\mathbf{y}) \, \mathrm{d}\theta, \qquad (3.13)$$

and by minimizing (3.13) with respect to $a$, we obtain a posterior Bayes action.

## 3.5 MARKOV CHAIN MONTE CARLO

### 3.5.1 Inversion Sampling

Let $f(x)$ be the density function, and let $F(x)$ be the cumulative distribution function of random variable $X$. The question is how to simulate random samples from $f(x)$. Define a transformed random variable $U = F(X)$, and then $U$ follows a uniform distribution on $(0, 1)$; that is, $U \sim \mathrm{Unif}(0, 1)$. This property implies a simple way to sample from $f(x)$: First simulate a random sample $u$ from $\mathrm{Unif}(0, 1)$, and then solve $F(x) = u$ to obtain $x = F^{-1}(u)$ which is a sample from $f(x)$.

### 3.5.2 Rejection Sampling

Sometimes, it may not be easy to solve $x = F^{-1}(u)$, and thus the inversion sampling becomes very difficult. As an alternative, the rejection sampling provides an attractive way to simulate samples from $f(x)$. Let $g(x)$ be a probability density function that is easy to sample from. We construct an envelope function $Kg(x)$, where $K \geq 1$ is a constant such that $f(x) \leq Kg(x)$ for all $x$. The rejection sampling algorithm proceeds as follows:

- Sample $x$ from $g(x)$ and $u$ from $\mathrm{Unif}(0, 1)$.

- If $u \leq f(x)/Kg(x)$, accept $x$ as a realized value from $f(x)$; otherwise, reject the value of $x$ and go back to the sampling step.

Through such sampling and rejection/acceptance steps, we can generate i.i.d. samples from $f(x)$.

### 3.5.3 Gibbs Sampler

In practice, it is often needed to draw samples from a multivariate distribution, which may be complicated and nonstandard. Suppose that a vector of $K$ random variables $(X_1, \ldots, X_K)$ follows a multivariate distribution $f(x_1, \ldots, x_K)$. To circumvent the difficulty of directly sampling from $f(x_1, \ldots, x_K)$, the MCMC offers a straightforward approach to generating an ergodic Markov chain with $f(x_1, \ldots, x_K)$ as the stationary distribution.

Gibbs sampling is one of the most popular MCMC algorithms (Geman and Geman, 1984; Gelfand and Smith, 1990), which relies upon the availability of full conditional distributions; that is, the conditional distribution of each $X_k$ given the rest of the $X_j$'s $(j \neq k)$,

$$f(x_k | x_1, \ldots, x_{k-1}, x_{k+1}, \ldots, x_K), \quad k = 1, \ldots, K.$$

If all of the full conditional distributions are available, the multivariate sampling problem can be cast into a sequence of samples from a set of univariate conditional distributions. Under some mild conditions, this set of univariate conditional distributions uniquely determines the multivariate distribution of $(X_1, \ldots, X_K)$, and hence all the marginal distributions of $X_k$ for $k = 1, \ldots, K$.

The Gibbs sampler starts with a set of initial values $x_1^{(0)}, \ldots, x_K^{(0)}$, and proceeds as follows:

- Sample $x_1^{(1)}$ from $f(x_1 | x_2^{(0)}, x_3^{(0)}, \ldots, x_K^{(0)})$.

- Sample $x_2^{(1)}$ from $f(x_2 | x_1^{(1)}, x_3^{(0)}, \ldots, x_K^{(0)})$.

 $\vdots$

- Sample $x_K^{(1)}$ from $f(x_K | x_1^{(1)}, x_2^{(1)}, \ldots, x_{K-1}^{(1)})$.

These $K$ steps complete one iteration of the Gibbs sampler, and result in the first set of samples $x_1^{(1)}, \ldots, x_K^{(1)}$. After a large number of iterations, a Markov chain is produced, whose joint distribution converges to that of $(X_1, \ldots, X_K)$.

The trace plot of the samples is helpful to provide visual checking of the stationarity of the Markov chain, while more rigorous examinations of the MCMC convergence are also available (Geweke, 1992; Gelman and Rubin, 1992; Cowles and Carlin, 1996). There is often a burn-in period to discard the first hundreds or thousands of iterations before taking the "real" samples for inference. To reduce the autocorrelations among the samples, we may thin the Markov chain by recording one sample every a fixed number of iterations.

### 3.5.4 Metropolis–Hastings Algorithm

The Metropolis–Hastings algorithm is another widely used MCMC procedure to draw samples from a target distribution (Metropolis et al., 1953; Hastings,

1970; Gilks, Best, and Tan, 1995). If the target distribution $f(x)$ is not easy to sample from, we need to come up with a proposal distribution $p(x, y)$ in order to produce a Markov chain. The Metropolis–Hastings algorithm starts with an initial value $x^{(0)}$ and proceeds through the following transition:

- At step $i$, generate $y$ from $p(x^{(i)}, y)$ given $x = x^{(i)}$.

- At step $(i + 1)$, set

$$x^{(i+1)} = \begin{cases} y, & \text{with probability } \pi(x^{(i)}, y), \\ x^{(i)}, & \text{with probability } 1 - \pi(x^{(i)}, y), \end{cases}$$

where

$$\pi(x, y) = \min\left\{\frac{f(y)p(y, x)}{f(x)p(x, y)}, 1\right\}.$$

Each time, the new sample $y$ simulated from the proposal distribution may be accepted or rejected, and the optimal acceptance rate is around 23%. Repeating this procedure for a large number of iterations, a random sample is then generated from the density function $f(x)$.

## 3.6   SUMMARY

This chapter provides a statistical background for clinical trial designs that will be discussed in the forthcoming chapters. We introduced the estimation and inference procedures separately for the frequentist and Bayesian approaches. For more in-depth discussions on frequentist statistics, see Sen and Singer (1993), Casella and Berger (2001), and Hogg, McKean, and Craig (2005); for those on Bayesian statistics, see Gelman et al. (2003) and Carlin and Louis (2008).

In the frequentist clinical trial designs, the prior knowledge is informally utilized at the planning stage, such as specification of the effect size and variance for sample size calculation. Hypothesis testing mainly relies upon the maximum likelihood estimation, confidence intervals, and $p$-values. If a sequence of hypothesis tests is conducted during a trial, multiple testing issues arise, and the inference procedure must be adjusted to control the overall/familywise type I error rate. Moreover, the design should be equipped with sufficient power to detect the specified treatment difference.

In contrast, Bayesian clinical trial designs incorporate prior information in a more formal and natural way (Spiegelhalter, Abrams, and Myles, 2004). In the Bayesian paradigm, interim analysis is not subject to multiple comparison issues; that is, multiple "looks" of the data would not affect Bayesian decisions. Trial designs are typically based on posterior probabilities of prespecified rules, which must be carefully calibrated through simulation studies. In addition, using the predictive probability to forecast the future trial outcomes is a very useful and unique feature for Bayesian trial monitoring.

Designing a clinal trial is an interactive process between statisticians and physicians. Before a real trial is carried out, the design must be investigated thoroughly, with all the design parameters carefully calibrated and all the decision rules clearly specified in advance. The design properties may be explored extensively back and forth using computer simulations until it produces good operating characteristics. The simulated scenarios should be chosen broadly to match the real situation and cover all of the possibilities that may happen in reality. In summary, the goals of clinical trial designs are to save sample sizes and resources while still making correct decisions, which, for example, include to

- select excessively toxic doses with low probabilities and recommend the optimal dose with a high probability,

- drop nonworking or unsafe drugs as early as possible and select promising drugs sooner,

- treat more patients in the superior arms and fewer patients in the inferior arms, and

- preserve the type I error rate and achieve high statistical power.

## EXERCISES

**3.1**    Let $X$ and $Y$ be independent random variables with corresponding density functions $f_X(x)$ and $f_Y(y)$. Show that the probability density function of the random variable $Z = X + Y$ is given by

$$f_Z(z) = \int f_X(x) f_Y(z - x)\, \mathrm{d}x.$$

Also, prove that

$$P(X > Y) = \int f_X(x) F_Y(x)\, \mathrm{d}x,$$

where $F_Y(y)$ is the cumulative distribution function of $Y$.

**3.2**    For a continuous random variable $X$, let $F(x)$ denote its cumulative distribution function. Define $Y = F(X)$; show that the distribution of $Y$ is uniform on $(0, 1)$.

**3.3**    In the frequentist hypothesis testing framework, what is the distribution of the $p$-value under the null hypothesis?

**3.4**    Let $T$ denote the failure time, and let $S(t)$ denote the survival function. Show that

$$\mathrm{E}(T) = \int_0^\infty S(t)\,\mathrm{d}t.$$

**3.5**    The mean residual lifetime is the remaining life expectancy conditional on survival up to time $t$,

$$m(t) = \mathrm{E}(T - t | T > t) \quad \text{for } t \geq 0,$$

where $T$ is the failure time. Show that the mean residual lifetime has an explicit one-to-one correspondence to the survival function,

$$S(t) = \frac{m(0)}{m(t)} \exp\left\{ -\int_0^t \frac{1}{m(u)}\,\mathrm{d}u \right\}.$$

**3.6**    In survival analysis, suppose that the observed data are given as follows:

| Patient $i$ | $X_i$ | $\Delta_i$ | $Z_i$ |
|:---:|:---:|:---:|:---:|
| 1 | 0.3 | 1 | 0 |
| 2 | 0.1 | 1 | 0 |
| 3 | 0.2 | 0 | 1 |
| 4 | 0.4 | 1 | 0 |
| 5 | 0.5 | 0 | 1 |
| 6 | 0.6 | 1 | 1 |

where $X_i$ is the observed survival time, $\Delta_i$ is the censoring indicator, and $Z_i$ is the treatment indicator, for $i = 1, \ldots, 6$. Under the Cox proportional hazards model,

$$\lambda(t | Z_i) = \lambda_0(t) \exp(\beta Z_i),$$

we assume an exponential distribution with $\lambda_0(t) = \lambda$. Derive both the full and the partial likelihood, and find the corresponding MLE and the maximum partial likelihood estimator (may not exist). If an additional patient with ($X_7 = 0.2, \Delta_7 = 1, Z_7 = 1$) is added, find the MLEs of $\beta$ by maximizing the full and the partial likelihood functions, respectively; and also compare the efficiency based on the corresponding variance estimates.

**3.7**    Show that the inverse-Wishart distribution is a conjugate prior distribution for the covariance matrix of a multivariate normal distribution.

**3.8**    Under the linear random effects model (3.12), derive the conditional and marginal likelihood functions. In the Bayesian paradigm, derive the full conditional distribution for each model parameter.

# CHAPTER 4

# PHASE I TRIAL DESIGN

## 4.1 MAXIMUM TOLERATED DOSE

If a compound shows promising anti-disease activity through extensive preclinical research, a phase I clinical trial will be launched as the first step of drug testing in human subjects. The primary goal of a phase I trial is to determine the recommended dose for future phase II studies. Statistical issues in this phase include the ethics of the trial, selection of the starting dose, rapidity of dose escalation, the target toxicity probability, the number of patients, and the efficiency of the trial design.

The aims of a typical phase I oncology trial are to determine the maximum tolerated dose (MTD), assess the safety and tolerability, and investigate pharmacokinetics and pharmacodynamics of a new drug. The MTD is defined as the dose that has a toxicity probability closest to the target toxicity rate specified by the investigators. The recommended phase II dose may be the MTD or the dose of one level below the MTD. The dose-limiting toxicities (DLTs) refer to the drug-induced toxicities up to a certain level of severity so that no more of the treatment can be given to patients. For cytotoxic agents in cancer, DLTs are

*Clinical Trial Design.* By Guosheng Yin
Copyright © 2012 John Wiley & Sons, Inc.

drug-related severe adverse effects that are usually reversible, such as grade 3 nonhematologic toxicities and grade 4 hematologic toxicities.

## EXAMPLE 4.1

In a phase I trial with leukemia patients, a single agent, R7112, was investigated through oral administration. Predefined DLTs included any drug-related nonhematologic toxicity of grade 3, according to the Common Terminology Criteria for Adverse Events version 3.0, except for fatigue, anorexia, and alopecia. Nausea, vomiting, and diarrhea were also considered DLTs only if they reached grade 3 despite adequate supportive care measures. Toxicities that were not considered DLTs included grade 3–4 myelosuppression lasting less than six weeks or in the presence of persistent leukemia, grade 3 neutropenic fever without infection, cytopenias not resulting in death, grade 3 blood transfusions, and nausea and vomiting if manageable.

It is often assumed that as the dose of a drug increases, the induced toxicity becomes more severe, while at the same time the drug's efficacy is also expected to strengthen. The MTD is the most toxic dose that can still be tolerated by patients, so that the therapeutic effect of the drug can be maximized if patients are treated at the MTD. Finding the MTD is crucial because it is the dose that will be further investigated in the subsequent phase II or phase III trials. Misidentification of the MTD may result in many serious consequences. For example, if an over-toxic dose is identified as the MTD, an undesirably large number of patients might be treated at that excessively toxic dose in the follow-up studies. On the other hand, mistakenly selecting a dose with low toxicity (and also presumably negligible efficacy) as the MTD may cause a truly effective drug being overlooked. Therefore, in a phase I trial we need to identify the MTD accurately and efficiently, while exposing as few subjects as possible to suboptimal doses that are inefficacious or unsafe.

## EXAMPLE 4.2

A phase I dose-finding trial was designed to study the safety of INNO-406 in adult patients with imatinib-resistant or -intolerant Philadelphia chromosome-positive leukemia. The primary objective of the study was to determine the MTD of INNO-406 with a target toxicity probability of 33%; that is, at most one-third of the patients treated at the MTD are expected to experience the DLT.

## 4.2  INITIAL DOSE AND SPACING

In the early stage of drug development, relatively little is known about the new drug and its appropriate dosages on human subjects. Hence, a sequence of doses is screened to search for the MTD—the most toxic but still tolerable dose. The sample size of a phase I trial is small, usually ranging from 20 to 50 subjects. Dose finding in a phase I trial is adaptive by nature. Patients are sequentially enrolled into the study and are often treated in cohorts. The trial may start from the lowest or the physician-specified dose. If at a dose level an undesirably large number of patients have experienced the DLTs, the next cohort will be treated at a lower dose; and if a dose can be well-tolerated, the next cohort will be treated at a higher dose. Through adaptive dose escalation and de-escalation, each cohort of patients will be assigned to the most appropriate dose based on the data accrued in the trial thus far.

Figure 4.1 displays a typical dose-finding situation, in which six increasing doses are considered and the MTD is the fourth dose with a target toxicity rate of 33%. To identify the MTD, we need to collect the toxicity data by adaptively treating patients through dose escalation and de-escalation. Toxicity is expected to occur shortly after treatment such that the outcomes of previously treated patients can be observed timely for decision making. For safety, the doses of the study drug should start from a very low dose level, and gradually increase, so that the MTD is likely to be covered by the entire range of the considered doses. The doses selected for investigation are usually some fractions of the dose that causes harm in animal studies. For example, the lethal dose 10% ($LD_{10}$) of a drug is the dose that causes 10% of death in the animals that received the drug. To be conservative, the first human trial for a new drug may start at one-tenth of the rodent $LD_{10}$, after adjusting for the body surface area.

Due to discreteness of dose preparation, the MTD may not exactly match the target toxicity probability, say 33%. The MTD should be the dose that has

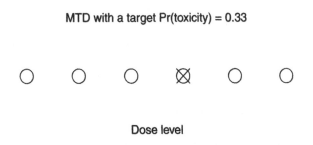

Dose level

**Figure 4.1**    Dose finding for the MTD in a phase I clinical trial with six dose levels. The cross indicates the MTD with a target toxicity probability of 33%.

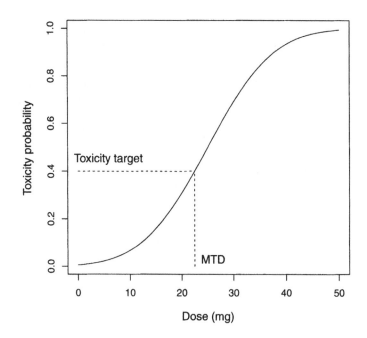

**Figure 4.2** Dose–toxicity curve with a target toxicity probability of 40%.

the toxicity probability closest to the target level. Doses may be prepared in an escalation scheme following a sequence of Fibonacci numbers: Starting from 0 and 1, each subsequent number is the sum of the two preceding numbers; that is, 0, 1, 1, 2, 3, 5, 8, . . ., and the ratio of consecutive Fibonacci numbers converges to the golden ratio $(1 + \sqrt{5})/2 \approx 1.618$. In practice, a modified Fibonacci sequence is often used, in which the percentages of dose increment for succeeding dose levels are 100%, 65%, 52%, 40%, 29%, 33%, 33%, . . ., and followed by 33% for all the remaining dose levels. For simplicity, dose escalation may increase the adjacent doses with a fixed percentage of 33%, or with a constant increment of the actual dose, say, 10 mg.

As remarked earlier, dose finding is the main theme of a phase I clinical trial. Figure 4.2 shows a typical dose–toxicity curve that monotonically increases with respect to the dose. Suppose that the target toxicity rate is 40%, and we search over the prespecified doses from 10 mg up to 50 mg with a constant increment of 10 mg. In this case, the dose of 20 mg is expected to be claimed as the MTD. However, the true dose–toxicity curve is unknown in reality. To search for the MTD, many statistical methods are developed, which can be generally classified as algorithm-based or model-based approaches. The algorithm-based

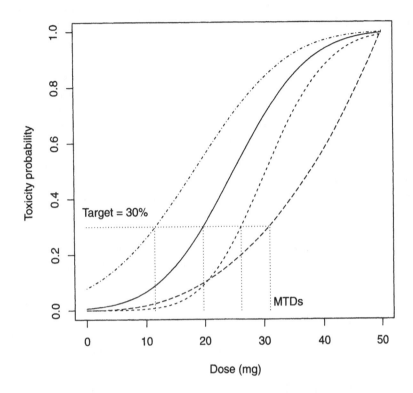

**Figure 4.3**    Different dose–toxicity curves lead to different maximum tolerated doses (MTDs). The solid line is the true dose–toxicity curve, while others are hypothetical curves.

methods, such as the $3 + 3$ design (Storer, 1989) and the biased coin dose-finding design (Stylianou and Flournoy, 2002), can be viewed as "nonparametric" or model-free methods. These nonparametric methods do not explicitly assume a dose–toxicity curve, while dose escalation and de-escalation rigorously follow a set of prespecified rules. Other examples include a family of random walk rules for dose finding (Durham, Flournoy, and Rosenberger, 1997), a curve-free method using a product of beta priors (Gasparini and Eisele, 2000), and dose finding based on toxicity probability intervals (Ji, Li, and Yin, 2007; Ji, Li, and Bekele, 2007).

By contrast, model-based dose-finding methods typically assume a parametric dose–toxicity relationship to pool the information across different doses for decision making. However, these parametric approaches are subject to model misspecification, because the true dose–toxicity curve is unknown. Figure 4.3

shows that for the same target toxicity probability of 30%, the identified MTD may vary dramatically under different dose–toxicity curves. Hence, if the dose–toxicity curve is specified incorrectly, the MTD would be likely misidentified. Among a variety of model-based designs, the continual reassessment method (CRM) is a very popular dose-finding approach (O'Quigley, Pepe, and Fisher, 1990). The practical performance of the CRM may be improved by assigning one cohort instead of one patient to each dose level and also limiting dose escalation by one dose level at a time (Faries, 1994; Goodman, Zahurak, and Piantadosi, 1995). Other extensions of the CRM are described as follows. Møller (1995) applies a preliminary up-and-down design to reach the neighborhood of the target dose during successive dose escalation. Piantadosi, Fisher, and Grossman (1998) propose using a simple dose–toxicity model to guide data interpolation and grouping three patients into a cohort to stabilize the estimates. Heyd and Carlin (1999) develop a further refinement for the CRM by allowing the trial to stop earlier when the width of the 95% posterior probability interval for the MTD becomes sufficiently narrow. Ishizuka and Ohashi (2001) propose monitoring a posterior density function of toxicity to reduce the number of patients treated at doses higher than the MTD. Leung and Wang (2002) apply decision theory to optimize the number of patients allocated to the highest dose with tolerable toxicity. Yuan, Chappell, and Bailey (2007) develop a quasi-likelihood approach to accommodating multiple toxicity grades. To resolve the CRM's sensitivity to the prespecified toxicity probabilities, Yin and Yuan (2009a) propose using multiple sets of toxicity probabilities and integrating the toxicity estimates through the Bayesian model averaging procedure. Along a similar line, Daimon, Zohar, and O'Quigley (2011) apply posterior maximization and averaging for the CRM working model. Cheung (2011) provides detailed discussions on dose-finding methodologies using the CRM. Apart from the CRM framework, Whitehead and Brunier (1995) introduce a Bayesian decision-theoretic approach to dose finding. To prevent patients from experiencing excessive toxicity, Babb, Rogatko, and Zacks (1998) develop a dose escalation scheme that directly controls the probability of overdosing. For comprehensive coverage of various dose-finding methods in phase I clinical trials, see Chevret (2006) and Ting (2006).

## 4.3  3 + 3 DESIGN

In a phase I dose-finding study, dose escalation should proceed cautiously to avoid overshooting the MTD so that patients can be protected from overly toxic doses. On the other hand, the dose needs to be escalated quickly to avoid treating too many patients at ineffective doses that are far below the MTD. In light of these two guidelines, the standard 3 + 3 design provides an algorithm-based approach to dose finding that typically finds the MTD as the highest dose with a

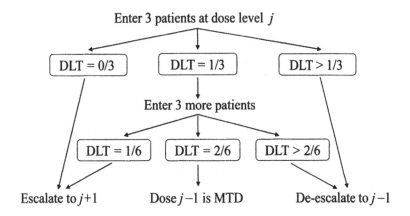

Enter 3 patients at dose level $j$

| DLT = 0/3 | DLT = 1/3 | DLT > 1/3 |

Enter 3 more patients

| DLT = 1/6 | DLT = 2/6 | DLT > 2/6 |

Escalate to $j+1$          Dose $j-1$ is MTD          De-escalate to $j-1$

**Figure 4.4**  Diagram of the standard 3 + 3 design.

toxicity probability less than 33% (Storer, 1989). Due to its simplicity and ease of implementation, the 3 + 3 design is widely used in practice.

Apparently by the design's name, patients are treated with a cohort size of 3 after entering the trial sequentially. The toxicity outcomes of the enrolled patients should be completely observed before any more patients enter the trial. The first cohort is treated at the lowest dose level or the one specified by physicians. Figure 4.4 exhibits the diagram of the 3 + 3 design, which is described in detail as follows:

(1) Suppose that the current dose level is $j$, at which 3 patients are treated and evaluated for toxicity.

(2) If none of the 3 patients experiences the DLT, escalate to dose level $j + 1$, and go back to step (1).

(3) If 1 out of 3 patients develops the DLT, then 3 more patients will be treated at the same dose level $j$ and the trial proceeds as follows:

   (i) If 1 out of 6 patients experiences the DLT, escalate to dose level $j + 1$ provided that dose level $j + 1$ has not exceeded the MTD.

   (ii) If 2 out of 6 patients experience the DLT, then the trial is finished and the dose at the next lower level $j - 1$ is declared as the MTD.

   (iii) If more than 2 patients experience the DLT, the current dose level $j$ has exceeded the MTD, and 3 more patients will be treated at dose level $j - 1$ provided that fewer than 6 patients have been treated at that dose level.

(4) If 2 or 3 patients experience the DLT (the dose level has exceeded the MTD), 3 more patients will be treated at dose level $j - 1$ provided that fewer than 6 patients have been treated at that dose level.

If 2 or 3 DLTs are observed among the first 3 patients in the $3+3$ design, the trial will be stopped early without selecting the MTD, which is called an inconclusive trial.

Following this set of rules, the MTD is defined as the highest dose at which 6 patients have been treated with none or one occurrence of the DLT (the incidence rate of the DLT is less than 33%). A more aggressive definition for the MTD is the highest dose at which 6 patients are treated and 2 or fewer patients have developed the DLT (the incidence rate of the DLT may be equal to 33%). If there are $J$ doses under investigation, the maximum number of patients required for a $3+3$ design is $J \times 6$.

To investigate the operating characteristics of the $3+3$ design, we conducted simulation studies with five increasing doses. The first cohort was treated at the lowest dose level, and the maximum sample size was 30. We simulated four different scenarios as shown in Table 4.1, and for each scenario 10,000 trials were replicated.

**Table 4.1   Simulation Study Using the $3+3$ Design with Five Increasing Dose Levels**

| $3+3$ design | Dose level | | | | | Total # Toxicity | Total # Patients |
|---|---|---|---|---|---|---|---|
| | 1 | 2 | 3 | 4 | 5 | | |
| Scenario 1 | 0.30 | 0.40 | 0.55 | 0.60 | 0.65 | | |
| Selection % | **44.2** | 20.9 | 2.9 | 0.2 | 0.0 | | |
| # Patients | 4.8 | 2.4 | 0.6 | 0.1 | 0.0 | 2.8 | 7.9 |
| Scenario 2 | 0.10 | 0.20 | 0.30 | 0.40 | 0.50 | | |
| Selection % | 18.9 | 33.8 | **28.5** | 12.7 | 1.4 | | |
| # Patients | 4.0 | 4.2 | 3.1 | 1.5 | 0.4 | 3.0 | 13.2 |
| Scenario 3 | 0.02 | 0.06 | 0.10 | 0.20 | 0.30 | | |
| Selection % | 1.6 | 5.8 | 18.2 | 32.2 | **11.8** | | |
| # Patients | 3.2 | 3.5 | 3.9 | 4.0 | 2.7 | 2.2 | 17.3 |
| Scenario 4 | 0.20 | 0.30 | 0.60 | 0.70 | 0.75 | | |
| Selection % | 37.8 | **42.0** | 5.3 | 0.1 | 0.0 | | |
| # Patients | 4.6 | 3.6 | 1.4 | 0.1 | 0.0 | 2.9 | 9.7 |

Under each scenario, the first row represents the true toxicity probabilities of the five considered doses. The selection percentages for the probability of toxicity of 30% are in boldface.

Under each scenario, we present the true toxicity probability, the dose selection percentage and the number of patients treated at each dose, the number of DLTs and the total number of patients in the trial. For example, in scenario 1, 44.2% of the simulated trials selected dose 1 as the MTD, on average approximately 5 patients were treated at dose level 1, and a total of 8 patients were treated in the entire trial and 3 DLTs were observed. The 3 + 3 design does not have a specific toxicity probability target; it often selects the MTD as a dose with a toxicity probability less than 33%. In scenarios 1 and 4, the dose with a toxicity probability 30% was selected with the highest percentages, while in scenarios 2 and 3, the 3 + 3 design tended to select the dose with a toxicity probability of 20% as the MTD. Due to inconclusive trials, the sum of the selection percentages at all of the dose levels may not be 1.

The 3 + 3 design may be modified as a two-stage dose-finding procedure: The first stage takes single-patient dose escalation until the first DLT is observed, and the second stage switches to the usual 3 + 3 design afterwards. Stage 1 aims to use as few patients as possible to reach the dose-action neighborhood; once within the vicinity of the MTD, stage 2 applies the standard 3 + 3 design to locate the MTD.

Despite the popularity, the 3 + 3 design has some limitations that may affect its practical performance (O'Quigley and Chevret, 1991; O'Quigley and Shen, 1996). First, the 3 + 3 design is "memoryless" because dose escalation or de-escalation is solely based on the toxicity data observed at the current dose level with no regard to other dose levels. Second, this design does not have any statistical convergence property and also has no specific toxicity target to aim for. Finally, the 3 + 3 design tends to be conservative and is only suitable for a trial with the target toxicity probability less than 33%.

## 4.4  A + B DESIGN

The 3 + 3 design can be extended to a more general A + B design (Lin and Shih, 2001), in which the cohort size may not always be 3. The schema of the A + B design is shown in Figure 4.5 and described below.

(1) Suppose that the current dose level is $j$, at which A patients are treated and evaluated for toxicity.

(2) If fewer than C out of A patients experience the DLT, escalate to dose level $j + 1$.

(3) If the number of DLTs is between C and D, the dose will stay the same, and B more patients will be treated at dose level $j$. After A + B patients are treated at dose level $j$, the design proceeds as follows:

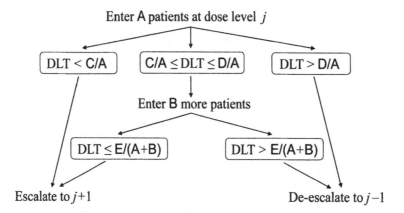

Enter A patients at dose level $j$

| DLT < C/A | C/A ≤ DLT ≤ D/A | DLT > D/A |

Enter B more patients

| DLT ≤ E/(A+B) |     | DLT > E/(A+B) |

Escalate to $j+1$                                  De-escalate to $j-1$

**Figure 4.5**   Diagram of the A + B design.

- If the number of DLTs is more than E, de-escalate to dose level $j - 1$ provided that only A patients have been treated at that dose level. However, if A + B patients have already been treated at dose level $j - 1$, that dose will be claimed as the MTD.

- Otherwise, escalate to dose level $j + 1$.

(4) If more than D out of A patients experience the DLT (D ≥ C), de-escalate to dose level $j - 1$. That is, the next cohort of B patients will be treated at dose level $j - 1$ provided that only A patients have been treated at that dose level. However, if A + B patients have already been treated at dose level $j - 1$, that dose will be claimed as the MTD.

The standard 3+3 design is a special case of the A+B design with A = B = 3 and C = D = E = 1. For practical use, there may be several modifications to the A + B design as follows:

- The starting dose level may not necessarily be the lowest one; instead the investigator may specify the starting dose level.

- In steps (3) and (4) of the A + B algorithm, the current dose $j$ instead of dose $j - 1$ may be declared as the MTD.

- The design may be divided into two stages: In stage 1, one or two patients are treated per dose level until minor toxicities or DLTs occur, and stage 2 follows the A + B design.

## 4.5  ACCELERATED TITRATION DESIGN

### 4.5.1  Acceleration and Escalation

If a new drug has never been used previously in humans, we can only rely upon preclinical data to select the testing doses for a phase I trial. In this circumstance, the starting doses are often set at very low levels to ensure patients' safety. The MTD may be located at the higher dose range, and thus it will take a long time and a large number of patients to reach the MTD area if using a cohort size of 3 as in the $3 + 3$ design. Hence, a large number of patients, especially most of the early participants, might be treated at doses far below the biologically active level of the drug. In addition, the $3 + 3$ design provides little information on inter-patient variability or cumulative toxicity. To address these issues, the accelerated titration design (ATD) is developed through rapid intra-patient dose escalation (Simon et al., 1997). The ATD dramatically reduces the number of patients treated at subtherapeutic dose levels, shortens the duration of the trial, and acquires substantially more information on inter-patient variability and cumulative toxicity.

Starting from the lowest or the physician-specified dose, the ATD is composed of two sequential stages: an acceleration stage and an escalation stage. During the acceleration stage, one patient is treated at each dose level, and the dose is escalated until the first DLT is observed. Then the design switches to a traditional dose-escalation scheme, such as the $3+3$ design, by treating 2 additional patients at the dose that has triggered the switch. From then on, 3 patients are treated in the subsequent cohorts at each dose level. This approach offers the possibility of speeding up the trial at the beginning of dose escalation and reducing the number of patients assigned to the doses that are far below the MTD and are presumably therapeutically ineffective.

Cancer therapy often involves multiple courses of treatment. The ATD may allow within-patient dose escalation depending on the toxicities observed in the previous course of treatment. For the same patient, we may escalate the dose if grade 0 or grade 1 toxicity is observed, and de-escalate the dose if grade 3 or higher toxicity is observed at the previously administered dose. The accelerated phase ends until one patient experiences the DLT or two patients experience moderate toxicity (usually grade 2) during the first course of treatment. Afterwards, the dose assignment for new patients follows the same rule as that in the standard $3 + 3$ design.

### 4.5.2  Modeling Toxicity with Random Effects

Similar to a longitudinal study with repeated measurements, each subject in the trial is treated for multiple courses over time. Rather than identifying the MTD as in the $3 + 3$ design, the ATD applies the random effects model to all of the toxicity data (including toxicity experienced in the subsequent treatment courses) to select the dose for the following phase II trial. More specifically, let $y_{ik}$ be an unobserved continuous variable representing the underlying toxicity level, let $d_{ik}$ be the dose administered to patient $i$ in treatment course $k$, and let $D_{ik}$ be the cumulative dose administered to patient $i$ up to, but not including, treatment course $k$. Under this setup, the random effects model takes the form of

$$y_{ik} = \log(d_{ik} + \alpha D_{ik}) + \beta_i + \epsilon_{ik},$$

for $i = 1, \ldots, n$ and $k = 1, \ldots, K$. Here, $\alpha$ is the treatment effect of the cumulative dose; $\beta_i$ is the random effects representing the inter-patient variability, $\beta_i \sim N(0, \sigma_\beta^2)$; and $\epsilon_{ik}$ is the error characterizing the intra-patient variability, $\epsilon_{ik} \sim N(0, \sigma_\epsilon^2)$. The unobserved (latent) variable $y_{ik}$ can be cast into discrete toxicity levels using three additional cutoff parameters, $c_1 < c_2 < c_3$, which divide the continuous toxicity measurement into four intervals: minimal toxicity (usually grade 0 or 1), moderate toxicity, DLT, and unacceptable toxicity. Based on the observed toxicity data, the model parameters $(\alpha, \sigma_\beta^2, \sigma_\epsilon^2, c_1, c_2, c_3)$ can be estimated using the maximum likelihood approach. The probabilities of observing the moderate toxicity and DLT at different dose levels can thereby be estimated, which will be used as the basis for recommending a phase II dose. The ATD effectively reduces the number of patients who are undertreated, and it speeds up the completion of a phase I trial. These advantages are accomplished through the accelerated dose escalation in stage 1, which, however, may sacrifice relatively more patients with grade 3 or 4 toxicities.

**EXAMPLE 4.3**

As an example, a phase I clinical trial was designed using the ATD to study a novel triplatinum complex, BBR3464 (Sessa et al., 2000). The objective of the trial was to find the MTD of BBR3464 and determine the associated toxicity and pharmacokinetic profile. The starting dose of BBR3464 was 0.03 mg/m$^2$ per day, which corresponded to $1/10$ of the mouse equivalent MTD. The DLTs included short-lasting neutropenia and late-onset diarrhea. The MTD was defined as the dose at which one-third of the patients developed the DLT after the first treatment cycle. Fourteen patients received BBR3464 on a daily $\times$ 5 schedule every 28 days, among them five patients were in the acceleration phase and nine in the standard phase. During the acceleration stage, only one patient per cohort was treated until one patient experienced the DLT or two patients experienced toxicities of grade $\geq 2$. The dose was escalated from 0.03, 0.06, 0.12, 0.14, up to 0.17 mg/m$^2$ per day, and eventually the MTD of BBR3464 identified by the trial was 0.12 mg/m$^2$.

## 4.6  BIASED COIN DOSE-FINDING METHOD

The biased coin design (BCD) has a long history in the sequential allocation of patients through randomization; see Section 7.6. The BCD aims to balance the number of patients in each treatment arm by hypothetically tossing a biased coin which has an unequal probability of landing on a head or a tail. With an extension of the BCD to dose finding, Durham, Flournoy, and Rosenberger (1997) introduce a family of random walk rules.

Let $\phi_T$ denote the target toxicity probability. Starting from the lowest dose level, the biased coin dose-finding design proceeds as follows:

- *In the case of $\phi_T \leq 0.5$:*
  At any stage of the trial, if the previously treated patient has experienced the DLT, de-escalate the dose to one level lower; if no DLT is observed for the previous patient, escalate the dose to one level higher with probability $\phi_T/(1 - \phi_T)$ and the dose stays at the same level with probability $(1 - 2\phi_T)/(1 - \phi_T)$.

- *In the case of $\phi_T > 0.5$:*
  At any stage of the trial, if the previously treated patient has experienced the DLT, de-escalate the dose to one level lower with probability $(1 - \phi_T)/\phi_T$ and the dose stays at the same level with probability $(2\phi_T - 1)/\phi_T$; if no DLT is observed for the previous patient, escalate the dose to one level higher.

At the lowest and the highest dose levels, appropriate adjustments are made so that treatment always remains within the prespecified dose range. For example, if the current dose is the lowest while the decision is to de-escalate the dose, or if the current dose is the highest while the decision is to escalate the dose, then the next patient will still be treated at the current dose. Stylianou and Flournoy (2002) further explore the biased coin dose-finding procedures using the maximum likelihood method, weighted least-squares approach, sample averages, and isotonic regression. However, dose-finding methods that involve random dose assignment are typically not preferred, especially when using toxicity alone as the primary endpoint.

In oncology, the target toxicity probability is usually less than 0.5. Therefore, for $\phi_T \leq 0.5$, if no DLT is observed for the patient treated at the current dose level, the probabilities of dose escalation and dose staying at the same level (no change) for the next patient are given below.

| Toxicity Target $\phi_T$ | 0.10 | 0.20 | 0.25 | 0.30 | 0.33 | 0.35 | 0.40 |
|---|---|---|---|---|---|---|---|
| Pr(dose escalation) | 0.11 | 0.25 | 0.33 | 0.43 | 0.50 | 0.54 | 0.67 |
| Pr(dose no change) | 0.89 | 0.75 | 0.67 | 0.57 | 0.50 | 0.46 | 0.33 |

Often, the algorithm-based designs as aforementioned are closely related to the family of up-and-down designs (Gezmu and Flournoy, 2006). In the general up-and-down design, let $j$ be the dose level at which the most recent cohort is treated, and let $t_j$ be the number of patients who have experienced the DLT at dose level $j$. We denote the cohort size by $s$, and specify two cutoff integers $c_L$ and $c_U$, satisfying $0 \leq c_L \leq c_U \leq s$. The group up-and-down design assigns the next cohort of patients to

- dose level $j - 1$, if $t_j \geq c_U$; while if the current dose is at the lowest level, the next dose remains the same;

- dose level $j + 1$, if $t_j \leq c_L$; while if the current dose is at the highest level, the next dose remains the same; and

- dose level $j$, if $c_L < t_j < c_U$.

## 4.7  CONTINUAL REASSESSMENT METHOD

### 4.7.1  Probability Model

As we have seen, algorithm-based approaches to dose finding simply follow a set of prespecified rules. Often, dose assignment only depends on the data observed at the current dose level, while there is no modeling or borrowing information across other doses. By contrast, model-based dose-finding methods assume a certain parametric model for the underlying dose–toxicity curve. In particular, the continual reassessment method (CRM) links the true toxicity probability at each dose with the prespecified toxicity probability through a single-parameter model. During the trial, as the toxicity data are accumulated, the CRM continuously updates the estimates of the toxicity probabilities of all the doses. Each new cohort of patients will be sequentially assigned to the most appropriate dose based on the updated toxicity probabilities, and eventually the MTD will be identified when the total sample size is exhausted.

Typically, toxicity is assumed to monotonically increase with respect to the dose. Let $p_1 < \cdots < p_J$ be the prespecified toxicity probabilities of a set of $J$ doses for the drug under consideration, which is often known as the skeleton of the CRM. Let $\phi_T$ be the target toxicity probability specified by the investigator. The CRM assumes a working dose–toxicity model; that is, for $j = 1, \ldots, J$,

$$\Pr(\text{toxicity at dose level } j) = \pi_j(\alpha) = p_j^{\exp(\alpha)}, \qquad (4.1)$$

where $\alpha$ is the only unknown parameter (O'Quigley and Shen, 1996). Figure 4.6 displays dose–toxicity curves for different values of $\alpha$ under model (4.1).

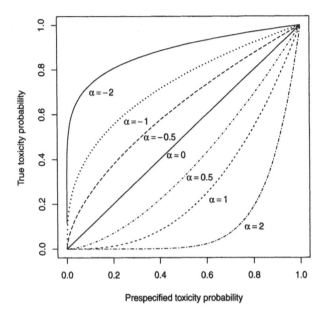

**Figure 4.6**    Dose–toxicity curves with different values of $\alpha$ under the CRM power function.

The CRM may take a different model structure other than the power function in (4.1), such as a logistic model with a fixed intercept of $-3$,

$$\pi_j(\alpha) = \frac{\exp(-3 + \alpha d_j)}{1 + \exp(-3 + \alpha d_j)},$$

where $d_j$ is the standardized dose at dose level $j$, or a hyperbolic tangent function,

$$\pi_j(\alpha) = \left\{ \frac{\tanh(d_j) + 1}{2} \right\}^\alpha = \left\{ \frac{(e^{2d_j} - 1)/(e^{2d_j} + 1) + 1}{2} \right\}^\alpha.$$

Figure 4.7 shows possible dose–toxicity curves for different values of $\alpha$ under the logistic and hyperbolic tangent functions, respectively.

### 4.7.2  Likelihood and Posterior

Suppose that $y_j$ patients have experienced the DLT among the $n_j$ patients treated at dose level $j$, for $j = 1, \ldots, J$. Let $D$ denote the observed data, then the

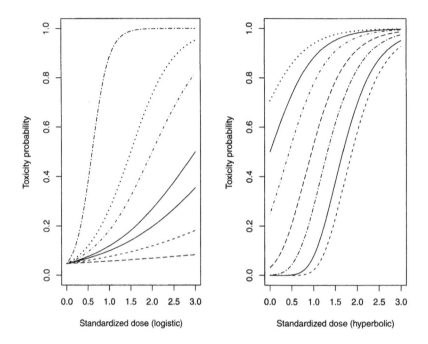

**Figure 4.7**    Dose–toxicity curves with different values of $\alpha$ under the CRM logistic and hyperbolic tangent functions, respectively.

likelihood function is given by

$$L(D|\alpha) \propto \prod_{j=1}^{J} \{p_j^{\exp(\alpha)}\}^{y_j} \{1 - p_j^{\exp(\alpha)}\}^{n_j - y_j}.$$

Let $f(\alpha)$ denote a prior distribution for $\alpha$, for example, $\alpha \sim N(0, \sigma^2)$. Using Bayes' theorem, the toxicity probability at dose level $j$ can be estimated by the posterior mean,

$$\hat{\pi}_j = \int p_j^{\exp(\alpha)} \frac{L(D|\alpha)f(\alpha)}{\int L(D|\alpha)f(\alpha)\,\mathrm{d}\alpha}\,\mathrm{d}\alpha.$$

After each cohort is treated, in light of the newly updated toxicity data including all the patients enrolled thus far, we re-calculate the posterior means of the toxicity probabilities at all the dose levels. The dose that has a toxicity probability closest to the target $\phi_T$ may be recommended to treat the next cohort. Whereas for safety, it is typically required no dose skipping during dose escalation or de-escalation, and thus each time dose assignment only moves one level up or down toward the target. The trial continues until the total sample size is exhausted, and finally the dose with a toxicity probability closest to $\phi_T$ is selected as the MTD.

In the CRM, we may specify the prior mean toxicity probabilities, $(\tilde{p}_1, \ldots, \tilde{p}_J)$, instead of $(p_1, \ldots, p_J)$. The skeleton $(p_1, \ldots, p_J)$ can then be obtained through

$$\tilde{p}_j = E\{p_j^{\exp(\alpha)}\} = \int p_j^{\exp(\alpha)} f(\alpha)\,d\alpha, \quad j = 1, \ldots, J. \tag{4.2}$$

Because $p_j$ and $\tilde{p}_j$ are one-to-one related, whichever specified would not affect the trial performance much. It is worth noting that $(p_1, \ldots, p_J)$ is the intrinsic component of the CRM model, which is not part of the prior distributions as in the usual Bayesian sense.

### 4.7.3 Dose-Finding Algorithm

In practice, patients are often treated in a cohort size of three. To be conservative, dose escalation or de-escalation is restricted by one dose level of change at a time. The CRM dose-finding procedure is described as follows:

(1) Treat the first cohort of patients at the lowest or the physician-specified dose level.

(2) Denote the current dose level as $j^{\mathrm{curr}}$. Based on the data observed thus far, we obtain the posterior means of the toxicity probabilities for all the doses under consideration; that is, $\hat{\pi}_1, \ldots, \hat{\pi}_J$. We find the dose level $j^*$ that has a toxicity probability closest to $\phi_T$,

$$j^* = \operatorname*{arg\,min}_{j \in \{1, \ldots, J\}} |\hat{\pi}_j - \phi_T|,$$

and

- if $j^{\mathrm{curr}} > j^*$, de-escalate to dose level $j^{\mathrm{curr}} - 1$;
- if $j^{\mathrm{curr}} < j^*$, escalate to dose level $j^{\mathrm{curr}} + 1$;
- otherwise, the dose stays at the same level for the next cohort of patients.

(3) Once the maximum sample size is reached, the dose with the toxicity probability closest to $\phi_T$ is selected as the MTD.

In addition, if the lowest dose is still too toxic, as noted by

$$\Pr(\pi_1 > \phi_T | D) = \int_{-\infty}^{\log\{\log(\phi_T)/\log(p_1)\}} f(\alpha | D)\,d\alpha > 0.9, \tag{4.3}$$

the trial will be terminated for safety. In (4.3), the threshold value 0.9 may be adjusted according to the trial's operating characteristics.

**Table 4.2    Simulation Study Using the CRM with Five Doses and a Target Toxicity Probability of $\phi_T = 30\%$**

| CRM | Dose level | | | | | Total # Toxicity | Total # Patients |
|---|---|---|---|---|---|---|---|
| | 1 | 2 | 3 | 4 | 5 | | |
| Scenario 1 | 0.30 | 0.40 | 0.55 | 0.60 | 0.65 | | |
| Selection % | **70.6** | 27.7 | 1.7 | 0.0 | 0.0 | | |
| # Patients | 20.6 | 8.2 | 1.2 | 0.0 | 0.0 | 10.1 | 30 |
| | | | | | | | |
| Scenario 2 | 0.10 | 0.20 | 0.30 | 0.40 | 0.50 | | |
| Selection % | 2.9 | 37.2 | **44.3** | 14.0 | 1.6 | | |
| # Patients | 5.6 | 11.8 | 9.1 | 3.0 | 0.5 | 7.1 | 30 |
| | | | | | | | |
| Scenario 3 | 0.02 | 0.06 | 0.10 | 0.20 | 0.30 | | |
| Selection % | 0.0 | 0.5 | 9.3 | 39.3 | **50.9** | | |
| # Patients | 3.2 | 4.2 | 6.1 | 8.7 | 7.8 | 5.0 | 30 |
| | | | | | | | |
| Scenario 4 | 0.20 | 0.30 | 0.60 | 0.70 | 0.75 | | |
| Selection % | 29.6 | **66.3** | 4.1 | 0.0 | 0.0 | | |
| # Patients | 12.3 | 14.8 | 2.8 | 0.1 | 0.0 | 8.6 | 30 |

### 4.7.4    Simulation Study

We conducted simulation studies to investigate the practical performance of the CRM. As shown in Table 4.2, we considered five increasing dose levels with monotonically increasing toxicity. The target toxic probability was $\phi_T = 30\%$, and the prespecified toxicity probabilities were $(p_1, \ldots, p_5) = (0.1, 0.2, 0.3, 0.4, 0.5)$. We took the prior distribution $\alpha \sim N(0, \sigma^2)$ with $\sigma = 1.34$. The first cohort was treated at the lowest dose level, and the maximum sample size was 30. For comparison with the $3 + 3$ design, we intentionally simulated the same four scenarios as those listed in Table 4.1, and for each scenario 10,000 trials were replicated.

Under each scenario, we present the true toxicity probability, the selection percentage, the number of patients treated at each dose, the total number of observed DLTs, and the total number of patients treated in the trial. Unlike the $3 + 3$ design which does not target any specific toxicity probability, the CRM had a target toxicity probability of $\phi_T = 30\%$. As an illustration, we interpret the simulation results of scenario 1, in which the first dose is the MTD. Because the early stopping rule in (4.3) was not invoked, each of the simulated trials under scenario 1 ran until exhausting the maximum sample size of 30. On average, there were 10 patients experiencing the DLT in each trial, approximately 21 patients were treated at the MTD, and there was a more than 70% of chance that the true MTD would be selected. Other three scenarios also demonstrated that the selection percentages of the MTD using the CRM were substantially higher than those in the $3 + 3$ design; see Table 4.1.

Regression models with more unknown parameters are typically more flexible in terms of model fitting. However, model flexibility might not help dose finding due to the small number of patients and the sequential nature of the CRM. In particular, at the beginning of a trial, the data are really sparse; for example, only three patients are involved for the first decision making. In general, dose-finding methods would work well as long as the model provides an adequate local fit around the current treating dose, because the dose assignment is only allowed to change by one dose level at a time. If the sample size is large, the CRM is consistent and the recommended dose converges to the true MTD (Shen and O'Quigley, 1996). Nevertheless, such asymptotic behaviors might not be very relevant due to the small sample size in a typical phase I clinical trial.

## 4.8 BAYESIAN MODEL AVERAGING CONTINUAL REASSESSMENT METHOD

### 4.8.1 Skeleton of the CRM

Despite its superior performance over the $3 + 3$ design, the CRM suffers from the arbitrariness and subjectivity in the prespecification of the skeleton $(p_1, \ldots, p_J)$. This is mainly due to a lack of toxicity information on the new drug. If the elicited $p_j$'s deviate far from the true dose–toxicity curve, the estimates of the toxicity probabilities may not be accurate. Such model misspecification often leads to poor performance of a trial design, which may end up selecting a wrong dose as the MTD. Of greater consequence is that an undesirably large number of patients may be treated at excessively toxic doses. Because the underlying true toxicity profile for a new drug is unknown in practice, there is no information to justify whether a specific skeleton is reasonable.

To enhance the robustness of the design, multiple CRM models may be used in parallel, each equipped with a different skeleton (Yin and Yuan, 2009a). Different skeletons represent different prior guesses of the toxicity profile of the drug. We assign a discrete prior probability mass to each CRM model, and accommodate model uncertainty through the Bayesian model averaging (BMA) procedure (Raftery, Madigan, and Hoeting, 1997; Hoeting et al., 1999). BMA produces more robust estimates of the toxicity probabilities based on the posterior model probability weighting. In other words, instead of using a single CRM for the trial conduct, we carry out multiple parallel CRMs. The BMA-CRM adaptively assigns a larger weight to a model of a better fit, and thus automatically ensures the estimated toxicity probabilities to be always close to the best estimates among all the candidate models.

### 4.8.2 BMA-CRM

Let $M_k$ denote the CRM probability model associated with the $k$th skeleton $(p_{k1}, \ldots, p_{kJ})$, for $k = 1, \ldots, K$. Under the working model $M_k$, the toxicity probability at dose level $j$ is given by

$$\pi_{kj}(\alpha_k) = p_{kj}^{\exp(\alpha_k)}, \quad j = 1, \ldots, J,$$

where $\alpha_k$ is the unknown parameter associated with model $M_k$. Suppose that at a certain stage of the trial, $y_j$ patients have experienced toxicity among the $n_j$ patients treated at dose level $j$. Based on the observed data $D$, the likelihood function under model $M_k$ is

$$L(D|\alpha_k, M_k) \propto \prod_{j=1}^{J} \{p_{kj}^{\exp(\alpha_k)}\}^{y_j} \{1 - p_{kj}^{\exp(\alpha_k)}\}^{n_j - y_j}.$$

Let $P(M_k)$ be the prior probability that model $M_k$ is the true model. We take a discrete uniform distribution for the prior model probability; that is, $P(M_k) = 1/K$, if there is no preference *a priori* for any single CRM model. Let $f(\alpha_k|M_k)$ denote the prior distribution of $\alpha_k$ under model $M_k$. The marginal likelihood of model $M_k$, $L(D|M_k)$, is obtained by integrating out $\alpha_k$ with respect to the corresponding prior distribution,

$$L(D|M_k) = \int L(D|\alpha_k, M_k) f(\alpha_k|M_k) \, d\alpha_k,$$

and the posterior model probability for $M_k$ is

$$P(M_k|D) = \frac{L(D|M_k)P(M_k)}{\sum_{i=1}^{K} L(D|M_i)P(M_i)}.$$

As a result, the BMA estimate of the toxicity probability at dose level $j$ is given by

$$\bar{\pi}_j = \sum_{k=1}^{K} \hat{\pi}_{kj} P(M_k|D), \quad j = 1, \ldots, J,$$

where $\hat{\pi}_{kj}$ is the posterior mean of the toxicity probability at dose level $j$ under model $M_k$,

$$\hat{\pi}_{kj} = \int p_{kj}^{\exp(\alpha_k)} \frac{L(D|\alpha_k, M_k) f(\alpha_k|M_k)}{\int L(D|\alpha_k, M_k) f(\alpha_k|M_k) d\alpha_k} \, d\alpha_k.$$

By assigning $\hat{\pi}_{kj}$ a weight of $P(M_k|D)$, the BMA estimator $\bar{\pi}_j$ automatically favors the best fitting model. The decision on dose escalation or de-escalation is based upon $\bar{\pi}_j$ as opposed to $\hat{\pi}_{kj}$. The BMA-CRM no longer regards the prior guesses of the toxicity probabilities as fixed; instead, they are associated with model fitting adequacy.

In contrast to model averaging, Bayesian model selection (BMS) finds the best fitting model according to a suitable criterion among all the candidate models (e.g., see Spiegelhalter et al., 2002). Clearly, the higher the posterior model probability, the better the model fit. In the resultant BMS-CRM, we naturally select the CRM model associated with the highest posterior model probability to determine dose assignment.

### 4.8.3 Dose-Finding Algorithm

Let $\phi_T$ be the prespecified target toxicity probability. Patients are treated in a cohort size of three. Dose escalation or de-escalation is restricted by one dose level of change at a time. The BMA-CRM dose-finding algorithm is described as follows:

(1) Treat the first cohort of patients at the lowest or the physician-specified dose level.

(2) Suppose that the current dose level is $j^{\mathrm{curr}}$. Based on the accumulated data $D$, we obtain the BMA estimates of the toxicity probabilities for all the doses under consideration; that is, $\bar{\pi}_1, \ldots, \bar{\pi}_J$. We find the dose level $j^*$ that has a toxicity probability closest to $\phi_T$,

$$j^* = \underset{j \in \{1,\ldots,J\}}{\arg\min} |\bar{\pi}_j - \phi_T|,$$

and

- if $j^{\mathrm{curr}} > j^*$, de-escalate to dose level $j^{\mathrm{curr}} - 1$;
- if $j^{\mathrm{curr}} < j^*$, escalate to dose level $j^{\mathrm{curr}} + 1$;
- otherwise, the dose stays at the same level for the next cohort of patients.

(3) Once the maximum sample size is reached, the dose with the toxicity probability closest to $\phi_T$ is selected as the MTD.

In addition, if the lowest dose is still too toxic, as noted by

$$\sum_{k=1}^{K} \Pr(\pi_{k1} > \phi_T | M_k, D) P(M_k | D) > 0.9,$$

the trial will be terminated early for safety.

### 4.8.4 Simulation Study

We investigated the operating characteristics of the BMA-CRM through simulation studies. We considered eight doses with the target toxicity probability

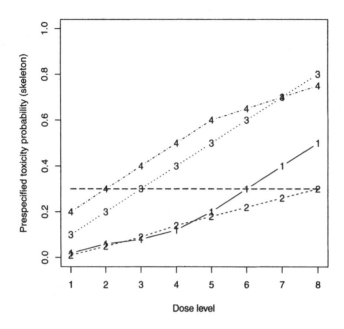

**Figure 4.8**    Four different skeletons in the BMA-CRM with a target toxicity probability of $\phi_T = 30\%$.

$\phi_T = 30\%$, and we prepared four sets of initial guesses of the toxicity probabilities:

$$(p_1, \ldots, p_8) = \begin{cases} (.02, .06, .08, .12, .20, .30, .40, .50), & \text{skeleton 1,} \\ (.01, .05, .09, .14, .18, .22, .26, .30), & \text{skeleton 2,} \\ (.10, .20, .30, .40, .50, .60, .70, .80), & \text{skeleton 3,} \\ (.20, .30, .40, .50, .60, .65, .70, .75), & \text{skeleton 4.} \end{cases}$$

As shown in Figure 4.8, these four skeletons represent quite different prior opinions on the dose–toxicity curve, which are expected to capture the true dose–toxicity relationship more effectively using the BMA procedure. In the first skeleton, toxicity increases slowly at the low doses but increases quickly at the high doses; the second skeleton is more concentrated at the low toxicity levels; the toxicity probabilities in the third skeleton are evenly spread over the range of 0.1 to 0.8; and the fourth skeleton starts at 0.2, and increases quickly at the low doses before leveling off at the high doses. The individual CRM using each single skeleton is referred to as CRM 1 to CRM 4. We took the prior distribution $\alpha \sim N(0, 2^2)$, and a discrete uniform prior model probability $P(M_k) = 1/4$ for $k = 1, \ldots, 4$. The maximum sample size was 30, and patients were treated in a cohort size of 3. The first cohort was treated at the lowest dose level, and for each scenario 10,000 trials were replicated.

In Table 4.3, under each scenario we present the true toxicity probability, the selection percentage of the MTD, the number of patients treated at each dose, and the total number of patients experiencing toxicity averaged over the 10,000 simulated trials. In scenario 1, the seventh dose is the MTD; the selection percentages of the MTD using four individual CRMs were very different: CRM 2 had the lowest MTD selection percentage of only 30.8%, but incorrectly selected the eighth dose with the highest percentage of 56.9%. By contrast, the BMA-CRM and the BMS-CRM selected the MTD with 51.5% and 50.5%, respectively. The number of patients treated at each dose was similar across these designs, except that CRM 2 treated almost twice as many as patients at dose level 8 compared with other designs. Therefore, if skeleton 2 had been used in the trial conduct, the eighth dose would have been very likely chosen as the MTD, which, however, was overly toxic with a toxicity probability of 0.5. Scenario 2 has the MTD at the sixth dose level, and the MTD selection using the BMA-CRM was the second highest among all the designs. The worst skeleton corresponded to CRM 2, which yielded a less than 30% selection of the MTD. Interestingly, in this scenario we intentionally matched the skeleton in CRM 1 with the true toxicity probabilities. As expected, CRM 1 yielded the highest MTD selection percentage, and that of the BMA-CRM was only 2% lower. In scenario 3, the MTD is the third dose; CRM 1 behaved the worst by selecting the MTD less than 50%, compared with more than 60% of the MTD selection for the other three CRMs.

Overall, both the BMA-CRM and BMS-CRM indeed enhance the robustness of the dose-finding procedure. Although the CRM with a certain skeleton may not perform well due to model misspecification, simultaneously using multiple skeletons would reduce the chance of such underperformance. These two methods carry the essence of model averaging and model selection by adaptively balancing among competing skeletons, and thus offer more reliable and more robust estimates for the toxicity probabilities. The BMA-CRM and BMS-CRM typically cannot beat the best-performing single-skeleton CRM, while their performances are always close to that best CRM and can be much better than the worst one.

Figure 4.9 presents the posterior model probability for the individual CRM after each cohort was sequentially accrued under scenarios 1 to 3, respectively. The posterior model probabilities of the four CRM models started diverging after approximately 4 to 8 cohorts, and eventually they reached the stabilized values in an order correctly matching with their performances. Hence, the BMA-CRM automatically distinguishes model fitting as more data are collected in the trial, and assign a higher posterior model probability to a better-performing CRM. For example, in scenario 1, the BMA procedure selected CRM 3 as the best-fitting model and CRM 2 as the worst after approximately 15 cohorts, which exactly

**Table 4.3    Simulation Study Comparing the CRM, BMA-CRM, and BMS-CRM with Eight Doses and a Target Toxicity Probability of $\phi_T = 30\%$**

| Design | \multicolumn{8}{c}{Selection Percentage at Dose Level} | | | | | | | | Total # Toxicity |
|---|---|---|---|---|---|---|---|---|---|
| | 1 | 2 | 3 | 4 | 5 | 6 | 7 | 8 | |
| Scenario 1 | 0.02 | 0.03 | 0.04 | 0.06 | 0.08 | 0.10 | 0.30 | 0.50 | |
| CRM 1 | 0.0 | 0.0 | 0.0 | 0.1 | 1.4 | 16.0 | **52.6** | 29.9 | |
| # Patients | 3.2 | 3.0 | 3.0 | 3.1 | 3.6 | 4.7 | 5.7 | 3.6 | 4.7 |
| CRM 2 | 0.0 | 0.0 | 0.0 | 0.1 | 1.0 | 11.2 | **30.8** | 56.9 | |
| # Patients | 3.2 | 3.0 | 3.1 | 3.1 | 3.2 | 3.5 | 4.3 | 6.6 | 5.6 |
| CRM 3 | 0.0 | 0.0 | 0.0 | 0.8 | 4.6 | 22.1 | **59.3** | 13.1 | |
| # Patients | 3.2 | 3.0 | 3.2 | 3.5 | 4.1 | 5.2 | 6.4 | 1.4 | 3.9 |
| CRM 4 | 0.0 | 0.0 | 0.0 | 0.6 | 3.6 | 18.0 | **44.8** | 33.0 | |
| # Patients | 3.2 | 3.0 | 3.1 | 3.5 | 3.8 | 4.2 | 5.2 | 3.8 | 4.7 |
| BMA-CRM | 0.0 | 0.0 | 0.0 | 0.2 | 1.5 | 16.2 | **51.5** | 30.6 | |
| # Patients | 3.2 | 3.0 | 3.1 | 3.2 | 3.5 | 4.4 | 6.3 | 3.2 | 4.7 |
| BMS-CRM | 0.0 | 0.0 | 0.0 | 0.1 | 1.5 | 19.2 | **50.5** | 28.6 | |
| # Patients | 3.2 | 3.0 | 3.1 | 3.2 | 3.6 | 4.5 | 5.4 | 4.0 | 4.8 |
| | | | | | | | | | |
| Scenario 2 | 0.02 | 0.06 | 0.08 | 0.12 | 0.20 | 0.30 | 0.40 | 0.50 | |
| CRM 1 | 0.0 | 0.0 | 0.0 | 2.9 | 23.9 | **43.6** | 22.7 | 6.9 | |
| # Patients | 3.2 | 3.1 | 3.2 | 3.6 | 6.3 | 6.6 | 3.0 | 0.8 | 5.9 |
| CRM 2 | 0.0 | 0.0 | 0.3 | 4.3 | 17.1 | **28.4** | 25.5 | 24.4 | |
| # Patients | 3.2 | 3.1 | 3.4 | 3.8 | 4.6 | 4.8 | 3.8 | 3.2 | 6.5 |
| CRM 3 | 0.0 | 0.0 | 0.6 | 6.3 | 32.6 | **40.8** | 18.1 | 1.6 | |
| # Patients | 3.2 | 3.1 | 3.6 | 4.8 | 6.9 | 5.7 | 2.4 | 0.2 | 5.2 |
| CRM 4 | 0.0 | 0.0 | 0.4 | 7.5 | 27.8 | **35.3** | 20.7 | 8.2 | |
| # Patients | 3.2 | 3.1 | 3.6 | 4.9 | 6.4 | 4.8 | 2.9 | 1.0 | 5.5 |
| BMA-CRM | 0.0 | 0.0 | 0.3 | 4.3 | 23.9 | **41.6** | 22.7 | 7.3 | |
| # Patients | 3.2 | 3.1 | 3.4 | 4.3 | 5.9 | 5.8 | 3.3 | 0.8 | 5.7 |
| BMS-CRM | 0.0 | 0.0 | 0.2 | 3.8 | 26.1 | **38.4** | 21.2 | 10.3 | |
| # Patients | 3.2 | 3.1 | 3.4 | 4.1 | 6.3 | 5.4 | 3.1 | 1.3 | 5.8 |
| | | | | | | | | | |
| Scenario 3 | 0.06 | 0.15 | 0.30 | 0.55 | 0.60 | 0.65 | 0.68 | 0.70 | |
| CRM 1 | 0.9 | 27.8 | **48.5** | 21.0 | 1.5 | 0.2 | 0.0 | 0.0 | |
| # Patients | 4.3 | 7.4 | 9.7 | 6.5 | 1.9 | 0.2 | 0.0 | 0.0 | 9.1 |
| CRM 2 | 0.2 | 22.6 | **60.8** | 15.1 | 1.0 | 0.2 | 0.0 | 0.0 | |
| # Patients | 3.9 | 7.5 | 11.7 | 5.1 | 1.5 | 0.3 | 0.0 | 0.0 | 8.8 |
| CRM 3 | 0.3 | 19.6 | **65.1** | 14.4 | 0.6 | 0.0 | 0.0 | 0.0 | |
| # Patients | 4.1 | 7.2 | 13.0 | 5.0 | 0.6 | 0.0 | 0.0 | 0.0 | 8.4 |
| CRM 4 | 0.4 | 19.3 | **65.6** | 14.2 | 0.5 | 0.0 | 0.0 | 0.0 | |
| # Patients | 4.1 | 7.2 | 12.7 | 5.2 | 0.7 | 0.1 | 0.0 | 0.0 | 8.5 |
| BMA-CRM | 0.3 | 20.6 | **62.0** | 16.1 | 0.9 | 0.0 | 0.0 | 0.0 | |
| # Patients | 4.1 | 7.2 | 12.2 | 5.6 | 0.8 | 0.1 | 0.0 | 0.0 | 8.6 |
| BMS-CRM | 0.2 | 20.0 | **64.9** | 13.7 | 1.0 | 0.1 | 0.0 | 0.0 | |
| # Patients | 4.1 | 7.2 | 12.4 | 5.2 | 1.0 | 0.1 | 0.0 | 0.0 | 8.6 |

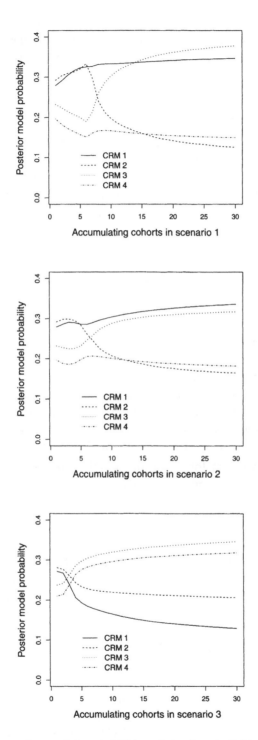

**Figure 4.9** Posterior model probabilities of the four individual CRMs versus the accumulating number of cohorts under scenarios 1–3, respectively.

matched with the order of the performance of the individual CRMs. For scenarios 1 and 2, the true toxicity probabilities at the first several dose levels are extremely low, and thus very few patients would experience toxicity at the beginning of the trial. This in turn requires a larger number of cohorts to discriminate the model fitting.

### 4.8.5   Sensitivity Analysis

To examine how the number of skeletons affects the practical performance of the BMA-CRM, we considered another scenario with the true toxicity probabilities $(\pi_1, \ldots, \pi_8) = (0.10, 0.20, 0.30, 0.40, 0.50, 0.60, 0.70, 0.80)$. We increased the number of skeletons from one to six, by successively adding one skeleton at a time in the original order of skeletons 1–4, while the fifth and sixth skeletons are given by

$$(p_1, \ldots, p_8) = \begin{cases} (.08, .15, .21, .29, .37, .44, .51, .58), & \text{skeleton 5,} \\ (.05, .10, .20, .25, .30, .40, .47, .55), & \text{skeleton 6.} \end{cases}$$

As shown in Figure 4.10, the CRM using only the first skeleton yielded the lowest selection percentage of the MTD, and adding the second and the third skeleton steadily improved the results, while using three to six skeletons did not affect the design performance much.

The remaining question is how to specify the skeletons, and whether different ways of specification would have an impact on the performance of the design. Generally speaking, the skeletons should be chosen in a way to cover a reasonable range of dose–toxicity relationships, while avoiding redundant skeletons. The two skeletons, $(p_{i1}, \ldots, p_{iJ})$ and $(p_{k1}, \ldots, p_{kJ})$, are equivalent if one can be expressed as a power transformation of the other; that is, $p_{ij} = p_{kj}^{\exp(\gamma)}$ for $j = 1, \ldots, J$, where $\gamma$ is a constant. This can be written as

$$\frac{\log(p_{i1})}{\log(p_{k1})} = \cdots = \frac{\log(p_{iJ})}{\log(p_{kJ})} = \exp(\gamma),$$

and thus we may use the variability of the ratios of the log probabilities as a measure of "dissimilarity" between skeletons $i$ and $k$. A larger value of this variance indicates a higher level of dissimilarity between the two skeletons. In practice, the investigator often gives a range of toxicity probabilities for each dose, say, $[p_{j,L}, p_{j,U}]$ for dose level $j$. For example, the toxicity probability at dose level 1 may range from 0.1 to 0.3, that at dose level 2 from 0.25 to 0.4, and so on. We can naturally construct three skeletons by grouping $p_{j,L}$, $p_{j,U}$, and $(p_{j,L} + p_{j,U})/2$ across all the dose levels, respectively.

The BMA-CRM is intuitive, coherent, and easy to implement using the Gaussian quadrature or the Markov chain Monte Carlo (MCMC) method to approximate the posterior integrals. The BMA-CRM software and many others to be

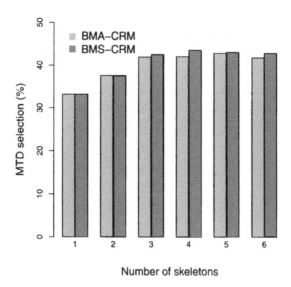

**Figure 4.10**    Selection percentage of the MTD as the number of skeletons increases.

introduced in the forthcoming chapters can be freely downloaded from the website of the Department of Biostatistics at the University of Texas M. D. Anderson Cancer Center:

http://biostatistics.mdanderson.org/SoftwareDownload/

In the BMA-CRM software, the prespecified toxicity probabilities are the prior mean values of the considered doses as defined in (4.2). If only one set of prior mean toxicity probabilities is specified, the BMA-CRM reduces to the original CRM.

## 4.9  ESCALATION WITH OVERDOSE CONTROL

Escalation with overdose control (EWOC) is another model-based Bayesian dose-finding method (Babb et al., 1998). The EWOC design directly controls the toxicity percentage in a trial such that patients are protected from over-toxic doses. Each time, the dose is selected in a way that the predicted proportion of patients who will receive overdoses equals a predetermined threshold.

For the $i$th patient treated at dose $x_i$, let $y_i = 1$ if the patient experienced the DLT and $y_i = 0$ otherwise. The relationship between $y_i$ and $x_i$ can be modeled

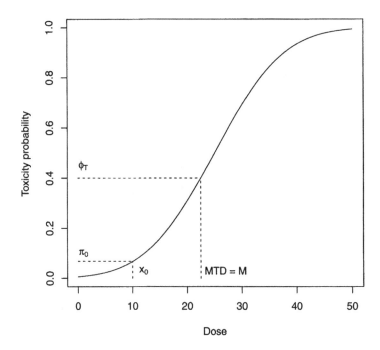

**Figure 4.11**    A typical dose–toxicity curve with the lowest dose $x_0$ and the MTD $M$ in the EWOC design.

as

$$\Pr(y_i = 1|\text{dose} = x_i) = F(\beta_0 + \beta_1 x_i),$$

where $F(\cdot)$ is a prespecified cumulative distribution function, and $\beta_0$ and $\beta_1$ are unknown parameters with $\beta_1 > 0$ to maintain the dose–toxicity monotonic order. Suppose that $n$ subjects have been enrolled in the trial, and given the observed data $\mathbf{y} = (y_1, \dots, y_n)$ the likelihood function is

$$L(\mathbf{y}|\beta_0, \beta_1) = \prod_{i=1}^{n} F(\beta_0 + \beta_1 x_i)^{y_i} \{1 - F(\beta_0 + \beta_1 x_i)\}^{1-y_i}. \tag{4.4}$$

Figure 4.11 shows a typical dose–toxicity curve, which monotonically increases with respect to the dose. Let $\phi_T$ denote the target toxicity probability, let $M$ denote the MTD, and let $\pi_0$ denote the toxicity probability of the lowest dose $x_0$. Then, we have

$$\phi_T = \Pr(y = 1|\text{dose} = M) = F(\beta_0 + \beta_1 M),$$

and

$$\pi_0 = \Pr(y = 1|\text{dose} = x_0) = F(\beta_0 + \beta_1 x_0).$$

As a result, the unknown parameters $(\beta_0, \beta_1)$ can be linked with $(M, \pi_0)$ through

$$\beta_1 = \frac{F^{-1}(\phi_T) - F^{-1}(\pi_0)}{M - x_0},$$

$$\beta_0 = F^{-1}(\pi_0) - \beta_1 x_0.$$

If we assume $F^{-1}(x) = \text{logit}(x) = \log\{x/(1-x)\}$, we have

$$F(\beta_0 + \beta_1 x) = \frac{\exp\left[\text{logit}(\pi_0) + \{\text{logit}(\phi_T) - \text{logit}(\pi_0)\}\left(\dfrac{x - x_0}{M - x_0}\right)\right]}{1 + \exp\left[\text{logit}(\pi_0) + \{\text{logit}(\phi_T) - \text{logit}(\pi_0)\}\left(\dfrac{x - x_0}{M - x_0}\right)\right]}.$$

After plugging $F(\beta_0 + \beta_1 x)$ into the likelihood function in (4.4) and specifying the prior distributions for $M$ and $\pi_0$, we can derive the joint posterior distribution of $M$ and $\pi_0$. The next dose can be determined using the marginal distribution of $M$. Let $G(x|\mathbf{y})$ denote the posterior cumulative distribution function of $M$; that is,

$$G(x|\mathbf{y}) = \Pr(M \leq x|\mathbf{y}),$$

which is in fact the probability of an overdose given the data available in the trial. The dose $x$ recommended for the next patient satisfies $G(x|\mathbf{y}) = \alpha$; that is, the predicted probability that the chosen dose exceeds the MTD must equal a prespecified threshold $\alpha$. Hence, after the posterior distribution of the MTD is obtained, the next patient will be treated at the dose $x = G^{-1}(\alpha|\mathbf{y})$.

Once the trial is completed, the EWOC design selects the dose that has a minimal posterior expected loss,

$$\int \mathcal{L}_\alpha(x, M) \, dG(M|\mathbf{y}),$$

where the asymmetric loss function takes the form of

$$\mathcal{L}_\alpha(x, M) = \begin{cases} \alpha(M - x), & \text{if } x \leq M \text{ (underdose)}, \\ (1 - \alpha)(x - M), & \text{if } x > M \text{ (overdose)}. \end{cases}$$

This loss function implies that the loss incurred by treating a patient above the MTD is $(1 - \alpha)/\alpha$ times more than that associated with treating the patient at the same distance below the MTD.

## 4.10  BAYESIAN HYBRID DESIGN

### 4.10.1  Algorithm- versus Model-Based Dose Finding

As discussed in Section 4.2, algorithm-based dose-finding methods typically follow a set of dose-finding rules without imposing any modeling structure for the underlying dose-toxicity curve. By contrast, model-based approaches explicitly postulate the dose-toxicity relationship, which, however, would be vulnerable to model misspecification. In practice if the assumed model is wrong, it may yield inappropriate dose movement during escalation and de-escalation. For example, the CRM may continue treating patients at the same dose when 3 out of 3 patients have experienced the DLT; escalate the dose when 2 out of 3 patients have experienced the DLT; or de-escalate the dose when there is no DLT among 6 treated patients. These inappropriate dose assignments are not allowed if using algorithm-based approaches, such as the $3+3$ design. However, the $3+3$ design does not borrow information across different dose levels, and thus may result in efficiency loss.

The Bayesian hybrid dose-finding method takes a compromise between the algorithm- and model-based designs, which inherits advantages from both the nonparametric and parametric approaches by adaptively selecting one of them for decision making (Yuan and Yin, 2011a). The intuition behind the hybrid dose-finding method is that, if the data observed at the current dose provide adequate information on whether this dose is below or above the MTD, there is no need to enforce a parametric dose–toxicity model to borrow information or strength from other doses; and if the information at the current dose is not strong enough for such decision making, we resort to a parametric model to pool information from all other doses.

### 4.10.2   Bayesian Hypothesis Testing

Suppose that the current dose level is $j$, and let $\pi_j$ denote its toxicity probability. We formulate three complementary hypotheses to gauge how close $\pi_j$ is to the target toxicity probability $\phi_T$,

$$
\begin{aligned}
H_1 &: \pi_j < \phi_T - \delta, \\
H_2 &: \phi_T - \delta \le \pi_j \le \phi_T + \delta, \\
H_3 &: \pi_j > \phi_T + \delta,
\end{aligned}
$$

where $\delta$ is a prespecified tolerance margin, for example, $\delta = 0.03$. As displayed below, the hypotheses $H_1$, $H_2$, and $H_3$ represent the situations that dose level $j$ is below, in the vicinity of, and above the MTD, respectively.

Toxicity probability at dose level $j$: $\pi_j$

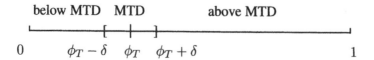

Under each hypothesis, we take a uniform prior distribution for $\pi_j$,

$$
\begin{aligned}
\pi_j | H_1 &\sim \text{Unif}(0, \phi_T - \delta), \\
\pi_j | H_2 &\sim \text{Unif}(\phi_T - \delta, \phi_T + \delta), \\
\pi_j | H_3 &\sim \text{Unif}(\phi_T + \delta, 1).
\end{aligned} \tag{4.5}
$$

Suppose that $y_j$ patients have experienced DLTs among the $n_j$ patients treated at dose level $j$. Considering the information at dose level $j$ only, the posterior probability of each hypothesis is given by

$$
P(H_k | y_j) = \frac{P(H_k)}{P(H_1)\text{BF}_{1,k} + P(H_2)\text{BF}_{2,k} + P(H_3)\text{BF}_{3,k}},
$$

where $\text{BF}_{i,k} = P(y_j | H_i)/P(y_j | H_k)$ is the Bayes factor for testing hypothesis $i$ versus hypothesis $k$, for $i, k = 1, 2, 3$. The marginal distribution of $y_j$ under $H_1$ is given by

$$
\begin{aligned}
P(y_j | H_1) &= \int_0^{\phi_T - \delta} \binom{n_j}{y_j} \pi_j^{y_j} (1 - \pi_j)^{n_j - y_j} \frac{1}{\phi_T - \delta} \, \mathrm{d}\pi_j \\
&= \frac{F(\phi_T - \delta; y_j + 1, n_j - y_j + 1)}{(\phi_T - \delta)(n_j + 1)},
\end{aligned}
$$

where $F(c; \alpha, \beta)$ is the cumulative distribution function of a beta distribution with the shape and scale parameters $\alpha$ and $\beta$, evaluated at $c$. Similarly, the marginal distributions of $y_j$ under $H_2$ and $H_3$ are given by

$$
\begin{aligned}
P(y_j | H_2) = \frac{1}{2\delta(n_j + 1)} \{ &F(\phi_T + \delta; y_j + 1, n_j - y_j + 1) \\
&- F(\phi_T - \delta; y_j + 1, n_j - y_j + 1) \}
\end{aligned}
$$

and

$$
P(y_j | H_3) = \frac{1 - F(\phi_T + \delta; y_j + 1, n_j - y_j + 1)}{(1 - \phi_T - \delta)(n_j + 1)},
$$

respectively. With no favor of any hypothesis *a priori*, we take a discrete uniform prior distribution for the three hypotheses: $P(H_1) = P(H_2) = P(H_3) = 1/3$. Hence, the posterior probability for hypothesis $k$ is simplified as

$$
P(H_k | y_j) = \frac{1}{\text{BF}_{1,k} + \text{BF}_{2,k} + \text{BF}_{3,k}}. \tag{4.6}
$$

Based on Jeffreys' (1961) interpretation of Bayes factors (see Section 3.4.6), if $\log_{10}(\text{BF}_{1,2}) > 1/2$ and $\log_{10}(\text{BF}_{1,3}) > 1/2$, which is equivalent to $P(H_1 | y_j) > 0.61$, there is substantial evidence in favor of $H_1$ against both $H_2$ and $H_3$. This suggests that dose level $j$ is far below the MTD, and thus we should escalate to dose level $j + 1$, without the need of borrowing any information from other doses. Similarly, if $P(H_3|y_j) > 0.61$, we should de-escalate to dose level $j - 1$ as there is substantial evidence supporting that dose level $j$ is far above the MTD. Finally, if $P(H_2|y_j) > 0.61$, the next cohort of patients will be treated at the same dose level, since dose $j$ is within the $\delta$-neighborhood of the MTD.

However, it may happen that $P(H_k|y_j) \leq 0.61$ for all $k$; that is, the information at dose level $j$ alone is not adequate to determine any action. In this case, we invoke a parametric dose–toxicity model, such as the CRM, to pool information across all the doses to determine the next dose assignment. The working model in the CRM takes the form of

$$\pi_j(\alpha) = p_j^{\exp(\alpha)}, \quad j = 1, \ldots, J, \tag{4.7}$$

where the $p_j$'s are the prespecified toxicity probabilities of the considered $J$ doses and $\alpha$ is an unknown parameter. Recall that dose $j$ is the currently treating dose, which is now denoted as $j^{\mathrm{curr}}$ for clarity. Under the three hypotheses, the uniform prior distributions for $\pi_{j^{\mathrm{curr}}}$ in (4.5) can be transformed into the prior distributions for $\alpha$ in (4.7):

$$f(\alpha|H_1) = -\frac{\log(p_{j^{\mathrm{curr}}})}{\phi_T - \delta} p_{j^{\mathrm{curr}}}^{\exp(\alpha)} \exp(\alpha),$$

for $\alpha > \log\{\log(\phi_T - \delta)/\log(p_{j^{\mathrm{curr}}})\}$;

$$f(\alpha|H_2) = -\frac{\log(p_{j^{\mathrm{curr}}})}{2\delta} p_{j^{\mathrm{curr}}}^{\exp(\alpha)} \exp(\alpha),$$

for $\log\{\log(\phi_T + \delta)/\log(p_{j^{\mathrm{curr}}})\} \leq \alpha \leq \log\{\log(\phi_T - \delta)/\log(p_{j^{\mathrm{curr}}})\}$; and

$$f(\alpha|H_3) = -\frac{\log(p_{j^{\mathrm{curr}}})}{1 - \phi_T - \delta} p_{j^{\mathrm{curr}}}^{\exp(\alpha)} \exp(\alpha),$$

for $\alpha < \log\{\log(\phi_T + \delta)/\log(p_{j^{\mathrm{curr}}})\}$. Let $\mathbf{y} = (y_1, \ldots, y_J)$ denote the observed data at all of the doses. The marginal distribution of $\mathbf{y}$ under $H_k$ is given by

$$P(\mathbf{y}|H_k) = \int \left[ \prod_{j=1}^{J} \binom{n_j}{y_j} \{p_j^{\exp(\alpha)}\}^{y_j} \{1 - p_j^{\exp(\alpha)}\}^{n_j - y_j} \right] f(\alpha|H_k)\, d\alpha,$$

for $k = 1, 2, 3$. The posterior distribution of $H_k$ given $\mathbf{y}$ takes the same form as (4.6), and Jeffereys' rule will again be used for decision making, but now based on all the data $\mathbf{y}$. If still none of the decisions can be reached under the CRM model, the next cohort of patients will be treated at the same dose level $j^{\mathrm{curr}}$ to accumulate more information.

### 4.10.3 Dose-Finding Algorithm

Patients are treated in a cohort size of three. To be conservative, dose escalation or de-escalation is restricted by one dose level of change at a time. The Bayesian hybrid dose-finding algorithm is described as follows:

(1) Treat the first cohort of patients at the lowest or the physician-specified dose level.

(2) Let $j^{\mathrm{curr}}$ denote the current dose level, and suppose that $y_{j^{\mathrm{curr}}}$ patients have experienced the DLT among the $n_{j^{\mathrm{curr}}}$ patients treated at dose level $j^{\mathrm{curr}}$. We calculate $P(H_k|y_{j^{\mathrm{curr}}})$ for $k = 1, 2, 3$, and

- if $P(H_1|y_{j^{\mathrm{curr}}}) > 0.61$, escalate to dose level $j^{\mathrm{curr}} + 1$;
- if $P(H_3|y_{j^{\mathrm{curr}}}) > 0.61$, de-escalate to dose level $j^{\mathrm{curr}} - 1$;
- if $P(H_2|y_{j^{\mathrm{curr}}}) > 0.61$, the dose stays at the same level as $j^{\mathrm{curr}}$ for the next cohort of patients.

(3) Otherwise, we switch to the CRM model to calculate $P(H_k|\mathbf{y})$ based on all the observed data $\mathbf{y}$, and apply the same decision rules as in step (2) but based on $P(H_k|\mathbf{y})$.

(4) Once the maximum sample size is exhausted, the dose with the toxicity probability closest to $\phi_T$ is selected as the MTD.

### 4.10.4 Simulation Study

We investigated the Bayesian hybrid design through simulation studies under four scenarios. We considered six doses with the target toxicity probability $\phi_T = 30\%$. The maximum sample size was 24 and patients were treated in a cohort size of 3. We compared the Bayesian hybrid design with two CRMs: One had an arbitrary skeleton $(p_1, \ldots, p_6) = (0.14, 0.20, 0.25, 0.30, 0.35, 0.40)$ which was also used in the hybrid design, and the other with the $p_j$'s equal to the true toxicity probabilities of each scenario (denoted as the true CRM). The true CRM is certainly not available in practice, while it may serve as the optimal case for comparison. In the hybrid design, we took the tolerance margin $\delta = 0.03$, and under each scenario we simulated 10,000 trials.

Figure 4.12 shows the selection percentage of the MTD under each scenario. As expected, the true CRM indeed performed the best, because the dose–toxicity model is correctly specified. The hybrid design outperformed the CRM with a higher selection percentage of the MTD in all scenarios. Moreover, the hybrid design is much safer than the CRM, as the number of patients treated at the doses above the MTD was reduced by almost a half.

Since the CRM always enforces a parametric dose–toxicity model to fit all the data, it may underestimate or overestimate the dose toxicity probabilities if the

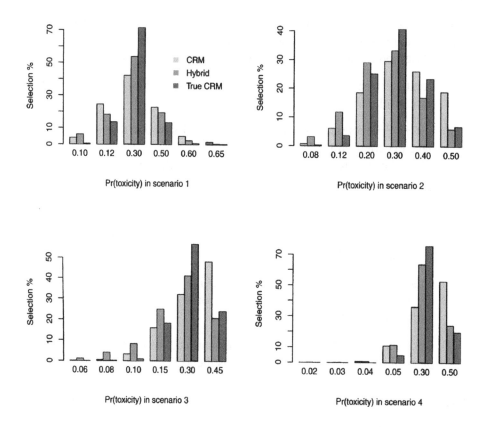

**Figure 4.12** Selection percentages of the MTD using the CRM, Bayesian hybrid design and true CRM under scenarios 1–4.

assumed model is wrong. As a consequence, the CRM may lead to some practically inappropriate dose escalation or de-escalation. For example, the CRM might still escalate the dose when 2 out of 3 patients have experienced toxicity at the current dose (the $3 + 3$ design would de-escalate the dose immediately), de-escalate the dose when only 1 out of 9 patients has experienced toxicity, or continue treating patients at the same dose when 3 out of 3 patients have experienced toxicity. In Table 4.4, we present the percentages of the simulated trials that had such inappropriate dose assignments using the CRM. By properly choosing nonparametric or parametric models, the hybrid design substantially improves dose finding and trial safety and, more importantly, none of the simulated trials had such inappropriate dose actions. In the hybrid design, the switch from the nonparametric to the parametric dose-finding scheme depends on the

**Table 4.4   Percentages of the Trials Having Practically Inappropriate Dose Movement Under the CRM**

| Dose Action | # Toxicity / # Patients | Scenario | | | |
|---|---|---|---|---|---|
| | | 1 | 2 | 3 | 4 |
| Escalation | 2/3 | 7.4 | 12.9 | 8.0 | 12.7 |
| De-escalation | 0/6 | 0.6 | 0.2 | 0.1 | 0.0 |
| | 1/6 | 5.1 | 2.8 | 0.8 | 0.4 |
| | 1/9 | 0.1 | 0.1 | 0.0 | 0.0 |
| Staying the same | 3/3 | 2.5 | 3.2 | 1.8 | 4.6 |
| | 5/6 | 0.0 | 0.3 | 0.5 | 1.9 |
| | 0/6 | 6.5 | 4.0 | 3.0 | 2.7 |
| | 0/9 | 0.5 | 0.2 | 0.3 | 0.2 |
| | 1/9 | 4.0 | 2.0 | 2.3 | 1.5 |

Note: The first row with (# Toxicity / # Patients) = 2/3 means that the decision is to escalate the dose when two out of three patients have experienced toxicity .

adequacy of the information at the current treating dose, which is adaptively triggered in order to borrow strength across other doses.

## 4.11   SUMMARY

In oncology, the toxicity and side effects of most cancer treatments, especially those of the cytotoxic agents, are severe. The main theme of a phase I oncology trial is to determine the MTD of an experimental drug; that is to find the maximum tolerable dose, while expecting that the drug's therapeutic effect can be maximized. A phase I clinical trial is single-arm (uncontrolled), and the sample size is small.

Among a variety of statistical methods for dose finding, the 3 + 3 design is widely used in practice due to its ease of implementation. This design is more appropriate for use if a broad range of doses of the new drug is screened to identify the MTD that is not too toxic (often the toxicity probability is less than 33%). The 3 + 3 design is relatively conservative and usually requires a smaller sample size than other dose-finding methods. For patient safety, the starting dose of a new drug is often prepared at a very low level. If the dose spacing is also conservative, the lower range of the doses may be far below the MTD. Thus, using a cohort size of three in the 3 + 3 design may have to treat a large number of patients before the dose is escalated up to the neighborhood of the MTD. However, the sample size is small, and patients may be used up before reaching the MTD. To alleviate this difficulty, the accelerated titration design speeds up the dose-finding process to avoid wasting many patients at very low and presumably inefficacious doses, which is particularly suitable for drugs that are undergoing the first-human test. In the acceleration stage, the accelerated titration design continues dose escalation with a cohort size of one until the first DLT is observed, afterwards the design switches to the standard $3 + 3$ algorithm. The algorithm-based designs, which also include the $A + B$ design and the biased coin dose-finding design, may be viewed as nonparametric approaches, because they do not impose any parametric model structure but fully rely upon a set of explicitly specified rules.

Due to the small sample size in a typical phase I trial, model-based designs may be preferred because they can borrow information or strength across all the doses. The CRM, which imposes a parametric dose–toxicity model with a single unknown parameter, has gained much popularity in dose-finding studies due to its superior performance over the $3 + 3$ design. However, the CRM is sensitive to the prespecified toxicity probabilities (skeleton) for the considered doses, and the skeleton is often arbitrary and subjective. To enhance the robustness of the design, the BMA-CRM specifies multiple skeletons and applies the Bayesian model averaging mechanism to update the posterior estimates of the toxicity probabilities in a coherent way. As long as one skeleton in the BMA-CRM is reasonable, the design would perform well. Model-based phase I trial designs are dominated by Bayesian methods, because they are more flexible and can naturally incorporate prior information or historical data. These Bayesian phase I designs, such as the CRM, BMA-CRM, and hybrid designs, often have good operating characteristics and plausible statistical properties and specifically target the MTD on the dose–toxicity curve. Whereas, the Bayesian dose-finding methods are relatively more complicated, requiring more intensive computations and closer collaborations between statisticians and physicians.

## EXERCISES

**4.1**  Explain why the maximum number of patients required for the $3 + 3$ design is $J \times 6$, where $J$ is the number of doses under investigation.

**4.2**  The $3 + 3$ dose-escalation design is similar to the standard $3 + 3$ design except that it does not allow dose de-escalation, which is described as follows:

- Treat the first cohort of patients at the lowest or the physician-specified dose.

- If no DLT is observed in any of the 3 subjects, escalate to the next higher dose.

- If 1 DLT is observed among the 3 subjects, treat 3 additional subjects at the same dose level. If none of the 3 additional subjects experiences the DLT, escalate to the next higher dose; otherwise, stop the trial.

- If 2 or more DLTs are observed among the 3 subjects, stop the trial.

For a given sequence of five doses with the true toxicity probabilities:

$$(\pi_1, \ldots, \pi_5) = (0.1, 0.2, 0.3, 0.4, 0.5),$$

compute the probability of dose escalation and the probability that the trial stops at each dose level, respectively.

**4.3** Consider a phase I clinical trial with 6 doses. Under the continual reassessment method, the true toxicity probability at dose level $j$ is

$$\pi_j(\alpha) = p_j^{\exp(\alpha)}, \quad j = 1, \ldots, 6,$$

where $(p_1, \ldots, p_6) = (0.1, 0.2, 0.3, 0.4, 0.5, 0.6)$. Suppose that the observed data are given by

| Dose Level | 1 | 2 | 3 | 4 | 5 | 6 |
|---|---|---|---|---|---|---|
| Number of DLTs | 0 | 1 | 2 | 1 | 0 | 0 |
| Number of Patients | 3 | 6 | 9 | 3 | 0 | 0 |

Given a normal prior distribution, $\alpha \sim N(0, 2^2)$, derive the posterior distribution for $\alpha$, and apply the MCMC procedure to draw the posterior samples of $\alpha$. Compare the posterior mean of each $\pi_j$ based on the MCMC with that using the Gaussian quadrature approximation.

**4.4** Download the BMA-CRM software from the website of M. D. Anderson Cancer Center. Let the target toxicity probability be $\phi_T = 30\%$.

(1) Using a single skeleton, run 10,000 simulations for the following three scenarios with true toxicity probabilities:

| Dose Level | 1 | 2 | 3 | 4 | 5 |
|---|---|---|---|---|---|
| Scenario 1 | 0.10 | 0.25 | 0.33 | 0.45 | 0.60 |
| Scenario 2 | 0.10 | 0.20 | 0.30 | 0.50 | 0.65 |
| Scenario 3 | 0.02 | 0.07 | 0.10 | 0.15 | 0.29 |

Summarize and explain the simulation results.

(2) Sequentially adding one skeleton at a time up to a total of five skeletons, run 10,000 simulations for each case and compare the results.

**4.5**   Using the BMA-CRM software with the default three skeletons, conduct a trial with seven prespecified doses: $(10, 20, 30, 40, 50, 60, 70)$ mg. The target toxicity probability is $\phi_T = 40\%$ and the cohort size is 3 with a total of 12 cohorts. If a patient experiences the DLT, we take the toxicity outcome $y = 1$, and otherwise $y = 0$. The sequence of the observed toxicity data is given as follows:

| Cohort | Toxicity Outcome | | |
|:------:|:-----:|:-----:|:-----:|
|        | $y_1$ | $y_2$ | $y_3$ |
| 1  | 0 | 0 | 0 |
| 2  | 0 | 1 | 0 |
| 3  | 1 | 0 | 0 |
| 4  | 0 | 0 | 0 |
| 5  | 0 | 1 | 0 |
| 6  | 0 | 0 | 1 |
| 7  | 0 | 1 | 1 |
| 8  | 1 | 0 | 0 |
| 9  | 0 | 1 | 1 |
| 10 | 1 | 0 | 0 |
| 11 | 1 | 0 | 0 |
| 12 | 1 | 0 | 0 |

In cohort 1, all three patients did not experience the DLT, and in cohort 2 there was one DLT observed among three patients, and so on. Describe how the trial was conducted; that is, at which dose each cohort was treated, and which dose was finally selected as the MTD.

# CHAPTER 5

# PHASE II TRIAL DESIGN

Following phase I trials for the initial assessment of safety and tolerability of the experimental drug, phase II trials focus on the evaluation of the drug's therapeutic effects and how well the drug works at the recommended dose. If a new drug fails during its developmental process, this usually happens in a phase II trial where the drug is discovered not working as expected or being overly toxic. The primary endpoint in a phase II clinical trial is often short-term and dichotomous, characterizing the patient clinical response to treatment. If the new drug shows sufficient efficacious effects, it will be carried forward to a long-term phase III study for confirmatory testing. Phase II trials can be either single-arm comparing the new treatment with the standard response rate or historical data, or multi-arm with patients randomized among different treatments.

Compared with the small sample size in a phase I trial, that in a phase II trial is relatively large, typically ranging from 30 to 200 subjects. Phase II trials are sometimes further classified as phase IIa and phase IIb studies. Phase IIa trials evaluate whether the drug has any anti-disease activity that warrants further investigation, and they are often used when there is no existing standard therapy for comparison. Phase IIb trials, which more resemble phase III trials, are designed to study the drug's effectiveness, and they entail a comparison with at least one standard treatment.

The goal of a typical phase II oncology trial is to screen new agents based on their short-term efficacy effects. The patient clinical response is often characterized by the drug's anti-tumor activity, which may be measured as the difference in the sum of the longest diameter of the target lesions pre- and post-treatment. Accordingly, patient status may be classified as

- complete response, if all of the target lesions are no longer detectable;

- partial response, if there has been a decrease of 30% or more in the target lesions;

- progressive disease, if one or more new lesions have appeared or if there has been an increase of 20% or more in the target lesions; or

- stable disease, if there is neither sufficient tumor shrinkage to qualify as partial response, nor sufficient tumor growth to qualify as progressive disease.

The clinical response should be measurable within a short period of time following the treatment so that a phase II trial can be finished quickly to make a decision on whether to carry out a large-scale phase III trial.

In a single-arm phase II trial, two- or multi-stage designs may be used to improve the trial efficiency by allowing for early termination if the treatment is deemed ineffective after partial data have been observed. This strategy offers an opportunity to examine whether the trial should continue to use up all of the planned subjects, or should stop early due to futility. Alone this direction, Gehan (1961) proposes that if no response is observed in the first stage, the trial is terminated for futility; otherwise, an additional number of patients will be enrolled in the second stage to provide more information for estimating the response rate. Simon (1989) develops an optimal and a minimax two-stage design by controlling both the type I and type II errors in a frequentist hypothesis testing framework. Fleming (1982) and Chang et al. (1987) study multiple testing and group sequential methods for phase II trial designs. In the Bayesian paradigm, Thall and Simon (1994) provide practical guidelines on how to implement a phase II trial design by continuously monitoring every new outcome. At any time during the trial conduct, the accumulated data may indicate that the experimental drug is promising, nonpromising, or the trial should continue to enroll the next patient due to a lack of evidence to support any decision. As one step further, Lee and Liu (2008) develop Bayesian predictive probability monitoring rules for single-arm phase II trials. The decision to continue or to stop the trial is made according to the strength of the predictive probability, which is the probability of rejecting the null hypothesis should the trial be conducted to the maximum sample size given the observed data. In an extension to randomized phase II studies, Yin, Chen, and Lee (2011) bridge predictive probability monitoring and adaptive randomization, and provide a detailed comparison with group sequential methods in a two-arm trial.

Conventionally, phase I and phase II trials are conducted separately in a sequential order; each requires all the necessary planning and review processes. After the maximum tolerated dose (MTD) or the recommended phase II dose (RP2D) is identified in phase I trials, a completely new phase II trial will be initiated. There is typically a "white" space or time lag between these two consecutive phases. Although phase I dose finding focuses on the drug's toxicity, patients might not be interested in participating in a trial if there is no hope for a cure. Moreover, drugs' toxicity and efficacy effects often interact with each other. Hence, dose finding solely based on toxicity while ignoring efficacy may not be the best strategy to evaluate a new drug. In a phase II trial, patients are treated at the MTD or RP2D to assess the drug's therapeutic effect, while toxicity is still closely monitored. As a result, there is a growing trend of bridging phase I and phase II trials by jointly evaluating drugs' toxicity and efficacy. Gooley et al. (1994) consider two dose-outcome curves using simulation as a design tool. Conaway and Petroni (1996) consider a compromise between treatment safety and anti-tumor activity. Thall and Russell (1998) propose phase I/II trial monitoring and dose finding based on both efficacy and adverse outcomes. O'Quigley, Hughes, and Fenton (2001) study viral failure, viral success, and toxicity for early-phase dose-finding trials in HIV. Braun (2002) generalizes the continual reassessment method to model two competing outcomes. Thall and Cook (2004) develop toxicity and efficacy trade-off contours for dose finding. Bekele and Shen (2005) investigate a joint distribution of a binary and a continuous outcome by introducing latent variables in a probit model. Yin, Li, and Ji (2006) propose Bayesian adaptive phase I/II designs based on toxicity and efficacy odds ratios. In an extension, Yuan and Yin (2009) develop survival models for the bivariate times to toxicity and efficacy, in which the unobserved events are naturally censored but still contribute to the likelihood.

The rest of this chapter will first introduce Gehan's and Simon's two-stage designs for single-arm phase II trials, which are based on frequentist hypothesis testing procedures. Then we will discuss phase II designs from Bayesian perspectives, including trial monitoring with posterior probabilities, and trial designs using predictive probabilities, adaptively randomized phase II trials, phase II designs with multivariate outcomes, and seamless phase I/II trial designs.

## 5.1  GEHAN'S TWO-STAGE DESIGN

The intuition behind a two-stage design is to conduct a futility analysis in the middle of the trial rather than waiting till the end to examine the drug's efficacy. If it is discovered that a drug is not working as effectively as expected, it would be unethical to continue treating patients with this futile drug. Instead, the trial should be stopped early to allow the remaining patients to seek better treatment options.

Following this route, Gehan (1961) proposes a two-stage trial design:  14 patients are treated in stage 1; if there is no response among the first 14 patients, the trial stops for futility; and if there is at least one response, the trial proceeds to stage 2 to accrue more patients.  The number of 14 patients is obtained as follows.  Suppose that in a phase II trial the target response rate is 20%, which is the lowest response rate considered clinically meaningful.  The treatment is likely to be ineffective if there is no single response after an adequately large number of patients are treated in stage 1, say $n_1$ patients.  Let $X_i$ denote a dichotomous outcome, which takes a value of 1 if subject $i$ has responded to the treatment, and 0 otherwise.  Let $p$ denote the probability of response of the experimental drug; that is, $p = \Pr(X_i = 1)$.  Clearly, the number of clinical responses observed out of the first $n_1$ patients follows a binomial distribution, $Y = \sum_{i=1}^{n_1} X_i \sim \mathrm{Bin}(n_1, p)$.  If $p \geq 0.2$, then the probability of no response among the first $n_1$ patients is

$$\Pr(Y = 0|p) = (1 - p)^{n_1} \leq 0.8^{n_1}.$$

We set $\Pr(Y = 0|p = 0.2)$ equal to a very small number; for example, let $\Pr(Y = 0|p = 0.2) = 0.05$, then $n_1 \approx 14$.  If the experimental treatment is active enough (e.g., the probability of response $p \geq 0.2$), there would be an approximately 95% chance of observing at least one response among the first 14 subjects, and thus the trial would proceed to stage 2.  The total sample size, including patients in both stage 1 and stage 2, can be calculated to achieve a specified level of accuracy for the estimated response rate.

In a more general setting, let $p$ denote the minimally acceptable response rate, which may not be 0.2, then the number of patients required for stage 1 is

$$n_1 = \frac{\log(0.05)}{\log(1 - p)}.$$

If there is no response among the first $n_1$ patients, the trial will be terminated to claim that the treatment is not promising; otherwise, an additional number of subjects will be recruited to ensure a certain degree of accuracy for the estimated response rate.

### EXAMPLE 5.1

Suppose that in a phase II trial $p = 0.2$ is of the minimal clinical interest. The estimation precision of the response rate is expected to be within $\pm 0.1$; that is, the standard error (SE) of the estimated response rate $\hat{p}$ is 0.1. Based on the data from stage 1, we have $\hat{p}_1 = y_1/n_1$ and $\widehat{\mathrm{SE}} = \sqrt{\hat{p}_1(1 - \hat{p}_1)/n_1}$.

To be conservative, we may take $\hat{p} = \hat{p}_1 + 1.15 \times \widehat{SE}$, which is the upper bound of the 75% confidence interval of $p$, and we set

$$\sqrt{\frac{\hat{p}(1 - \hat{p})}{n}} = 0.1,$$

to solve for the total sample size $n = n_1 + n_2$. If there are $y_1 = 5$ responses among the first $n_1 = 14$ subjects in stage 1, then $\hat{p}_1 = 5/14$ and $\hat{p} \approx 0.504$. Therefore, stage 2 needs to enroll additional $n_2 = 11$ patients, which leads to a total sample size of $n = 25$.

## 5.2  SIMON'S TWO-STAGE DESIGN

The optimal and minimax two-stage designs proposed by Simon (1989) are very popular in single-arm phase II trials. The trial design is cast in a hypothesis testing framework with specification of the type I and type II error rates. In stage 1, a fixed number of patients are enrolled and if the number of responses is low, the trial stops and claims the drug nonpromising. If there is an adequate number of responses observed in stage 1, an additional fixed number of patients will be enrolled in stage 2. After the trial is finished, if there is a sufficient number of responses in the two stages combined, the study drug is considered promising; otherwise it is considered nonpromising.

Let $p$ denote the response rate of the test drug, let $p_0$ denote a clinically uninteresting response rate, and let $p_1$ ($p_1 > p_0$) denote a clinically desired response rate. The null hypothesis is that $p$ is at most $p_0$; and the alternative hypothesis is that $p$ is at least $p_1$,

$$H_0: p \leq p_0 \quad \text{versus} \quad H_1: p \geq p_1.$$

If there are $r_1$ or fewer responses observed from the $n_1$ subjects enrolled in stage 1, the trial is terminated to accept $H_0$ that the drug is not promising. If more than $r_1$ responses are observed in stage 1, the trial moves on to stage 2 by enrolling $n_2$ additional subjects. At the conclusion of the trial, if the total number of responses is $r$ or fewer, we accept $H_0$ to claim that the drug is not clinically interesting; otherwise, we reject $H_0$ to claim that the drug is promising enough to warrant further investigation.

More specifically, let $Y_1 = y_1$ be the number of responses among $n_1$ patients in the first stage, and let $Y_2 = y_2$ be that among $n_2$ patients in the second stage. Obviously, $Y_1$ and $Y_2$ are independent binomial random variables,

$$Y_1 \sim \text{Bin}(n_1, p) \quad \text{and} \quad Y_2 \sim \text{Bin}(n_2, p).$$

The experimental treatment is claimed to be

- nonpromising, if $y_1 \leq r_1$ or $(y_1 > r_1) \cap (y_1 + y_2 \leq r)$; or

- promising, if $(y_1 > r_1) \cap (y_1 + y_2 > r)$.

Nevertheless, there is an extreme case that the number of responses observed in the first stage is already greater than $r$ (i.e., $y_1 > r$), then there is no need to have the second stage, and the treatment can be declared promising immediately after the first stage.

Based on the specified type I and type II error rates (denoted as $\alpha$ and $\beta$, respectively), the hypothesis testing needs to satisfy

$$\Pr(\text{the treatment is declared promising} \mid p \le p_0) \le \alpha,$$
$$\Pr(\text{the treatment is declared promising} \mid p \ge p_1) \ge 1 - \beta.$$

For ease of computation, the type I and type II error constraints can be computed at the boundary values; that is,

$$\Pr\{(y_1 > r_1) \cap (y_1 + y_2 > r) \mid p = p_0\} = \alpha,$$
$$\Pr\{(y_1 > r_1) \cap (y_1 + y_2 > r) \mid p = p_1\} = 1 - \beta,$$

(5.1)

where by the independence of $Y_1$ and $Y_2$,

$$\Pr\{(y_1 > r_1) \cap (y_1 + y_2 > r) \mid p\}$$
$$= \sum_{y_1 > r_1} \sum_{y_2 > r - y_1} P(y_1 \mid p) P(y_2 \mid p)$$
$$= \sum_{y_1 > r_1} \sum_{y_2 > r - y_1} \binom{n_1}{y_1} p^{y_1} (1 - p)^{n_1 - y_1} \binom{n_2}{y_2} p^{y_2} (1 - p)^{n_2 - y_2}.$$

However, many sets of values of $(n_1, n_2, r_1, r)$ may be found to satisfy the two constraints in (5.1). To uniquely determine the design parameters, we need to specify an additional optimality criterion to select the most suitable set of design parameters.

Under the type I and type II error constraints, the four design parameters $(n_1, n_2, r_1, r)$ can be calibrated to meet one of the following two optimality criteria:

- The optimal two-stage design minimizes $E(N|H_0)$, the expected sample size given that the regimen has low anti-disease activity.

- The minimax two-stage design minimizes the maximum sample size, $n = n_1 + n_2$, in the trial.

Given that the drug does not work, the expected sample size is given by

$$E(N|H_0) = n_1 + n_2 \times \Pr(\text{proceed to stage 2} \mid H_0)$$
$$= n_1 + n_2 \times \Pr(r_1 + 1 \le y_1 \le r \mid p = p_0).$$

By enumerating all the possible values of $(n_1, n_2, r_1, r)$, the two-stage design selects the final design parameters according to either the optimal or the minimax criterion.

**Table 5.1    Illustration of Simon's Optimal and Minimax Two-Stage Designs with Two Separate Sets of Design Parameters:** $(\alpha, \beta, p_0, p_1) = (0.05, 0.1, 0.1, 0.3)$ **and** $(0.1, 0.1, 0.2, 0.4)$

| $(\alpha, \beta, p_0, p_1)$ | (0.05, 0.1, 0.1, 0.3) | | (0.1, 0.1, 0.2, 0.4) | |
|---|---|---|---|---|
| Two-Stage Design | Optimal | Minimax | Optimal | Minimax |
| First-stage sample size $n_1$ | 18 | 22 | 17 | 19 |
| Drug is not promising if $y_1 \leq$ | 2 | 2 | 3 | 3 |
| Maximum sample size $n$ | 35 | 33 | 37 | 36 |
| Drug is not promising if $y \leq$ | 6 | 6 | 10 | 10 |
| Expected sample size under $p_0$ | 22.5 | 26.2 | 26.0 | 28.3 |
| Pr(trial early stopping $\mid p_0$) | 0.73 | 0.62 | 0.55 | 0.46 |

Note: $y_1$ is the number of responses in stage 1, and $y$ and $n$ are the total numbers of responses and patients in the trial, respectively.

**EXAMPLE 5.2**

To demonstrate Simon's two-stage designs, we first specify the type I and type II error rates: The probability of accepting a "bad" drug is $\alpha = 0.05$, and the probability of rejecting a "good" drug is $\beta = 0.1$; that is, the test power is 90%. In addition, the response rate of a "bad" drug is $p_0 = 0.1$, which is not of clinical interest, and the response rate of a "good" drug is $p_1 = 0.3$, which is considered clinically meaningful. Finally, the upper bound of the sample size is set as 100, so that the two-stage design would enumerate all the possible values of the design parameters $(n_1, n_2, r_1, r)$ within this range. If the upper limit of the sample size is too small, the numerical algorithm may fail to find an optimal or a minimax design that satisfies both the type I and type II error constraints. We also present the case with the trial specification of $(\alpha = 0.1, \beta = 0.1, p_0 = 0.2, p_1 = 0.4)$ for the two-stage designs.

Table 5.1 shows the operating characteristics of the optimal and minimax two-stage designs. For illustration, we interpret the optimal two-stage design under the first scenario with $(\alpha = 0.05, \beta = 0.1, p_0 = 0.1, p_1 = 0.3)$ as follows. The design parameters of Simon's optimal two-stage design are $(n_1 = 18, n_2 = 17, r_1 = 2, r = 6)$. If 2 or fewer responses are observed among the first 18 patients treated in stage 1, the trial will stop and claim the drug nonpromising; otherwise, the trial will proceed to stage 2 to accrue 17 more patients. At the end of stage 2, if 6 or fewer patients have responded among a total of 35 patients, the drug will be declared nonpromising; otherwise, the drug will be claimed promising.

## 5.3  BAYESIAN PHASE II DESIGN WITH POSTERIOR PROBABILITY

Starting from this section, we will switch from frequentist to Bayesian phase II trial designs. Thall and Simon (1994) provide Bayesian practical guidelines on how to implement a single-arm phase II trial by examining the drug's anti-disease activity. During the trial, the data are monitored continuously, and decisions are made adaptively, until the maximum sample size, $N$, is reached. Based on the accumulated data as the trial proceeds, the experimental drug may be claimed promising, not promising, or the information accrued in the trial is not adequate to deliver any conclusion, so more data are needed.

Let $p_E$ denote the response rate of the experimental drug. For each subject, we observe a dichotomous outcome taking a value of 1 with probability $p_E$, and 0 with probability $1 - p_E$. In a single-arm trial, the experimental drug is compared with the response rate of the standard treatment, denoted by $p_S$. For both $p_E$ and $p_S$, we take beta prior distributions:

$$p_E \sim \text{Beta}(\alpha_E, \beta_E) \quad \text{and} \quad p_S \sim \text{Beta}(\alpha_S, \beta_S),$$

where $\alpha_E, \beta_E, \alpha_S$, and $\beta_S$ are the hyperparameters. If there exist historical data for the standard treatment, we may center the prior mean of $p_S$ at its empirical estimate, but enlarge the prior variance to discount the historical data. In general, the prior distribution of $p_E$ should have a larger variance than that of $p_S$ because much less is known about the new drug. For example, we may take a vague prior distribution for the experimental drug, $p_E \sim \text{Beta}(0.4, 1.6)$, which contains as much information as two observations only. If the historical data had eight responses among 40 treated subjects, we fix the prior mean of $p_S$ at the estimated historical response rate, but inflate the prior variance; for example, we may take $p_S \sim \text{Beta}(4, 16)$ as the prior distribution for the standard drug, which corresponds to 20 patients' information.

At a certain stage of the trial, let $Y$ be the number of responses among $n$ patients treated by the experimental drug, then $Y \sim \text{Bin}(n, p_E)$. Due to the conjugate property between beta and binomial distributions, the posterior of $p_E$ given $Y = y$ is still a beta distribution,

$$p_E | y \sim \text{Beta}(\alpha_E + y, \beta_E + n - y).$$

If we denote the probability density function of $p \sim \text{Beta}(\alpha, \beta)$ by $f(p; \alpha, \beta)$ and the cumulative distribution function by $F(p; \alpha, \beta) = \int_0^p f(x; \alpha, \beta)\, dx$, then

$$\Pr(p_E > p_S + \delta | y)$$
$$= \int_0^{1-\delta} \{1 - F(p + \delta; \alpha_E + y, \beta_E + n - y)\} f(p; \alpha_S, \beta_S)\, dp,$$

where $0 < \delta < 1$ is the minimally acceptable increment of the response rate for the experimental drug compared with the standard drug.

Let $\theta_U$ and $\theta_L$ be the prespecified upper and lower probability cutoffs, typically, $\theta_U \in [0.95, 0.99]$ and $\theta_L \in [0.01, 0.05]$. Subsequently, we determine the upper and lower decision boundaries based on the number of observed responses.

- Let $U_n$ be the smallest integer of $y$ satisfying $\Pr(p_E > p_S|y) \geq \theta_U$.

- Let $L_n$ be the largest integer of $y$ satisfying $\Pr(p_E > p_S + \delta|y) \leq \theta_L$.

The decision rule after observing $y$ responses out of $n$ patients is described as follows:

- If $y \geq U_n$, terminate the trial and declare the experimental drug promising.

- If $y \leq L_n$, terminate the trial and declare the experimental drug not promising.

- If $L_n < y < U_n$ and $n < N$, continue the trial to treat the next patient.

If $y$ does not cross any stopping boundary until reaching the total number of subjects with $n = N$, the trial is considered inconclusive: the effectiveness of the experimental agent is undetermined.

Although the stopping rule requires that the trial be terminated to declare the experimental drug promising if $y \geq U_n$, investigators rarely stop the trial in such a case so that more patients are allowed to benefit from the "good" drug. Therefore, the stopping rule for superiority of the drug is often not implemented in a single-arm phase II trial.

**EXAMPLE 5.3**

We present two examples to illustrate how to use the Bayesian posterior probability to monitor a phase II trial. In the first trial design, we take beta prior distributions for the response rates of the standard drug and the experimental drug, $p_S \sim \text{Beta}(15, 35)$ and $p_E \sim \text{Beta}(0.6, 1.4)$. We specify $\theta_L = 0.05$ and $\delta = 0$ for futility stopping, and the maximum sample size $N = 40$. The trial is monitored on a one-by-one patient basis. Under this setup, the stopping boundaries are given by

| $L_n$ | 0 | 1 | 2 | 3 | 4 | 5 | 6 |
|-------|---|---|----|----|----|----|----|
| $n$ | 6 | 13 | 18 | 24 | 29 | 35 | 40 |

where $L_n$ is the number of responses and $n$ is the number of patients in the trial. The paired values of $L_n/n$ indicate to stop the trial if the number of responses after treating $n$ patients is less than or equal to $L_n$. For example, $L_n/n = 2/18$ suggests that if there are 2 or fewer responses in the first 18 treated patients, the trial will be terminated for a lack of efficacy.

In the second example, we take beta prior distributions for $p_S$ and $p_E$ as $p_S \sim \text{Beta}(10, 40)$ and $p_E \sim \text{Beta}(0.4, 1.6)$, respectively. We specify the maximum sample size $N = 30$, $\theta_L = 0.05$, and $\delta = 0$. The stopping boundaries for the number of responses are given by

| $L_n$ | 0 | 1 | 2 | 3 |
|---|---|---|---|---|
| $n$ | 7 | 19 | 29 | 30 |

That is, if there is no response among the first 7 treated patients, if there is only 1 response among the first 19 patients, or if there are 2 or fewer responses among the first 29 patients, the trial would be terminated early for futility. If the trial runs to the maximum sample size 30, and 3 or fewer responses have been observed, we claim the experimental drug not promising.

## 5.4 BAYESIAN PHASE II DESIGN WITH PREDICTIVE PROBABILITY

In the Bayesian paradigm, the posterior predictive distribution characterizes the distribution of the future data conditional on the observed data. Using the posterior predictive probability for decision making in the middle of a trial, we can produce the probability distribution of the statistic that has not been observed yet. Frequentist predictive methods usually obtain the probability of the future data by conditioning on a particular value of the model parameter, whereas Bayesian predictive methods average these probabilities over the parameter space given the observed data. Based on the accumulated data in a trial, we can compute the predictive probability of either claiming the experimental drug promising or not promising at the conclusion of the study. In other words, the predictive probability characterizes the future trial conclusion given the strength of the currently observed data.

Consider a single-arm phase II trial as before. Let $p_E$ denote the probability of response for the experimental drug. During the trial conduct, the data are accumulated as more patients are enrolled. Let $n$ be the number of patients who have entered the trial thus far, $1 \leq n \leq N$, where $N$ is the maximum sample size planned for the entire trial. Let $Y$ denote the number of responses among $n$ treated patients, then $Y \sim \text{Bin}(n, p_E)$. We specify a beta prior distribution for $p_E$; that is, $p_E \sim \text{Beta}(\alpha_E, \beta_E)$. At the interim analysis, if we observe $Y = y$ responses out of $n$ treated patients, the posterior distribution of $p_E$ is

$$p_E | y \sim \text{Beta}(\alpha_E + y, \beta_E + n - y).$$

The number of patients to be recruited in the future is $N - n$, among which let $X$ denote the number of patients who would respond. The probability of $X = x$ given the current data $y$ follows a beta-binomial distribution,

$$X | y \sim \text{Beta-Bin}(N - n, \alpha_E + y, \beta_E + n - y),$$

with the probability mass function of

$$
\begin{aligned}
P(x|y) &= \int_0^1 \binom{N-n}{x} p^x (1-p)^{N-n-x} \frac{p^{\alpha_E+y-1}(1-p)^{\beta_E+n-y-1}}{B(\alpha_E+y, \beta_E+n-y)} \, dp \\
&= \binom{N-n}{x} \frac{B(\alpha_E+y+x, \beta_E+N-y-x)}{B(\alpha_E+y, \beta_E+n-y)},
\end{aligned}
$$

where the beta function $B(\alpha, \beta) = \Gamma(\alpha)\Gamma(\beta)/\Gamma(\alpha+\beta)$. By the end of the trial, suppose that we observe $X = x$, then the posterior distribution of the response rate given both $y$ and $x$ would be

$$
p_E|(y,x) \sim \text{Beta}(\alpha_E+y+x, \beta_E+N-y-x).
$$

Lee and Liu (2008) demonstrate how to monitor a phase II trial using the predictive probability. Given the current data $y$, if we observe the future data $X = x$ at the end of the trial, we would claim the experimental drug promising, if

$$
\Pr(p_E > p_S | y, x) \geq \theta_T,
$$

where $p_S$ is the standard response rate and $\theta_T$ is the prespecified target probability, e.g., $\theta_T \in [0.85, 0.95]$. Because $X$ is not observed, we take an average over all the possible outcomes in the future to define the predictive probability (PP) as

$$
\text{PP} = \sum_{x=0}^{N-n} P(x|y) I\{\Pr(p_E > p_S | y, x) \geq \theta_T\}, \tag{5.2}
$$

where $I\{\cdot\}$ is the indicator function. Let $\theta_U$ and $\theta_L$ denote the cutoff probabilities for decision making, which need to be calibrated through simulations to achieve desirable trial performance. The cutoff probability $\theta_L$ is chosen as a small constant, and $\theta_U$ as a large constant, between 0 and 1. Under the predictive probability monitoring, the trial proceeds as follows:

- If $\text{PP} > \theta_U$, stop the trial and claim the experimental drug promising.

- If $\text{PP} < \theta_L$, stop the trial and claim the experimental drug not promising.

- Otherwise, continue the trial until the number of treated patients reaches the maximum sample size $N$.

If there were no indicator function in (5.2), the PP simply reduces to the posterior probability after averaging out the unobserved $X$,

$$
\sum_{x=0}^{N-n} P(x|y) \Pr(p_E > p_S | y, x) = \Pr(p_E > p_S | y),
$$

which does not depend on the total sample size $N$. However, the predictive probability mimics the decision process of claiming the drug promising or non-promising at the completion of a trial, for which the sample size of the future data indeed makes a difference. Consider the following two situations: one trial with the maximum sample size $N = 25$, and the other with $N = 50$. Suppose that we have observed only one response among the first $n = 22$ treated patients, then we would be more certain that the drug is futile in the first case where there are only three subjects left to enroll compared with the second scenario in which there are still 28 subjects remaining in the pipeline.

## 5.5 PREDICTIVE MONITORING IN RANDOMIZED PHASE II TRIALS

Phase II trials provide an initial assessment of efficacy for new drugs, screen out ineffective treatments, and identify promising ones for further investigation. In reality, many "promising" drugs eventually fail in phase III trials although they have demonstrated potential efficacious effects in phase II trials. One of the main reasons for such drug failure is that the test drug is compared with the standard response rate or historical data in a single-arm phase II trial. Although single-arm trials are inherently comparative, they are less objective and can be biased, because there usually exist substantial differences in patient populations, study criteria, and medical facilities between the current and previous studies. For a better assessment, randomized phase II trials are becoming a common practice, in which the experimental drug is compared with the standard treatment (Ratain and Sargent, 2009). Randomization helps to eliminate potential bias and confounding effects, and balance patients' characteristics; more discussions on randomization are given in Chapter 7.

In a randomized phase II trial, the posterior predictive probability can be use to monitor a trial by predicting the outcome of the trial after all the patients are enrolled. If there is a high predictive probability that a definitive conclusion would be reached by the end of the study (e.g., superiority or futility), the trial could be stopped earlier. In a two-arm trial, let $p_k$ denote the response rate for treatment $k$, and we assign a beta prior distribution, $p_k \sim \text{Beta}(\alpha_k, \beta_k)$ for $k = 1, 2$. Let $N_k$ be the maximum sample size planned for arm $k$, and let $Y_k$ be the number of responses among $n_k$ treated patients, $1 \leq n_k \leq N_k$; so $Y_k \sim \text{Bin}(n_k, p_k)$. Following the conjugacy between beta and binomial distributions, the posterior distribution of $p_k$ is

$$p_k | y_k \sim \text{Beta}(\alpha_k + y_k, \beta_k + n_k - y_k), \quad k = 1, 2.$$

Let $X_k$ denote the number of responses among the remaining $N_k - n_k$ subjects in arm $k$. As discussed before, the posterior predictive distribution of $X_k$ given the current data $Y_k = y_k$ is beta-binomial,

$$P(x_k|y_k) = \binom{N_k - n_k}{x_k} \frac{B(\alpha_E + y_k + x_k, \beta_E + N_k - y_k - x_k)}{B(\alpha_E + y_k, \beta_E + n_k - y_k)}. \quad (5.3)$$

Suppose that we compare two treatments by formulating a frequentist hypothesis test with

$$H_0: p_1 = p_2 \quad \text{versus} \quad H_1: p_1 \neq p_2.$$

For each pair of the future data $(X_1 = x_1, X_2 = x_2)$, we can draw a conclusion of whether the hypothesis test would yield a significant treatment difference by the end of the trial. Summing over all the possible future outcomes $(x_1, x_2)$, the predictive probability of rejecting $H_0$ (i.e., there is a significant treatment difference) is given by

$$\Pr\,(\text{a significant difference at the end of the trial} \mid \text{data})$$

$$= \sum_{x_1=0}^{N_1-n_1} \sum_{x_2=0}^{N_2-n_2} P(x_1|y_1)P(x_2|y_2)I(\text{rejecting } H_0), \quad (5.4)$$

where the indicator function $I(\cdot)$ characterizes whether the usual binomial test for two proportions is significant. Based on both the current and future data, the estimate of the response rate for arm $k$ is

$$\hat{p}_k = \frac{y_k + x_k}{N_k}, \quad k = 1, 2.$$

Under the null hypothesis $H_0: p_1 = p_2 = p$, the pooled samples across the two arms produce an estimate of $p$ as

$$\hat{p} = \frac{y_1 + x_1 + y_2 + x_2}{N_1 + N_2}$$

and

$$\text{Var}(\hat{p}_1 - \hat{p}_2) = \frac{p_1(1-p_1)}{N_1} + \frac{p_2(1-p_2)}{N_2} = p(1-p)\left(\frac{1}{N_1} + \frac{1}{N_2}\right).$$

Using normal approximation, the frequentist two-sample statistic for testing two proportions is given by

$$Z = \frac{\hat{p}_1 - \hat{p}_2}{\sqrt{\hat{p}(1-\hat{p})(1/N_1 + 1/N_2)}},$$

which asymptotically follows the standard normal distribution under the null hypothesis. We would reject the null hypothesis if $|Z| \geq z_{\alpha/2}$, where $z_{\alpha/2}$ is the $100(1 - \alpha/2)$th percentile of the standard normal distribution. Given the interim data, the predictive probability of rejecting the null hypothesis at the end of the trial is

$$\sum_{x_1=0}^{N_1-n_1} \sum_{x_2=0}^{N_2-n_2} P(x_1|y_1)P(x_2|y_2)I(|Z| \geq z_\alpha).$$

The aforementioned interim monitoring scheme couples the Bayesian predictive probability with a frequentist hypothesis testing procedure. On the other hand, we can implement a fully Bayesian interim monitoring procedure using the predictive probability. Given both the current data $(y_1, y_2)$ and future data $(x_1, x_2)$, we calculate the posterior predictive probability,

$$\Pr(p_1 > p_2|y_1, y_2, x_1, x_2) = \int_0^1 \int_{p_2}^1 f(p_2|y_2, x_2)f(p_1|y_1, x_1)\, \mathrm{d}p_1\mathrm{d}p_2,$$

where $f(p_k|y_k, x_k)$ is the probability density function of $p_k$ with the beta distribution, $p_k \sim \text{Beta}(\alpha_k + y_k + x_k, \beta_k + N_k - y_k - x_k)$, for $k = 1, 2$. Treatment 1 is claimed to be superior to treatment 2 if

$$\Pr(p_1 > p_2|y_1, y_2, x_1, x_2) \geq \theta_T, \tag{5.5}$$

where the cutoff probability $\theta_T$ typically takes a value between 0.85 and 0.95, depending on how much certainty we have to claim superiority of treatment 1 based on (5.5). However, the future data $(x_1, x_2)$ have not been observed yet. Thus given the observed data $(y_1, y_2)$, the predictive probability of claiming treatment 1 superior to treatment 2 at the end of the trial is

$\Pr(\text{claiming superiority of treatment 1} \mid \text{data})$

$$= \sum_{x_1=0}^{N_1-n_1} \sum_{x_2=0}^{N_2-n_2} P(x_1|y_1)P(x_2|y_2)I\{ \Pr(p_1 > p_2|y_1, y_2, x_1, x_2) \geq \theta_T\}.$$

We demonstrate how to use the predictive probability for trial monitoring in a two-arm randomized trial. The planned sample size for each treatment arm is the same; that is, $N_1 = N_2 = N/2$. For the frequentist hypothesis testing, we use a two-sided binomial test at the significance level of $\alpha = 0.05$. For the Bayesian method, we take the prior distributions for $p_1$ and $p_2$ as $\text{Beta}(0.2, 0.8)$ and set the cutoff probability $\theta_T = 0.95$ in (5.5).

In Table 5.2, we present the total sample size $N$; the number of responses over the current number of subjects in arm $k$, $y_k/n_k$; and the predictive probabilities in favor of arm 1 or arm 2 using the frequentist and Bayesian approaches, respectively. As an illustration, we interpret the results with $N = 40$ in the first row. We planned to enroll 20 subjects in each arm to compare the two treatments. After 10 patients were treated in each arm, 5 patients responded in arm 1 and 2 patients responded in arm 2. At this point, the predictive probability of favoring treatment 1 at the conclusion of the trial is approximately 51% using

**Table 5.2    Illustration of Interim Monitoring with the Posterior Predictive Probability in a Two-Arm Randomized Phase II Trial**

| | Arm 1 | Arm 2 | Pr(favoring arm 1) | | Pr(favoring arm 2) | |
|---|---|---|---|---|---|---|
| $N$ | $y_1/n_1$ | $y_2/n_2$ | Frequentist | Bayesian | Frequentist | Bayesian |
| 40 | 5/10 | 2/10 | 0.5062 | 0.6702 | <0.0001 | <0.0001 |
| 60 | 5/10 | 2/10 | 0.6266 | 0.7225 | 0.0005 | 0.0013 |
| 80 | 5/10 | 2/10 | 0.6915 | 0.7567 | 0.0020 | 0.0037 |
| 100 | 5/10 | 2/10 | 0.7291 | 0.7815 | 0.0040 | 0.0065 |
| 100 | 10/20 | 4/20 | 0.8415 | 0.8999 | <0.0001 | <0.0001 |
| 100 | 15/30 | 6/30 | 0.9306 | 0.9735 | <0.0001 | <0.0001 |
| 100 | 20/40 | 8/40 | 0.9910 | 0.9993 | <0.0001 | <0.0001 |
| 100 | 10/20 | 8/20 | 0.2167 | 0.2821 | 0.0069 | 0.0120 |
| 100 | 10/20 | 9/20 | 0.1157 | 0.1573 | 0.0211 | 0.0328 |

Note: $N$ is the maximum sample size, $y_1$ and $n_1$ are the numbers of responses and patients in arm 1, respectively; $y_2$ and $n_2$ correspond to those in arm 2.

the frequentist two-sample test, and 67% using the fully Bayesian approach. In addition, the predictive probabilities of favoring treatment 2 are negligible using both methods. Because there may be no definitive prediction of favoring any treatment at the conclusion of the trial, the sum of the probabilities of favoring arm 1 and arm 2 is not equal to 1. From row 1 to row 4, there is an increasing trend for the predictive probability of favoring arm 1 as $N$ increases, which reaches a plateau quickly. In other words, if there are more data to collect in the future, the currently observed treatment difference may be enhanced.

The indicator function of (5.4) may take a frequentist hypothesis test or a Bayesian procedure for decision making. As will be discussed further in the next section, the design can continuously update the predictive probability of the trial outcome, such that early termination of a trial is possible for either superiority or futility.

## 5.6    PREDICTIVE PROBABILITY WITH ADAPTIVE RANDOMIZATION

### 5.6.1    Bayesian Adaptive Randomization

For a more objective comparison of different treatments, phase II trials are often randomized with multiple arms. Patients may be randomly allocated to each treatment arm with a fixed probability throughout the trial (e.g., equal randomization assigns patients to each arm with the same probability). Or, the randomization probability may be adaptively changing based on the accumulated data during the trial. Response- or outcome-based adaptive randomization (AR) tends to assign more trial participants to better treatments, as each new patient has a higher probability to receive the more effective treatment based on the data collected in the on-going trial.

Yin, Chen, and Lee (2011) naturally bridge the Bayesian AR and predictive probability for trial monitoring. More specifically, in a two-arm randomized trial, let $p_k$ denote the response rate for treatment $k$, and let $N_k$ denote the maximum sample size planned for arm $k$, $k = 1, 2$. Let $y_1$ and $y_2$ be the observed numbers of responses after treating $n_1$ and $n_2$ ($1 \leq n_k \leq N_k$) patients in arms 1 and 2, respectively. We assign a beta prior distribution to $p_k$; that is, $p_k \sim \text{Beta}(\alpha_k, \beta_k)$. Based on the binomial likelihood, the posterior of $p_k$ is still a beta distribution, $p_k|y_k \sim \text{Beta}(\alpha_k + y_k, \beta_k + n_k - y_k)$. As a result, we can compute $\lambda = \Pr(p_1 > p_2|y_1, y_2)$, and the next patient will be randomized to arm 1 with the probability

$$\pi(\lambda, \gamma) = \frac{\lambda^\gamma}{\lambda^\gamma + (1 - \lambda)^\gamma},$$

where the tuning parameter $\gamma$ often takes a value of 0.5 (Thall and Wathen, 2007). To prevent extreme imbalance between the two arms, the randomization probability may be constrained between 0.1 and 0.9. For stability, there is typically a prephase of equal randomization before the AR procedure takes place. More discussions on various randomization methods are given in Chapter 7.

### 5.6.2 Predictive Probability

Let $X_1 = x_1$ and $X_2 = x_2$ denote the unobserved numbers of responses among the future patients in arm 1 and arm 2, respectively. The posterior predictive distribution of $X_k$ given the current data $y_k$ is beta-binomial as in (5.3). To characterize the treatment difference, we specify a target probability $\theta_T$ and a threshold $\delta$. The two treatments are claimed to be nonequivalent (i.e., one treatment is superior to the other), if

$$\Pr(|p_1 - p_2| > \delta|y_1, x_1, y_2, x_2) \geq \theta_T.$$

The predictive probability (PP) can be computed by averaging out the randomness in $X_1$ and $X_2$,

$$\text{PP} = \sum_{x_1=0}^{N_1-n_1} \sum_{x_2=0}^{N_2-n_2} P(x_1|y_1)P(x_2|y_2)$$
$$\times I\{\Pr(|p_1 - p_2| > \delta|y_1, x_1, y_2, x_2) \geq \theta_T\}. \quad (5.6)$$

Let $\theta_U$ and $\theta_L$ denote the two cutoff probabilities for trial early stopping. The decision rules based on the predictive probability are described as follows.

**Table 5.3    Stage 1 Parameter Calibration for $\delta$ and $\theta_T$ (Fixing $\theta_L = 0$ and $\theta_U = 1$)**

| | Type I Error Rate | | | | | Power | | | | |
|---|---|---|---|---|---|---|---|---|---|---|
| $\delta \backslash \theta_T$ | 0.70 | 0.75 | 0.80 | **0.85** | 0.90 | 0.70 | 0.75 | 0.80 | **0.85** | 0.90 |
| 0.02 | 1.000 | 1.000 | .797 | .427 | .230 | 1.000 | 1.000 | .991 | .967 | .919 |
| 0.03 | .844 | .517 | .362 | .228 | .124 | .991 | .978 | .955 | .918 | .859 |
| 0.04 | .429 | .317 | .224 | .142 | .080 | .967 | .949 | .920 | .864 | .788 |
| **0.05** | .291 | .218 | .157 | **.097** | .053 | .945 | .912 | .875 | **.822** | .735 |
| 0.06 | .214 | .158 | .112 | .073 | .038 | .917 | .878 | .833 | .765 | .669 |
| 0.07 | .157 | .119 | .080 | .056 | .028 | .878 | .835 | .785 | .716 | .617 |
| 0.08 | .111 | .086 | .060 | .034 | .016 | .845 | .797 | .741 | .667 | .564 |
| 0.09 | .093 | .064 | .043 | .026 | .013 | .800 | .753 | .680 | .612 | .501 |

The staircase lines indicate the 10% type I error rate (left panel) and 80% power (right panel) boundaries, the shaded areas are the overlapping parameters that satisfy both the design constraints, and the final chosen values are in boldface.

- Superiority stopping: If $PP > \theta_U$, stop the trial to claim superiority of a treatment.

- Futility stopping: If $PP < \theta_L$, stop the trial to claim equivalence of two treatments.

To compute the PP, the maximum sample size in each arm must be given, which, however, becomes unknown due to the implementation of AR. If there is no early stopping, the total number of subjects remaining in the trial is known; that is, $m = N_1 + N_2 - n_1 - n_2$. Let $Z$ denote the number of subjects that will be assigned to arm 1, then $Z \sim \text{Bin}(m, \pi)$. We first average over $X_1$ and $X_2$ conditioning on $Z = z$, and then average over $Z$ according to the binomial distribution, which leads to

$$PP = \sum_{z=0}^{m} \sum_{x_1=0}^{z} \sum_{x_2=0}^{m-z} \binom{m}{z} \pi^z (1-\pi)^{m-z} P(x_1|y_1, z) P(x_2|y_2, z)$$
$$\times I\{\Pr(|p_1 - p_2| > \delta|y_1, x_1, y_2, x_2) \geq \theta_T\}.$$

Due to the additional marginalization over $Z$, the computation of the PP becomes intensive. As an approximation, we may use the expected number of subjects that will be assigned to each arm in (5.6); that is, $N_1 - n_1 = m\pi$ and $N_2 - n_2 = m(1 - \pi)$.

### 5.6.3   Parameter Calibration

The design needs to calibrate four parameters $(\delta, \theta_T, \theta_L, \theta_U)$ to ensure that the trial possesses the desired frequentist properties: That is to control the type I

**Table 5.4  Stage 2 Parameter Calibration for $\theta_L$ and $\theta_U$ Using Two Different Methods (Fixing $\delta = 0.05$ and $\theta_T = 0.85$)**

| | Method 1: Enumerating All Possible Future Sample Sizes | | | | | | | | | |
|---|---|---|---|---|---|---|---|---|---|---|
| | Type I Error Rate | | | | | Power | | | | |
| $\theta_U \backslash \theta_L$ | 0.00 | **0.05** | 0.10 | 0.15 | 0.20 | 0.00 | **0.05** | 0.10 | 0.15 | 0.20 |
| 0.95 | .126 | .116 | .112 | .106 | .095 | .839 | .823 | .792 | .783 | .747 |
| 0.96 | .120 | .120 | .105 | .107 | .096 | .828 | .815 | .799 | .772 | .739 |
| 0.97 | .115 | .106 | .097 | .092 | .092 | .827 | .813 | .791 | .765 | .734 |
| 0.98 | .107 | .105 | .092 | .091 | .082 | .827 | .814 | .791 | .764 | .734 |
| **0.99** | .105 | **.099** | .095 | .080 | .079 | .820 | **.803** | .796 | .766 | .723 |
| 1.00 | .101 | .097 | .088 | .083 | .074 | .822 | .806 | .789 | .755 | .733 |
| | Method 2: Approximation with Expected Future Sample Sizes | | | | | | | | | |
| 0.95 | .125 | .116 | .113 | .104 | .099 | .840 | .822 | .793 | .782 | .747 |
| 0.96 | .121 | .115 | .106 | .102 | .088 | .829 | .816 | .799 | .772 | .734 |
| 0.97 | .112 | .110 | .099 | .096 | .082 | .829 | .813 | .789 | .765 | .735 |
| 0.98 | .112 | .101 | .096 | .092 | .085 | .826 | .815 | .796 | .765 | .731 |
| **0.99** | .102 | **.096** | .087 | .076 | .071 | .819 | **.802** | .796 | .767 | .722 |
| 1.00 | .101 | .093 | .088 | .080 | .070 | .820 | .806 | .790 | .760 | .731 |

The staircase lines indicate the 10% type I error rate (left panel) and 80% power (right panel) boundaries, the shaded areas are the overlapping parameters that satisfy both the design constraints, and the final chosen values are in boldface.

error rate below 10% and achieve a power above 80%. We took a two-stage procedure to first calibrate the main design parameters $(\delta, \theta_T)$ and then the early termination parameters $(\theta_L, \theta_U)$. In stage 1, we explored different values of $\delta$ and $\theta_T$ while fixing $\theta_L = 0$ and $\theta_U = 1$, such that the trials would not be terminated early. We considered the null hypothesis, $H_0$: $p_1 = p_2 = 0.4$, and the alternative hypothesis, $H_1$: $p_1 = 0.4$ and $p_2 = 0.2$. We specified noninformative beta prior distributions for both $p_1$ and $p_2$. The total sample size was $N = 160$, with the first 40 patients equally randomized between the two arms prior to the initiation of the AR procedure. For each configuration, we simulated 10,000 trials and recorded the percentages of trials rejecting $H_0$.

Table 5.3 presents the null cases in the left panel and the alternative cases in the right panel. The type I error rates below the staircase line are 10% or less; and simultaneously, the power values above the boundary line are 80% or higher. The shaded areas meet both the type I error and power criteria, from which we chose $\delta = 0.05$ and $\theta_T = 0.85$.

In stage 2 of parameter calibration, we followed a similar procedure to determine the early termination parameters $(\theta_L, \theta_U)$, while fixing $\delta = 0.05$ and $\theta_T = 0.85$. Each trial was monitored for early termination due to superiority or

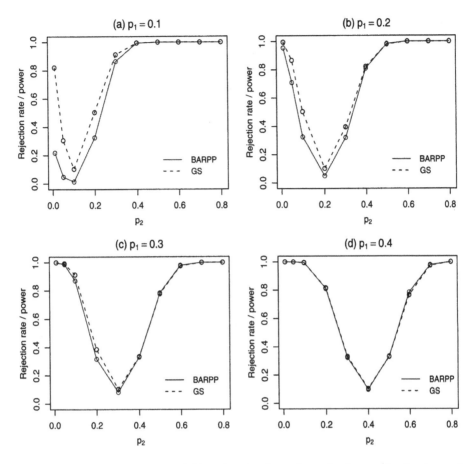

**Figure 5.1** Rejection rates of $H_0$ using the Bayesian adaptive randomization and predictive probability (BARPP) and group sequential (GS) methods at different values of $p_2$, while fixing $p_1 = 0.1, 0.2, 0.3$, and $0.4$, respectively.

equivalence after every 10 patients were enrolled. Table 5.4 presents the type I error rates and power values using two different computational methods for the PP: One is to enumerate all the possibilities of the future sample sizes and the other uses the expected future sample sizes. The results based on the two approaches are very close. There are multiple pairs of $(\theta_L, \theta_U)$ satisfying the design requirements, from which we chose $\theta_L = 0.05$ and $\theta_U = 0.99$.

### 5.6.4 Simulation Study

We examined the performance of the phase II design with the Bayesian adaptive randomization and predictive probability (BARPP) by exploring different scenarios. We varied $p_2$ from 0.01 to 0.8 while fixing $p_1$ at each value of

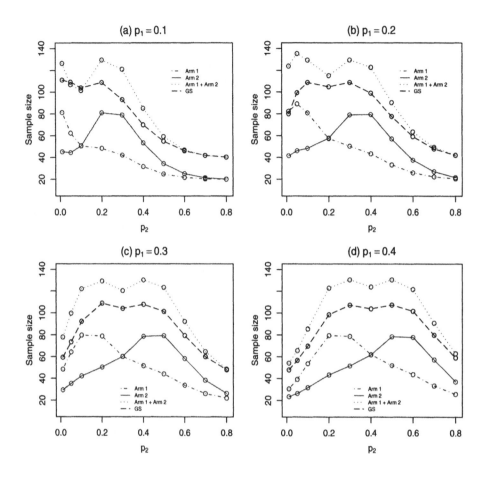

**Figure 5.2**    Sample size for each arm, the total sample size (arm 1 + arm 2) of the Bayesian adaptive randomization and predictive probability (BARPP) design and that of the group sequential (GS) method.

(0.1, 0.2, 0.3, 0.4), respectively.    For comparison, we also implemented the frequentist group sequential (GS) method with equal randomization using the O'Brien–Fleming superiority boundary (O'Brien and Fleming, 1979) and a futility stopping boundary; more discussions on group sequential methods are given in Chapter 6. Based on the type I error rate and power requirements, the maximum sample size for the GS method was 140 with a group size of 10. No early termination was allowed for the first 40 patients, and thereafter the superiority and futility stopping boundaries were regularly applied every 10 patients.

Figure 5.1 presents the percentage of the 10,000 simulated trials that rejected the null hypothesis; that is, the type I error rate under the null and power under the alternative hypothesis.    All of the curves are V-shaped with the minimum point at $p_1 = p_2$. Power increases as $p_2$ moves away from $p_1$ either to the left or to the right. In scenarios with $p_1 = 0.1$ or $0.2$, both the type I error rate and power of the GS method are higher than those under the BARPP design. In scenarios with $p_1 = 0.3$ or $0.4$, the two curves are almost identical. Figure 5.2 shows the sample sizes in arm 1 and arm 2, and the total sample sizes under different scenarios. When $p_1 = p_2$, patients were equally randomized to the two arms even using the AR procedure. When the difference between $p_1$ and $p_2$ was large, early stopping took place quickly after equal randomization and thus led to small sample sizes in both arms. Using the BARPP design, more patients were randomized to the better arm, while there incurs some loss of power due to imbalanced numbers of patients in the two arms, which, in turn, is reflected by a larger sample size compared with the GS method.

### 5.6.5   Posterior versus Predictive Trial Monitoring

To understand the difference between using the posterior probability and the predictive probability for trial monitoring, we consider the following two scenarios.

- Scenario 1: We observe 11 responses among 25 treated patients in arm 1, denoted as $11/25$; and 5 responses among 25 treated patients in arm 2, denoted as $5/25$.

- Scenario 2: We observe $10/25$ in arm 1, and $9/25$ in arm 2.

In the first situation, after 50 subjects were treated, we observe a substantial difference between the two arms: $11/25$ versus $5/25$. Given the observed data $D$ and $\delta = 0.05$, the posterior probability is $\Pr(|p_1 - p_2| > \delta | D) = 0.920$, which does not depend on the remaining number of subjects in the trial. By contrast, Figure 5.3 shows that the predictive probability first decays as the future sample size increases, and then it reaches a plateau after the future sample size becomes approximately 50. Here is the explanation for this phenomenon. If there are very few patients remaining in the enrollment pipeline, we may have a strong confidence that by the end of the trial, it is very likely to claim treatment 1 better than treatment 2; however, if there are still a large number of patients to recruit, the relative information collected thus far may not be as strong to claim superiority of treatment 1 as after reaching the maximum sample size. In other words, we make decisions based on the expected result at the end of the trial, which compromises the current information with the future sample size.

In the second case, the posterior probability is $\Pr(|p_1 - p_2| > \delta | D) = 0.706$. The predictive probability gradually increases with the increasing future sample size. This indicates that if there are still more data to collect and the trend continues, the current subtle difference between the two arms may become more "real" by the end of the trial. The predictive probability is a relatively conservative approach, which compromises the information contained in the

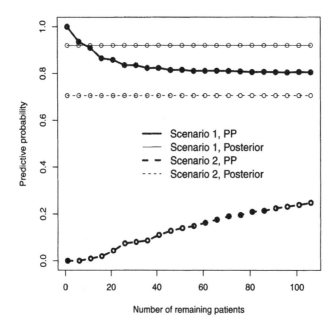

**Figure 5.3**   Predictive probability (PP) versus posterior probability when observing 11/25 and 5/25 responses in arm 1 and arm 2 (scenario 1), and 10/25 and 9/25 in arm 1 and arm 2 (scenario 2), respectively.

current data and the amount of future data. Using predictive probabilities to guide phase II trial designs is appealing, since it is desirable to terminate a trial if a definitive conclusion can be drawn in the course of a trial.

## 5.7   BAYESIAN PHASE II DESIGN WITH MULTIPLE OUTCOMES

### 5.7.1   Bivariate Binary Outcomes

Although phase II trials mainly focus on evaluation of efficacy, toxicity data are also collected in the study, because the toxicity information in phase I trials alone may not be adequate. By jointly modeling efficacy and toxicity data, we can borrow information across the bivariate outcomes for better decision making. Along this direction, Thall, Simon, and Estey (1995) present a Dirichlet-multinomial model to accommodate multivariate discrete outcomes arising in phase II trials.

Suppose that there are $K$ exclusive events that each patient may experience. For $k = 1, \ldots, K$, let $p_k$ be the probability associated with the occurrence of the $k$th event, satisfying $\sum_{k=1}^{K} p_k = 1$. If $n$ patients have been treated, let $y_k$ denote the number of subjects who have experienced event $k$, such that $\sum_{k=1}^{K} y_k = n$. Denote $\mathbf{p} = (p_1, \ldots, p_K)$ and $\mathbf{y} = (y_1, \ldots, y_K)$, and thus $\mathbf{y}$ follows a multinomial distribution with probability $\mathbf{p}$. If we take a Dirichlet prior distribution, $\mathbf{p} \sim \mathrm{Dir}(\alpha_1, \ldots, \alpha_K)$, then the posterior distribution of $\mathbf{p}$ is

$$\mathbf{p}|\mathbf{y} \sim \mathrm{Dir}(\alpha_1 + y_1, \ldots, \alpha_K + y_K).$$

In a phase II trial, we are often concerned with bivariate binary outcomes of toxicity and efficacy. There are four different possible events: observing both toxicity and efficacy $(T, E)$, observing toxicity but no efficacy $(T, E^c)$, observing efficacy but no toxicity $(T^c, E)$, and observing neither toxicity nor efficacy $(T^c, E^c)$. We may construct a $2 \times 2$ joint probability table:

|  | Toxicity ($p_T$) | No toxicity ($1 - p_T$) |
|---|---|---|
| Efficacy ($p_E$) | $p_{(T,E)}$ | $p_{(T^c,E)}$ |
| No efficacy ($1 - p_E$) | $p_{(T,E^c)}$ | $p_{(T^c,E^c)}$ |

Based on these four nonoverlapping events, we can compute the marginal probability for a "good" event such as efficacy, $p_E = p_{(T,E)} + p_{(T^c,E)}$, and that for a "bad" event such as toxicity, $p_T = p_{(T,E)} + p_{(T,E^c)}$. If we take the joint prior distribution of

$$\left( p_{(T,E)}, p_{(T,E^c)}, p_{(T^c,E)}, p_{(T^c,E^c)} \right) \sim \mathrm{Dir}\left( \alpha_{(T,E)}, \alpha_{(T,E^c)}, \alpha_{(T^c,E)}, \alpha_{(T^c,E^c)} \right),$$

then both $p_T$ and $p_E$ marginally follow beta distributions,

$$\begin{aligned} p_T &\sim \mathrm{Beta}\left( \alpha_{(T,E)} + \alpha_{(T,E^c)}, \alpha_{(T^c,E)} + \alpha_{(T^c,E^c)} \right), \\ p_E &\sim \mathrm{Beta}\left( \alpha_{(T,E)} + \alpha_{(T^c,E)}, \alpha_{(T,E^c)} + \alpha_{(T^c,E^c)} \right). \end{aligned} \tag{5.7}$$

### 5.7.2  Stopping Boundaries

In a single-arm phase II trial, we compare both toxicity and efficacy of the new treatment with the historical rates of the standard treatment. Let $\eta_T$ and $\eta_E$ denote the toxicity and efficacy rates of the standard treatment, for which we take beta prior distributions, $\eta_T \sim \mathrm{Beta}(\xi_T, \zeta_T)$ and $\eta_E \sim \mathrm{Beta}(\xi_E, \zeta_E)$, respectively. For the new treatment, the marginal prior distributions for toxicity and efficacy in (5.7) can be rewritten as

$$p_T \sim \mathrm{Beta}(\alpha_T, \beta_T) \quad \text{and} \quad p_E \sim \mathrm{Beta}(\alpha_E, \beta_E),$$

where $\alpha_T = \alpha_{(T,E)} + \alpha_{(T,E^c)}$, $\beta_T = \alpha_{(T^c,E)} + \alpha_{(T^c,E^c)}$, $\alpha_E = \alpha_{(T,E)} + \alpha_{(T^c,E)}$, and $\beta_E = \alpha_{(T,E^c)} + \alpha_{(T^c,E^c)}$.

Let $\mathbf{y} = \left( y_{(T,E)}, y_{(T,E^c)}, y_{(T^c,E)}, y_{(T^c,E^c)} \right)$ denote the observed data; that is, among $n$ treated patients, $y_{(T,E)}$ of them have experienced both toxicity and efficacy, $y_{(T,E^c)}$ have experienced toxicity only, $y_{(T^c,E)}$ have experienced efficacy only, and $y_{(T^c,E^c)}$ have neither experienced toxicity nor efficacy. The observed toxicity and efficacy data can be summarized in a $2 \times 2$ contingency table:

|  | $y_T$ | $n - y_T$ |
|---|---|---|
| $y_E$ | $y_{(T,E)}$ | $y_{(T^c,E)}$ |
| $n - y_E$ | $y_{(T,E^c)}$ | $y_{(T^c,E^c)}$ |

Let $0 \le \delta_E < 1$ denote the minimally acceptable increment in the response rate for the experimental drug compared with the standard drug, and let $0 \le \delta_T < 1$ denote the maximum tolerance for that of the toxicity rate. Then,

$$\Pr(p_E > \eta_E + \delta_E | y_E)$$
$$= \int_0^{1-\delta_E} \{1 - F(p + \delta_E; \alpha_E + y_E, \beta_E + n - y_E)\} f(p; \xi_E, \zeta_E) \, dp$$

and

$$\Pr(p_T > \eta_T + \delta_T | y_T)$$
$$= \int_0^{1-\delta_T} \{1 - F(p + \delta_T; \alpha_T + y_T, \beta_T + n - y_T)\} f(p; \xi_T, \zeta_T) \, dp,$$

where $f(p; \alpha, \beta)$ denotes the probability density function for $p \sim \text{Beta}(\alpha, \beta)$ and $F(p; \alpha, \beta)$ is the corresponding cumulative distribution function.

Let $\theta_U$, $\theta_L$, and $\theta_T$ denote the prespecified probability cutoffs, for example, $\theta_U, \theta_T \in [0.95, 0.99]$ and $\theta_L \in [0.01, 0.05]$. After $n$ subjects have been treated in a trial, we can determine the upper and lower decision boundaries as follows:

- Let $U_n$ be the smallest integer of $y_E$ satisfying $\Pr(p_E > \eta_E | y_E) \ge \theta_U$.

- Let $L_n$ be the largest integer of $y_E$ satisfying $\Pr(p_E > \eta_E + \delta_E | y_E) \le \theta_L$.

- Let $T_n$ be the smallest integer of $y_T$ satisfying $\Pr(p_T > \eta_T + \delta_T | y_T) \ge \theta_T$.

The decision rules after observing the multivariate data **y** from $n$ patients are then given as follows:

- If $y_E \ge U_n$, terminate the trial and declare the experimental drug promising.

- If $y_E \le L_n$, terminate the trial and declare the experimental drug not promising.

- If $y_T \ge T_n$, terminate the trial due to excessive toxicity of the experimental drug.

The first two stopping rules are constructed for efficacy, while the last one is for toxicity or patient safety. When calculating the stopping boundaries, the dependence between toxicity and efficacy is not relevant, and we can simply use the marginal beta distributions for the probabilities of toxicity and efficacy. However, when calculating the probability of stopping a trial due to crossing any of these boundaries, we must take into account the dependence between the bivariate binary outcomes by using the Dirichlet model.

**EXAMPLE 5.4**

We examine the operating characteristics of the phase II trial design accommodating both toxicity and efficacy. The prior distribution for the efficacy rate of the standard drug is taken as $\eta_E \sim \text{Beta}(3, 7)$, and that for the experimental drug is $p_E \sim \text{Beta}(0.6, 1.4)$. Correspondingly, the prior distribution for the toxicity rate of the standard drug is taken as $\eta_T \sim \text{Beta}(2, 8)$, and that for the experimental drug is $p_T \sim \text{Beta}(0.4, 1.6)$. The lower cutoff probability for efficacy is $\theta_L = 0.05$, and the upper cutoff for toxicity is $\theta_T = 0.95$, and $\delta_E = \delta_T = 0$. In practice, we set $\theta_U = 1$, because we typically do not implement an efficacy stopping bound for a promising drug in a single-arm trial. In other words, if the investigational drug appears to be effective, patient accrual will continue without interruption such that more patients would benefit from this "good" drug. The maximum sample size is $N = 30$, with a cohort size of 1.

Based on these design specifications, the stopping boundaries for response (efficacy) are given by

| $L_n$ | 0 | 1 | 2 |
|---|---|---|---|
| $n$ | 8 | 20 | 30 |

where $L_n$ is the number of responses and $n$ is the number of treated patients. The stopping boundaries for toxicity are given by

| $T_n$ | 3 | 4 | 5 | 5 | 6 | 7 | 8 | 8 | 9 | 10 | 11 | 12 | 12 | 13 | 14 | 15 |
|---|---|---|---|---|---|---|---|---|---|---|---|---|---|---|---|---|
| $n$ | 3 | 5 | 7 | 8 | 10 | 12 | 14 | 15 | 17 | 19 | 21 | 23 | 24 | 26 | 28 | 30 |

where $T_n$ is the number of toxicities observed among $n$ treated patients. We take the cases with $L_n/n = 0/8$ and $T_n/n = 5/8$ to illustrate how to implement the trial in practice. The trial would be stopped early if among the first eight treated patients, no response has been observed or the number of toxicities occurred is greater than or equal to five. Suppose that the trial runs to the maximum sample size (no early stopping). By the end of the trial, if there are two or fewer responses among 30 treated patients, the drug will be claimed nonpromising; if there are 15 or more patients experiencing toxicity, the drug will be considered unsafe. In either case, the drug should be "killed" at this developmental stage.

**Table 5.5   Phase II Trial Designs by Simultaneously Monitoring Toxicity and Efficacy for Six Scenarios**

| Sc. | True Joint Probabilities | | | | Number of | | |
| --- | --- | --- | --- | --- | --- | --- | --- |
| | $p_{(T,E)}$ | $p_{(T,E^c)}$ | $p_{(T^c,E)}$ | $p_{(T^c,E^c)}$ | Patients | Efficacy | Toxicity |
| 1 | 0.05 | 0.05 | 0.45 | 0.45 | 29.9 | 14.9 | 3.0 |
| 2 | 0.04 | 0.16 | 0.16 | 0.64 | 25.6 | 5.1 | 5.1 |
| 3 | 0.36 | 0.24 | 0.24 | 0.16 | 9.9 | 5.9 | 5.9 |
| 4 | 0.20 | 0.10 | 0.30 | 0.40 | 27.3 | 13.6 | 8.2 |
| 5 | 0.10 | 0.30 | 0.20 | 0.40 | 21.6 | 6.5 | 8.6 |
| 6 | 0.50 | 0.30 | 0.10 | 0.10 | 4.8 | 2.9 | 3.8 |

Note: Sc. stands for Scenario.

As shown in Table 5.5, we simulated six scenarios for phase II trials using the aforementioned design specifications. The first three scenarios generate the joint toxicity and efficacy probabilities by assuming the independence between the two endpoints, while the last three scenarios accommodate correlations between them. In scenario 1, almost one-half of the patients achieved the efficacy event, and approximately 10% of the patients experienced toxicity, which closely matched the marginal efficacy and toxicity rates, respectively. In scenarios 3 and 6, on average only ten and five patients were treated respectively, since the trials were likely to be terminated early due to excessive toxicities (the marginal toxicity rate is 60% in scenario 3 and 80% in scenario 6).

## 5.8   PHASE I/II DESIGN WITH BIVARIATE BINARY DATA

### 5.8.1   Motivation

As discussed in Chapter 4, the primary objective of a phase I trial is to find the MTD, for which toxicity is usually considered alone. In general, dose-finding studies need to locate the MTD accurately and efficiently, while exposing as few patients as possible to over-toxic or inefficacious doses. Subsequently in phase II trials, patients are often treated at the MTD to examine the short-term efficacy effect of the drug. In conventional settings, phase I and phase II trials are conducted separately without any kind of formal borrowing of information or strength across them. However, with limited resources and especially a small sample size, the MTD identified in the phase I trial might not be accurate, which certainly has an undesirable impact on the subsequent phase II and phase III studies. In addition, the ultimate goal of drug development is to find a cure. Therefore, it is critical to search for the optimum biologic dose of a drug that has the highest efficacy as well as tolerable toxicity.

To fully utilize the data collected in both phase I and phase II trials, toxicity and efficacy may be jointly evaluated for the drug's risk and benefit trade-offs. Following this route, the seamless phase I/II trial design works to

- speed up the drug developmental process by eliminating the gap between phase I and phase II clinical trials,

- improve the dose-finding procedure by maximizing the drug's efficacy as well as controlling its toxicity, and

- enlarge the sample size by pooling patients from phase I and phase II trials such as to produce more accurate estimates for toxicity and efficacy than would be achieved in each separate trial.

**EXAMPLE 5.5**

A multi-center, open-label, phase I/II dose-finding trial was designed to evaluate the efficacy, safety, and tolerability of RAD001, and to find the optimal biologic dose in combination with a standard 3-week cycle of docetaxel therapy for patients with metastatic breast cancer. RAD001 had three prespecified dose levels, and docetaxel was administered at a constant dose level. RAD001 was shown by *in vitro* and *in vivo* studies to be a potent inhibitor of tumor growth, which exerts its activity on interleukin and the growth-factor-dependent proliferation of cells through their high affinity for an intracellular receptor protein. Docetaxel takes its cytotoxic effect to prevent normal mitosis and alter the skeletal structure and functions of the cell. Dose-limiting toxicities were defined as grade 4 hematological toxicity, grade 3 or grade 4 nonhematological toxicity, or other well-defined serious adverse events. Efficacy of the combined treatments was assessed by tumor response. After docetaxel treatment was ceased, RAD001 continued to be administered alone till disease progression or appearance of unacceptable toxicity.

### 5.8.2 Likelihood and Prior

For $j = 1, \ldots, J$, let $p_j$ and $q_j$ denote the probabilities of toxicity and efficacy at dose level $j$ of the experimental drug, respectively. As to toxicity, a monotonic order is assumed with $p_1 < \cdots < p_J$, while there is no such a constraint imposed for $q_j$ because the treatment efficacy may plateau or even decrease as the dose increases. Figure 5.4 shows three possible patterns for efficacy: increasing, umbrella-shaped, and decreasing; but toxicity always monotonically increases with respect to the dose.

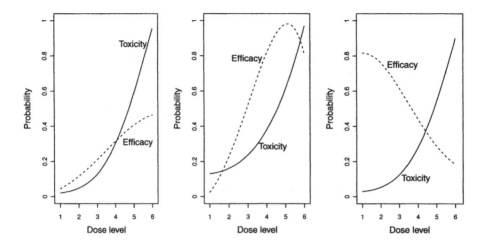

**Figure 5.4** Three possible patterns for efficacy and toxicity curves with six increasing doses.

Let $X_{ij}$ denote the binary toxicity outcome for subject $i$ treated at dose level $j$,

$$X_{ij} = \begin{cases} 1, & \text{with probability } p_j, \\ 0, & \text{with probability } 1 - p_j, \end{cases}$$

and similarly let $Y_{ij}$ denote the binary efficacy outcome of the same subject,

$$Y_{ij} = \begin{cases} 1, & \text{with probability } q_j, \\ 0, & \text{with probability } 1 - q_j. \end{cases}$$

The association between the bivariate binary outcomes can be measured by the global cross ratio (Dale, 1986),

$$\gamma_j = \frac{\pi_{j(00)}\pi_{j(11)}}{\pi_{j(01)}\pi_{j(10)}},$$

where $\pi_{j(xy)} = \Pr(X_{ij} = x, Y_{ij} = y)$ for $x = 0, 1$ and $y = 0, 1$. The joint toxicity and efficacy probabilities at dose level $j$, $\pi_{j(xy)}$, can be represented in a $2\times 2$ contingency table:

|  | $p_j$ | $1 - p_j$ |
|---|---|---|
| $q_j$ | $\pi_{j(11)}$ | $\pi_{j(01)}$ |
| $1 - q_j$ | $\pi_{j(10)}$ | $\pi_{j(00)}$ |

Given the marginal toxicity and efficacy probabilities $p_j$ and $q_j$, the joint probabilities are given by

$$
\pi_{j(11)} = \begin{cases} \dfrac{a_j - (a_j^2 + b_j)^{1/2}}{2(\gamma_j - 1)}, & \gamma_j \neq 1, \\ p_j q_j, & \gamma_j = 1, \end{cases}
$$
$$
\pi_{j(10)} = p_j - \pi_{j(11)},
$$
$$
\pi_{j(01)} = q_j - \pi_{j(11)}, \tag{5.8}
$$
$$
\pi_{j(00)} = 1 - p_j - q_j + \pi_{j(11)},
$$

where $a_j = 1 + (p_j + q_j)(\gamma_j - 1)$ and $b_j = -4\gamma_j(\gamma_j - 1)p_j q_j$. Let $\mathbf{p} = (p_1, \ldots, p_J)^\mathsf{T}$, and define $\mathbf{q}$ and $\boldsymbol{\gamma}$ similarly. Suppose that $n_j$ patients have been treated at dose level $j$, and $n_{j(11)}$ of them experienced both toxicity and efficacy, $n_{j(10)}$ with toxicity but no efficacy, $n_{j(01)}$ with efficacy but no toxicity, and $n_{j(00)}$ with neither toxicity nor efficacy. Let $D$ denote the observed data at all the dose levels, then the multinomial likelihood is given by

$$
L(D|\mathbf{p}, \mathbf{q}, \boldsymbol{\gamma}) \propto \prod_{j=1}^{J} \prod_{x=0}^{1} \prod_{y=0}^{1} \{\pi_{j(xy)}\}^{n_{j(xy)}}.
$$

In the Bayesian paradigm, parameter constraints often make the prior specification challenging. To incorporate the monotonic order for $p_j$, we define

$$
\xi_1 = \log\left(\frac{p_1}{1 - p_1}\right) \quad \text{and} \quad \xi_j = \log\left(\frac{p_j}{1 - p_j} - \frac{p_{j-1}}{1 - p_{j-1}}\right),
$$

for $j = 2, \ldots, J$, and then

$$
p_1 = \frac{e^{\xi_1}}{1 + e^{\xi_1}} \quad \text{and} \quad p_j = \frac{e^{\xi_1} + \cdots + e^{\xi_j}}{1 + e^{\xi_1} + \cdots + e^{\xi_j}},
$$

which automatically satisfy the order constraint. As for efficacy, we need not enforce such a monotonic ordering constraint, and thus define

$$
\zeta_1 = \log\left(\frac{q_1}{1 - q_1}\right) \quad \text{and} \quad \zeta_j = \log\left(\frac{q_j}{1 - q_j}\right) - \log\left(\frac{q_{j-1}}{1 - q_{j-1}}\right),
$$

which lead to

$$
q_1 = \frac{e^{\zeta_1}}{1 + e^{\zeta_1}} \quad \text{and} \quad q_j = \frac{e^{\zeta_1 + \cdots + \zeta_j}}{1 + e^{\zeta_1 + \cdots + \zeta_j}},
$$

for $j = 2, \ldots, J$. After such variable transformations, we can specify noninformative prior distributions on $(\mathbf{p}, \mathbf{q})$ by assigning multivariate normal prior distributions with zero means and large variances to $\boldsymbol{\xi} = (\xi_1, \ldots, \xi_J)^\mathsf{T}$ and $\boldsymbol{\zeta} = (\zeta_1, \ldots, \zeta_J)^\mathsf{T}$. For example, we consider five dose levels and take the

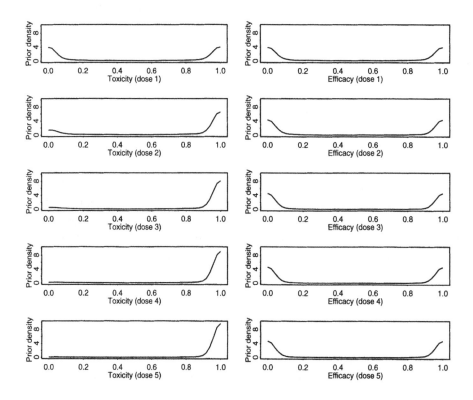

**Figure 5.5**    Prior distributions of the toxicity probabilities $p_j$ and the efficacy probabilities $q_j$, for $j = 1, \ldots, 5$.

marginal variances $\mathrm{Var}(\xi_j) = \mathrm{Var}(\zeta_j) = 100$ for $j = 1, \ldots, 5$. Figure 5.5 displays the prior distributions of the five paired probabilities of toxicity and efficacy. These prior distributions are indeed very flat in the middle range of $(0, 1)$, and there is an obvious trend of shifting to the right for toxicity due to the monotonic toxicity constraint. Subsequently, we can derive the joint posterior distribution and also the full conditional distributions for all the model parameters $(\boldsymbol{\xi}, \boldsymbol{\zeta}, \boldsymbol{\gamma})$, from which the posterior samples can be easily obtained by the usual Gibbs sampler.

### 5.8.3   Odds Ratio and Dose-Finding Algorithm

To facilitate dose finding, we construct toxicity–efficacy odds ratio trade-off contours in the two-dimensional probability domain. Figure 5.6 shows that for $j = 1, \ldots, J$ each dose $j$ corresponds to a point with the efficacy and toxicity probabilities $(q_j, p_j)$, and the optimal dose is the one that is closest

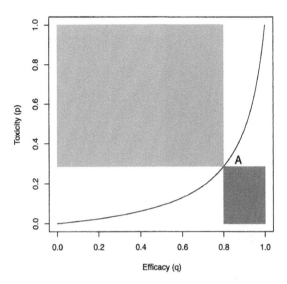

**Figure 5.6**    Two-dimensional toxicity–efficacy odds ratio contour with point A $(q_j, p_j)$ corresponding to dose level $j$.

to the lower-right corner $(1, 0)$. The horizontal and vertical lines crossing the dose with $(q_j, p_j)$, point A, partition the unit square into four rectangles. The toxicity–efficacy odds ratio $\omega_j$ at dose level $j$ is given by

$$\omega_j = \frac{p_j/(1 - p_j)}{q_j/(1 - q_j)} = \frac{p_j(1 - q_j)}{q_j(1 - p_j)},$$

which is exactly the ratio between the areas of the lower-right versus the upper-left rectangles. The smaller the value of $\omega_j$, the more desirable the corresponding dose. Figure 5.6 also presents a toxicity–efficacy odds ratio equivalence contour, along which all the points have the same value of $\omega_j$.

Nevertheless, $\omega_j$ is based on the marginal toxicity and efficacy probabilities $(q_j, p_j)$ without accounting for the correlation between them. To account for the correlation, we add a third dimension as shown in Figure 5.7:

$$\text{Pr(efficacy} \mid \text{no toxicity)} = \pi_{j(E|T^c)} = \frac{\pi_{j(01)}}{\pi_{j(01)} + \pi_{j(00)}}.$$

In this three-dimensional probability space, the optimal point is the lower-left corner, which corresponds to $(q_j, \pi_{j(E|T^c)}, p_j) = (1, 1, 0)$. The closer the dose to that point, the better. The horizontal and vertical planes crossing the dose

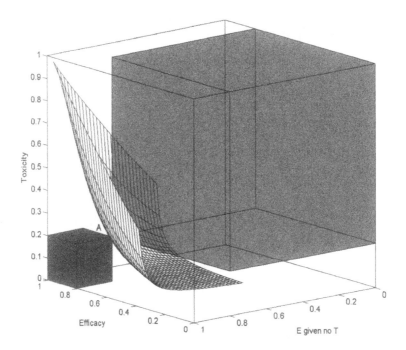

**Figure 5.7**    Three-dimensional toxicity–efficacy odds ratio trade-off incorporating the third axis of $\Pr(\text{efficacy} \mid \text{no toxicity})$, with point A $(q_j, \pi_{j(E|T^c)}, p_j)$ corresponding to dose level $j$.

with $(q_j, \pi_{j(E|T^c)}, p_j)$, point A, partition the unit cube into eight pieces. Along the diagonal line, the ratio between the volumes of the lower-left versus the upper-right cubes is

$$\Omega_j = \frac{p_j(1 - q_j)(1 - \pi_{j(E|T^c)})}{(1 - p_j)q_j\pi_{j(E|T^c)}} = \omega_j \frac{\pi_{j(00)}}{\pi_{j(01)}}.$$

The dose that yields the smallest value of $\Omega_j$ is considered the best. Figure 5.7 also presents an odds ratio equivalence surface across point A; that is, all the points on this smooth surface have the same value of $\Omega_j$. Hence, the dose-finding procedure may use either the two-dimensional or the three-dimensional toxicity–efficacy odds ratio as a selection criterion.

Let $\phi_T$ and $\phi_E$ be the prespecified maximum tolerable toxicity probability and the minimum acceptable efficacy probability, respectively. Define an admissible set $S$ that contains all the doses satisfying

$$\Pr(p_j < \phi_T | D) > \theta_T \quad \text{and} \quad \Pr(q_j > \phi_E | D) > \theta_E,$$

where $\theta_T$ and $\theta_E$ are fixed probability cutoffs that can be calibrated through simulation studies. For patients' safety, untried doses cannot be skipped during dose escalation. The phase I/II trial proceeds as follows:

(1) Treat the first cohort of patients at the lowest dose level.

(2) Let $p_{j\text{high}}$ denote the toxicity probability of the highest dose tried thus far, and let $\theta_T^*$ ($\theta_T^* > \theta_T$) denote the cutoff probability for dose escalation. If

$$\Pr(p_{j\text{high}} < \phi_T | D) > \theta_T^*, \tag{5.9}$$

we escalate to the lowest untried dose for the next cohort.

(3) Otherwise, treat the next cohort of patients at the most desirable dose selected from $S$ according to one of the odds ratio criteria.

(4) Once the maximum sample size is reached, the dose with the smallest toxicity–efficacy odds ratio in $S$ is recommended.

In practice, it may happen that (5.9) does not hold and $S$ is an empty set, then the trial would be terminated as an inconclusive study.

### 5.8.4 Numerical Comparison

For comparison, we introduce two other criteria for the drug's risk and benefit trade-offs. One is to select the dose with the largest joint probability of $\pi_{j(01)} = \Pr(\text{no toxcity}, \text{efficacy})$ given in (5.8), and the other constructs toxicity and efficacy trade-off contours in the two-dimensional probability space (Thall and Cook, 2004). The latter requires specification of three toxicity–efficacy equivalent points, based on which a concave trade-off contour can be constructed via a simple polynomial model. As shown in Figure 5.8, the straight line that connects each point of dose toxicity–efficacy probabilities with the lower-right point $(1, 0)$ crosses the equivalence contour. The desirability parameter for each dose $j$, $\delta_j$, is defined as the ratio of the Euclidean distance from the intersection point to $(1, 0)$ versus that from the dose point to $(1, 0)$. The larger the value of $\delta_j$, the more desirable the dose. Figure 5.8 shows that $\delta_1 = \text{AO/BO}$ and $\delta_2 = \text{CO/DO}$, and as $\delta_1 > \delta_2$ dose 1 is preferred to dose 2.

We compared the Bayesian phase I/II odds-ratio design and the dose-finding methods by using the $\pi_{j(01)}$ and $\delta_j$ criteria in the simulation study. We considered five doses with the maximum sample size of 60 and the cohort size of 3. The upper toxicity and lower efficacy probability limits were $\phi_T = \phi_E = 0.3$, and the cutoff probabilities were $\theta_T = 0.25$, $\theta_E = 0.1$, and $\theta_T^* = 0.5$. We used noninformative prior distributions for all the model parameters in the Markov chain Monte Carlo (MCMC) procedure.

Averaged over 1,000 simulated trials, Figure 5.9 exhibits the dose selection percentages using the two-dimensional odds ratio (2d-OR), three-dimensional

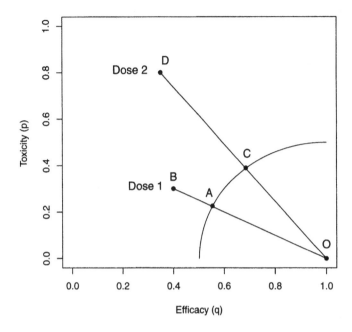

**Figure 5.8**   The $\delta_j$ criterion based on the toxicity–efficacy trade-off contour, with $\delta_1 = \mathrm{AO/BO}$ for dose 1 and $\delta_2 = \mathrm{CO/DO}$ for dose 2.

odds ratio (3d-OR), $\pi_{j(01)}$, and $\delta_j$ criteria under four scenarios, respectively. In scenario 1, toxicity increases substantially with respect to the dose while efficacy does not change as much. All the four designs selected the first dose over 50% and treated most of the patients at that dose as well. In scenario 2, toxicity is negligible but efficacy increases considerably over the dose. The 3d-OR criterion outperformed the 2d-OR, while the $\pi_{j(01)}$ design performed the best. The dose–response curve for efficacy in scenario 3 is not monotonic: Efficacy first increases and then decreases with the dose; and also the fourth and fifth doses are overly toxic. In that scenario, all of the designs selected the third dose the most, while the $\delta_j$ criterion appears to be slightly aggressive due to selecting dose 4 over 30%. In scenario 4, the 2d-OR design behaved the best. In conclusion, all of the four designs performed reasonably well by selecting the optimal dose with the highest percentage, at which most of the patients were also treated. The odds ratio equivalence contour between toxicity and efficacy is intuitive and meaningful, which allows for an objective quantification of trade-offs between toxicity and efficacy.

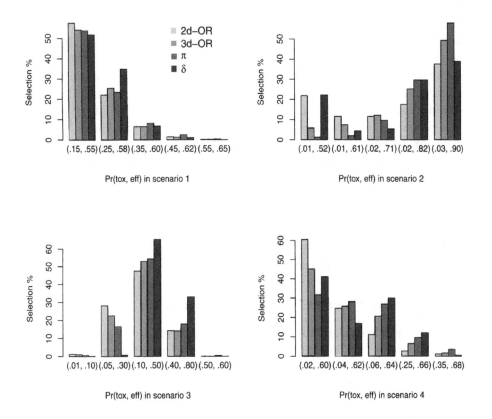

**Figure 5.9**   Dose selection percentages in the order of using the two-dimensional odds ratio (2d-OR), three-dimensional odds ratio (3d-OR), $\pi_{j(01)}$, and $\delta_j$ criteria, respectively.

## 5.9   PHASE I/II DESIGN WITH TIMES TO TOXICITY AND EFFICACY

In traditional phase I and phase II trials, toxicity and efficacy are often modeled as binary endpoints. Although such binary-outcome designs are simple and easy to implement, they ignore information of how soon patients experience toxicity or respond to treatment. By contrast, time-to-event data contain much more clinical information to discriminate drugs' therapeutic effects. For example, in addition to lowering the occurrence rate of toxicity, it is also desirable to delay the onset of such adverse events such that patients' quality of life could be improved. As an extreme case, if death is one of the severe adverse events, the longer the lag time to observe death, the better.

If the patient accrual is faster relative to the assessment of toxicity and efficacy, new participants may face delays in receiving treatment because the outcomes of the previous patients may still be unavailable what that information is needed. Under this circumstance, one choice is to suspend the enrollment until all the toxicity and efficacy data are completely observed, which, however, not only causes logistical inconvenience, but also results in a lengthy study duration. The other possibility is to choose the "best" dose based on the currently available data (i.e., discarding the missing data), so that each new cohort will be treated immediately upon arrival. Notwithstanding patients have not experienced toxicity by the decision-making time, they may experience toxicity later during the rest of the follow-up. Hence, ignoring the unobserved or censored data is likely to underestimate the toxicity probability; and consequently, dose escalation might be overly aggressive, leading to an undesirably large number of patients treated at over-toxic doses. On the other hand, if the response rate is underestimated due to the late onset of efficacy events, the trial may be inappropriately terminated early for futility. To accommodate possible delayed outcomes, both toxicity and efficacy can be modeled as time-to-event data (Yuan and Yin, 2009); patients who have not experienced the event by the decision-making time are naturally treated as censored, but still contribute partial information to the trial design.

### 5.9.1  Bivariate Times to Toxicity and Efficacy

The entire patient population may be viewed as a mixture of the subjects who would eventually experience the event of interest if a sufficient follow-up is taken and those who would never experience the event. For example, after intensive chemotherapy treatment, a substantial proportion of cancer patients become drug-resistant and will not respond to another therapy regardless of the dosage or the duration of treatment. In this regard, cure rate models are more suitable for the time-to-event data that need to incorporate a cure or insusceptible fraction. In contrast, toxicity will occur sooner or later if patients are treated with a sufficient amount of dosage, and thus there is typically no patient who would be insusceptible to toxicity.

Let $t_T$ and $t_E$ be the times from the initial treatment until occurrences of toxicity and efficacy events, respectively. Under the proportional hazards model (Cox, 1972), the hazard function for toxicity is

$$\lambda_T(t_T|Z) = \lambda_{0T}(t_T)\exp(\beta_T Z),$$

where $\lambda_{0T}(t_T)$ is the baseline hazard function and $Z$ represents the dose. Under a Weibull distribution with parameters $\alpha_T$ and $\eta_T$, $\lambda_{0T}(t_T) = \alpha_T \eta_T t^{\alpha_T - 1}$, and the survival function for times to toxicity is given by

$$S_T(t_T|Z) = \exp\{-\eta_T t_T^{\alpha_T} \exp(\beta_T Z)\}. \tag{5.10}$$

For efficacy, the mixture cure rate model (Berkson and Gage, 1952) is more appropriate such as to account for the proportion of patients who would never respond to treatment. Hence, the population survival function is given by

$$S_{E,\text{pop}}(t_E|Z) = 1 - \pi + \pi S_E(t_E|Z),$$

where $S_E(t_E|Z)$ is the usual survival function for susceptible subjects (potential responders), and $1 - \pi$ is the proportion of insusceptible patients (nonresponders) in the population. Similar to (5.10), under the proportional hazards assumption,

$$S_E(t_E|Z) = \exp\{-\eta_E t_E^{\alpha_E} \exp(\beta_E Z)\}.$$

In consideration of the correlation between the bivariate failure times $(t_T, t_E)$, the Clayton (1978) copula can be used to link the two marginal survival functions,

$$S(t_T, t_E|Z) = \{S_T(t_T|Z)^{-\gamma} + S_E(t_E|Z)^{-\gamma} - 1\}^{-1/\gamma},$$

where $\gamma > 0$ characterizes the association between $t_T$ and $t_E$. The larger the value of $\gamma$, the higher the correlation. The correlation approaches 1 as $\gamma \to \infty$, and $t_T$ and $t_E$ become independent as $\gamma \to 0$.

Let $t_{iT}$ be the time to toxicity for subject $i$, and let $u_i$ be the actual follow-up time. Due to censoring caused by decision making, we in fact observe the toxicity data $(y_{iT}, \Delta_{iT})$, where $y_{iT} = t_{iT}$ and $\Delta_{iT} = 1$ if the toxicity event has occurred, and $y_{iT} = u_i$ and $\Delta_{iT} = 0$ if the time to toxicity is censored. Similarly, define $(y_{iE}, \Delta_{iE})$ for efficacy. Based on the observed data $D$, the likelihood is given by

$$L(D|\beta_T, \alpha_T, \eta_T, \beta_E, \alpha_E, \eta_E, \pi, \gamma)$$

$$= \prod_{i=1}^n \left\{ \pi \frac{\partial^2 S(y_{iT}, y_{iE}|Z_i)}{\partial y_{iT} \partial y_{iE}} \right\}^{\Delta_{iT}\Delta_{iE}} \left\{ -\pi \frac{\partial S(y_{iT}, y_{iE}|Z_i)}{\partial y_{iE}} \right\}^{(1-\Delta_{iT})\Delta_{iE}}$$

$$\times \left\{ -(1-\pi) \frac{\partial S_T(y_{iT}|Z_i)}{\partial y_{iT}} - \pi \frac{\partial S(y_{iT}, y_{iE}|Z_i)}{\partial y_{iT}} \right\}^{\Delta_{iT}(1-\Delta_{iE})}$$

$$\times \left\{ (1-\pi) S_T(y_{iT}|Z_i) + \pi S(y_{iT}, y_{iE}|Z_i) \right\}^{(1-\Delta_{iT})(1-\Delta_{iE})},$$

where the first term is for both toxicity and efficacy observed, the second corresponds to toxicity censored but efficacy observed, the third stands for toxicity observed but efficacy censored, and the last term with both toxicity and efficacy censored. Because the efficacy event may be censored due to either insusceptibility or that the event has not occurred yet, the last two terms in the likelihood consist of two parts: One is for subjects who are insusceptible to efficacy, and the other is for those who may respond but the efficacy event is censored.

### 5.9.2 Areas Under Survival Curves

Toxicity and efficacy are typically evaluated within a fixed period of time $[0, \tau]$, where $\tau$ depends on the specific disease and the testing drug. Clinical events of

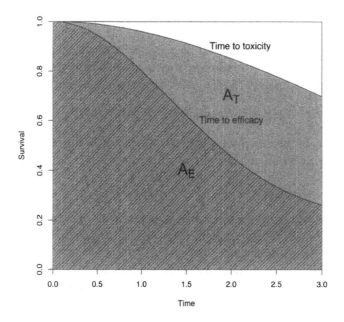

**Figure 5.10**    Areas under the survival curves for toxicity and efficacy, the AUSC ratio $= A_T/A_E$.

interest are expected to occur within $[0, \tau]$, and those happened after $\tau$ will not be relevant. Generally speaking, a desirable dose should induce more patients to achieve favorable responses quickly after treatment, and yet cause fewer patients to suffer from toxicity even long after treatment. As shown in Figure 5.10, a sharply declining survival curve for efficacy indicates that patients respond quickly to the treatment; and a slowly decaying survival curve for toxicity corresponds to the late onset of adverse events. By using the ratio of the areas under the survival curves (AUSCs), we simultaneously take into consideration the following two aspects of the treatment:

- both the toxicity and efficacy rates evaluated at the end of the follow-up time $\tau$, and

- how soon patients experience toxicity and how quickly they respond to treatment.

In contrast, dose selection in a binary-outcome design is solely based on the toxicity and efficacy rates, while ignoring the entire paths of the survival curves. For illustration, Figure 5.11(a) shows two survival curves for times to toxicity at a high and a low dose: Patients treated at the high dose would be more likely and also more quickly to experience toxicity, as the survival curve of the high dose consistently stays below that of the low dose. In this case, the low dose is preferred due to lower toxicity either based on the AUSC criterion or simply by comparing the toxicity rates at $\tau$. However, it may happen that the two doses have similar toxicity rates at the end of the follow-up, but the survival curve of the high dose declines much more sharply than that of the low dose because patients typically experience toxicity sooner when treated at a stronger dosage; see Figure 5.11(b). Under this situation, the AUSC criterion recommends the low dose as more desirable because patients' qualities of life would be improved due to delayed adverse events, whereas the two doses would be indistinguishable if the selection is solely based on the toxicity rates. In a dose-finding study, survival curves rarely cross; see Figure 5.11(c).

It is also critical to consider how quickly patients respond to treatment in order to discriminate drugs' therapeutic effects. For example, patients with leukemia are more likely to die if they cannot achieve partial or complete remission soon after treatment (Estey, Shen, and Thall, 2000). Hence, the dose that helps patients achieving quick remission is highly preferred. Given that the two doses have the same response rate at $\tau$, the AUSC criterion tends to select the dose that would induce a quicker response.

Let $A_T$ and $A_E$ denote the areas under the survival curves of toxicity and efficacy up to $\tau$, respectively; then

$$\frac{A_T}{A_E} = \frac{\alpha_T^{-1}(\eta_T e^{\beta_T Z})^{-1/\alpha_T}\Gamma(\alpha_T^{-1}, \eta_T \tau^{\alpha_T} e^{\beta_T Z})}{(1-\pi)\tau + \pi\alpha_E^{-1}(\eta_E e^{\beta_E Z})^{-1/\alpha_E}\Gamma(\alpha_E^{-1}, \eta_E \tau^{\alpha_E} e^{\beta_E Z})},$$

where $\Gamma(a, b)$ is the incomplete gamma function,

$$\Gamma(a, b) = \int_0^b x^{a-1}e^{-x}\,\mathrm{d}x.$$

When $\pi = 1$ and $\tau \to \infty$, $A_T/A_E$ has an important interpretation as the ratio of the mean survival times between toxicity and efficacy.

### 5.9.3  Dose-Finding Algorithm

Because there is limited information at the beginning of a trial, dose assignment is difficult for the first few patients in the accrual due to data sparsity. This is even more prominent if toxicity and efficacy events are of late onset. To facilitate the conduct of a trial, a prephase can be implemented prior to the initiation of the formal Bayesian time-to-event (TTE) dose-finding procedure.

During the start-up stage, no new patient will be treated until all the patients already in the trial are fully followed and evaluated. The prephase starts at the lowest dose level with a cohort size of 3. Suppose that the current dose level is $j$, and the trial proceeds as follows:

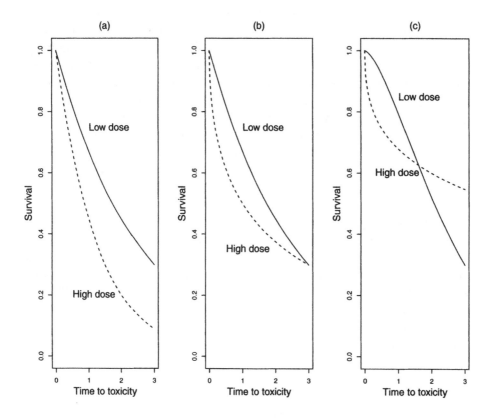

**Figure 5.11**   Three possible situations when comparing survival curves for the times to toxicity at a high and a low dose.

(1) If no patient experiences toxicity, escalate to dose level $j + 1$, while if $j = J$ (the highest dose level), switch to the Bayesian TTE dose-finding procedure at dose level $j$.

(2) If one patient experiences toxicity, switch to the Bayesian TTE dose-finding procedure at dose level $j$.

(3) If 2 or more patients experience toxicity, switch to the Bayesian TTE dose-finding procedure at dose level $j - 1$, while if $j = 1$, terminate the trial.

Let $\phi_T$ be the maximum toxicity rate that is acceptable, and let $\phi_E$ be the minimum efficacy rate that is clinically relevant. Furthermore, let $d_j$ denote the $j$th dose, and let $j^{\text{high}}$ denote the highest dose level tried thus far in the trial.

Based on the accumulated data $D$, the Bayesian TTE design is described as follows:

(1) If the probability of observing toxicity at dose level $j^{\text{high}}$ satisfies

$$\Pr\{1 - S_T(\tau | Z = d_{j^{\text{high}}}) < \phi_T | D\} > \theta_T^*,$$

where $\theta_T^*$ is the cutoff probability for dose escalation, say, $\theta_T^* = 0.85$, we escalate to dose level $j^{\text{high}} + 1$. If $j^{\text{high}} = J$, we treat the next cohort of patients at dose level $J$.

(2) Otherwise, we identify an admissible set $S$ that contains all of the doses satisfying

$$\begin{aligned} \Pr\{1 - S_T(\tau | Z = d_j) < \phi_T | D\} > \theta_T, \\ \Pr\{1 - S_{E,\text{pop}}(\tau | Z = d_j) > \phi_E | D\} > \theta_E, \end{aligned} \tag{5.11}$$

where $\theta_T$ ($\theta_T < \theta_T^*$) and $\theta_E$ are the fixed probability cutoffs that can be calibrated through simulations.

   (i) We treat the next cohort of patients at the (most desirable) dose in $S$, which has the largest value of the AUSC ratio, $A_T/A_E$.

   (ii) If $S$ is an empty set, we terminate the trial without dose selection, which leads to an inconclusive trial.

(3) Once the maximum sample size is reached, the dose that belongs to $S$ and maximizes $A_T/A_E$ will be recommended.

The admissible set $S$ defined by (5.11) serves for screening purposes to protect patients from excessively toxic doses, and also from futile doses.

Compared with the conventional binary-outcome design which potentially requires a full follow-up for each patient, the Bayesian TTE design naturally treats the unobserved toxicity data as censored data. As a consequence, the trial duration can be considerably shortened. However, this may result in more aggressive dose escalation because toxicity could be underestimated at the early stage of the trial when most of the observations are censored.

Dose finding is a sequential process by adaptively assigning patients to the most appropriate dose based on the data accumulated in the trial. When a new cohort arrives, the outcomes of the patients who previously entered the trial might still be unavailable. The Bayesian phase I/II TTE design fulfills the need of utilizing all the available data, especially the information of how soon the toxicity and efficacy events occur. Seamless transition between consecutive trial phases eliminates the "white" space between them, requires a single protocol, and gains statistical efficiency from using both data in a combined analysis.

## 5.10  SUMMARY

This chapter has covered many topics in phase II trial designs. For single-arm phase II trial designs, we introduced Gehan's two-stage design and Simon's optimal and minimax two-stage designs; both are cast in the frequentist hypothesis testing framework. From Bayesian perspectives, we discussed how to use posterior probabilities and predictive probabilities to monitor clinical trials. With the emergence of more randomized phase II trials, Bayesian posterior predictive probabilities provide very helpful guidance for trial conduct. In addition, adaptive randomization may be incorporated to phase II designs to enhance trial ethics by assigning more patients to better treatment arms. Phase II trials often collect multiple outcomes, such as both efficacy and toxicity measurements, which could be binary or time-to-event endpoints. For each case, we presented the trial design that accounts for the multivariate endpoints and also constructed the corresponding stopping rules.

## EXERCISES

**5.1**   In Simon's two-stage design, suppose that the design parameters are given as $(n_1 = 5, n_2 = 6, r_1 = 1, r = 3)$, where $n_1$ and $n_2$ are the respective numbers of patients in stages 1 and 2, $r_1$ is the number of responses in stage 1, and $r$ is the total number of responses at the end of the trial. Compute $\Pr\{(y_1 > r_1) \cap (y_1 + y_2 > r) \mid p\}$ under $H_0 \colon p = 0.2$ and under $H_1 \colon p = 0.4$, respectively. Compare these two probability values with the type I error rate $\alpha = 0.1$ and power 80%, and interpret the results. Repeat the calculation for another set of design parameters $(n_1 = 25, n_2 = 25, r_1 = 8, r = 21)$.

**5.2**   Download the software of Simon's two-stage design from the website of Biometric Research Branch of National Cancer Institute. Develop an optimal design and a minimax design with the type I error rate $\alpha = 0.1$, power 85%, $p_0 = 0.1$, and $p_1 = 0.35$, and describe the trial conduct.

**5.3**   In a single-arm trial, let $p$ denote the response rate of the investigational drug, with a prior distribution of $p \sim \text{Beta}(\alpha, \beta)$. Suppose that we observe $y$ responses out of $n$ subjects; that is, $Y|p \sim \text{Bin}(n, p)$. Derive the likelihood function, the posterior distribution of $p$, and the posterior predictive distribution of $Y$.

**5.4**   In a $K$-arm trial, let $p_k$ denote the response rate of treatment $k$, for $k = 1, \ldots, K$. Under Bayesian hierarchical modeling, the prior distribution for $p_k$ is $p_k \sim \text{Beta}(\alpha, \beta)$, with $\alpha \sim \text{Ga}(\eta, \eta)$ and $\beta \sim \text{Ga}(\eta, \eta)$. Suppose that we observe $y_k$ responses among $n_k$ subjects treated in arm $k$; that is, $Y_k|p_k \sim \text{Bin}(n_k, p_k)$. Derive the likelihood function, and the joint posterior distribution of the model parameters and their full conditional distributions.

**5.5**   Download the software for phase II trial monitoring with the Bayesian posterior probability from the Biostatistics website of M. D. Anderson Cancer Center.

  (1) For the standard treatment, we take a beta prior distribution for the response rate, $p_S \sim \text{Beta}(15, 35)$; and for the the experimental treatment, assign a prior distribution $p_E \sim \text{Beta}(0.6, 1.4)$. The total sample size is $N = 40$, the cohort size is 1, take $\theta_L = 0.05$ and $\delta = 0$. Under this setup, obtain the stopping boundaries for response.

  (2) Take $\theta_L = 0.1$ and $\delta = 0.02$ while keeping other design parameters the same as before, obtain the response stopping boundaries, and interpret the design's operating characteristics.

  (3) Consider jointly modeling both toxicity and efficacy in a phase II trial. The prior distributions for the efficacy and toxicity rates of the standard drug are $\eta_E \sim \text{Beta}(0.3, 0.7)$ and $\eta_T \sim \text{Beta}(0.2, 0.8)$, respectively; and those for the experimental drug are $p_E \sim \text{Beta}(0.6, 1.4)$ and $p_T \sim \text{Beta}(0.4, 1.6)$. The cutoff probability for efficacy is $\theta_L = 0.05$, and that for toxicity is $\theta_T = 0.95$, and $\delta_E = \delta_T = 0$. In practice, we set $\theta_U = 1$, because the efficacy stopping rule is typically not implemented for a promising drug. The maximum sample size is $N = 30$, and the cohort size is 1. Based on these design specifications, obtain both the efficacy and toxicity stopping boundaries.

**5.6**   Download the software of using the predictive probability to monitor a two-arm randomized trial from the Biostatistics website of M. D. Anderson Cancer Center. For the frequentist hypothesis testing, use a two-sided binomial test at a significance level of $\alpha = 0.05$. For the Bayesian approach, take a prior distribution $\text{Beta}(0.2, 0.8)$ for both the response rates of the two drugs in comparison. Set $\theta_T = 0.95$ to determine the superiority of treatment 1 over treatment 2 (see Section 5.5). Suppose that we observe 10 responses in arm 1 and 9 responses in arm 2 after 20 patients were treated in each arm. If we plan to enroll a total of 100 patients, compute the predictive probability of rejecting the null hypothesis at the end of the trial using the frequentist and Bayesian approaches, respectively.

# CHAPTER 6

# PHASE III TRIAL DESIGN

## 6.1 POWER AND SAMPLE SIZE

If an experimental agent exhibits adequate short-term therapeutic effects in a phase II trial, the drug will be moved forward to a phase III study for confirmative testing of its long-term effectiveness. Phase III clinical trials are randomized and controlled studies that directly compare the investigational drug with the current "gold standard" treatment or a placebo when there is no standard of care. The sample size of a phase III trial is large, usually ranging from hundreds up to thousands of participants. The typical endpoint in a phase III trial is a time-to-event measurement, such as progression-free survival or overall survival. Due to their enormous sizes, large scales, and long follow-ups, phase III trials are the most costly comparative studies to evaluate the drug's efficacy.

In a phase III trial, sample size calculation is the most critical component of the study design (Chow, Shao, and Wang, 2007; Julious, 2010). In the hypothesis testing framework, one needs to specify the type I error rate $\alpha$, the type II error rate $\beta$ (or power $1 - \beta$), and the effect size (including the treatment difference to be detected and the associated variance). The common practice is to compute the minimum sample size that is necessary to detect a clinically important treatment difference with sufficient power. If the sample size is inadequate, the trial may fail to discover a truly effective drug because the statistical test cannot reach the conventional significance level due to a lack of power. On the other hand, if the sample size is overestimated, enormous resources and efforts would be wasted and, more importantly, the drug development may be delayed because patient enrollment is often the bottleneck of a trial.

**EXAMPLE 6.1**

A multi-center two-arm randomized phase III trial was designed to compare the combination of gemcitabine and docetaxel versus gemcitabine alone for treating patients with advanced or metastatic unresectable soft tissue sarcoma. Each patient received up to four courses of chemotherapy, with each course lasting for six weeks. The goal of the study was to compare progression-free survival (the primary objective) and overall survival (the secondary objective) between the two treatment groups.

## 6.1.1  Statistical Hypothesis

For ease of exposition, we consider a two-arm clinical trial with dichotomous outcomes. Let $p_1$ denote the response rate of the experimental drug, and let $p_2$ denote that of the standard drug. In the hypothesis testing, the null hypothesis states that there is no difference between the two treatments, while the alternative hypothesis claims that there exists a clinically meaningful difference between them:

$$H_0: p_1 = p_2 \quad \text{versus} \quad H_1: p_1 \neq p_2.$$

If the data provide enough evidence to support $H_1$, we would reject $H_0$ and claim that there is a significant difference between the two treatments. A type I error is rejection of $H_0$ given $H_0$ is true; a type II error is acceptance of $H_0$ given $H_1$ is true. The probabilities of committing the type I and type II errors are given by

$$\alpha = \Pr(\text{reject } H_0 \mid H_0 \text{ is true}),$$

and

$$\beta = \Pr(\text{accept } H_0 \mid H_1 \text{ is true}),$$

respectively. Power is defined as

$$\text{power} \equiv 1 - \beta = \Pr(\text{reject } H_0 \mid H_1 \text{ is true}).$$

The $p$-value of a statistical test is the probability of observing the sample statistics at least as extreme as the test statistic based on the data, assuming that $H_0$ is true. In general, the significance level of hypothesis testing is set at 0.05. If the $p$-value is smaller than 0.05, we claim that the statistical test is significant and thus reject the null hypothesis; otherwise, we accept (or fail to reject) the null hypothesis.

### 6.1.2   Classification of Phase III Trials

Depending on the study goal, a phase III clinical trial may be designed to test for

- any treatment difference: $p_1 \neq p_2$,

- superiority: $p_1 > p_2$,

- noninferiority: $p_1 > p_2 - \delta_N$, or

- equivalence: $|p_1 - p_2| < \delta_E$,

where $\delta_N > 0$ and $\delta_E > 0$ are called the noninferiority and equivalence margins, respectively.

It is more intuitive to illustrate these four types of clinical trials using the 95% confidence interval of $p_1 - p_2$. When we are concerned with any difference between the two treatments regardless of which one is better, the hypothesis test is two-sided with

$$H_0: p_1 = p_2 \quad \text{versus} \quad H_1: p_1 \neq p_2. \tag{6.1}$$

If the 95% confidence interval of $p_1 - p_2$ does not contain zero along either direction, we claim that there is a significant difference between the two treatments.

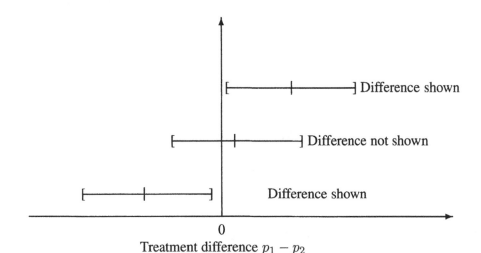

Treatment difference $p_1 - p_2$

Superiority trials aim to test whether the experimental drug is clinically superior to the standard treatment. Based on the one-sided hypothesis test,

$$H_0: p_1 \leq p_2 \quad \text{versus} \quad H_1: p_1 > p_2,$$

if the lower bound of the confidence interval of $p_1 - p_2$ does not cover zero, the experimental treatment is claimed to be superior to the standard treatment.

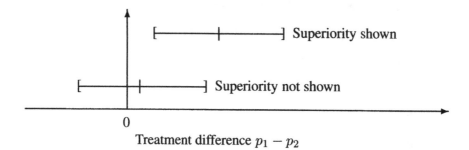

Treatment difference $p_1 - p_2$

Noninferiority trials intend to demonstrate that the therapeutic effect of the experimental treatment is not worse than that of the standard treatment by more than a prespecified noninferiority margin, $\delta_N > 0$. This corresponds to a one-sided hypothesis test with

$$H_0: p_1 \leq p_2 - \delta_N \quad \text{versus} \quad H_1: p_1 > p_2 - \delta_N.$$

In a noninferiority trial, the new treatment is expected to be at least similar to the existing therapy in terms of efficacy, while the advantages of the new treatment may include being more convenient to administer, inducing fewer side effects, or being less expensive.

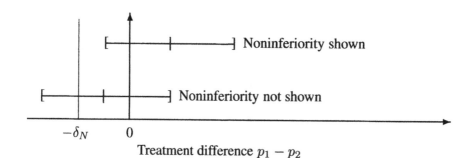

Treatment difference $p_1 - p_2$

To establish equivalence of two treatments, we need to specify the equivalence margin $\delta_E > 0$, which is the maximal difference between $p_1$ and $p_2$ that is considered clinically acceptable. In contrast to (6.1), the fundamental strategy for testing equivalence is to reverse the roles of the null and alternative hypotheses; that is,

$$H_0: |p_1 - p_2| \geq \delta_E \quad \text{versus} \quad H_1: |p_1 - p_2| < \delta_E.$$

The two treatments are claimed to be equivalent if the null hypothesis is rejected.

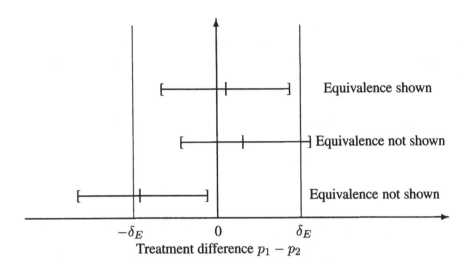

### 6.1.3  Superiority versus Noninferiority

Superiority and noninferiority often cause much confusion in clinical trial designs. A noninferiority trial is recommended for use only when the experimental treatment is not expected to be superior to the active control in a superiority trial. The use of a placebo is not allowed in a noninferiority trial. In general, noninferiority trials are more difficult to design, implement, and interpret, and they cannot be simply regarded as "underpowered" superiority trials.

In clinical trials, minimizing trial conduct errors and protocol deviations are of paramount importance. At the end of a superiority trial, the primary analysis is often based on the intent-to-treat (ITT) population, which consists of all the patients randomized regardless of their noncompliance, crossover, or dropouts. ITT analysis tends to draw the effectiveness of two treatments closer to each other; that is, the trial findings would be biased toward the null. On the other hand, the per-protocol (PP) analysis only includes the compliers who have strictly followed the protocol, which tends to exaggerate the treatment difference. In contrast to a superiority trial, the converse is true for a noninferiority trial: Misconduct such as patient noncompliance or missing data would bias the results toward the alternative. It is thus common to carry out both the ITT and PP analyses in the end, and expect the findings to be similar and interpretable. More discussions on ITT, PP, and other population-based analyses of clinical trials are given in Section 6.8.

In a noninferiority trial, if the 95% confidence interval for the treatment benefit excludes both the noninferiority margin and zero, we may directly claim superiority without the need to adjust for multiplicity due to the close testing principle (Moyé, 2003); see Section 6.6.1 for multiple testing issues. However, if a superiority trial fails to reject the null hypothesis, one cannot infer noninferiority as a backup. To claim noninferiority of an experimental therapy to the standard treatment, the noninferiority margin must be explicitly specified prior to the trial conduct. However, if a trial is designed as a superiority trial to begin with, there is no such a noninferiority margin specified in advance.

## 6.2  COMPARING MEANS FOR CONTINUOUS OUTCOMES

### 6.2.1  Testing for Equality

The sample size is calculated under the alternative hypothesis based on the type I error rate $\alpha$ and power $1 - \beta$. First of all, one needs to specify a clinically meaningful difference that is to be detected at the conclusion of the trial. Intuitively, if a small difference is expected between the two treatments in comparison, a large sample size would be required, and vice versa. Not only does the sample size estimation depend on the effect size, it also depends on the variance. The larger the variance, the harder it is to detect the difference and thus a larger sample size is needed.

Consider a two-sample comparison with continuous outcomes. Let $Y_{ik}$ be the observed outcome for the $i$th subject in the $k$th treatment arm, for $i = 1, \ldots, n_k$ and $k = 1, 2$. The outcomes in the two groups are assumed to be independent and normally distributed with different means but an equal variance $\sigma^2$,

$$Y_{ik} \sim \mathrm{N}(\mu_k, \sigma^2), \quad k = 1, 2.$$

Let $\theta = \mu_1 - \mu_2$, the difference in the mean between treatment 1 (the new therapy) and treatment 2 (the standard of care).

To test whether the effects of the two treatments are the same, we formulate the null and alternative hypotheses as

$$H_0: \theta = 0 \quad \text{versus} \quad H_1: \theta \neq 0.$$

Based on the observed data, we first construct a test statistic $T_n$ for discriminating $H_0$ and $H_1$, and then calculate the $p$-value by gauging the observed value of $T_n$ against its distribution under $H_0$. The hypothesis testing procedure assesses the strength of evidence contained in the data in favor of or against the null hypothesis. If the $p$-value is adequately small, say, less than 0.05 under a two-sided test, we reject the null hypothesis and claim that there is a significant difference between the two treatments; otherwise there is no significant difference.

More specifically, the sample mean for each group is given by

$$\bar{Y}_k = \frac{1}{n_k} \sum_{i=1}^{n_k} Y_{ik}, \quad k = 1, 2,$$

and the pooled-sample variance is

$$s_n^2 = \frac{1}{n_1 + n_2 - 2} \sum_{k=1}^{2} \sum_{i=1}^{n_k} (Y_{ik} - \bar{Y}_k)^2.$$

Then the two-sample $t$ test statistic is given by

$$T_n = \frac{\bar{Y}_1 - \bar{Y}_2}{s_n \sqrt{1/n_1 + 1/n_2}},$$

which follows a central $t_\nu$ distribution with $\nu = n_1 + n_2 - 2$ degrees of freedom under $H_0$, and a noncentral $t_\nu(c)$ distribution with a noncentrality parameter

$$c = \frac{\theta}{\sigma \sqrt{1/n_1 + 1/n_2}},$$

under $H_1$. The null hypothesis would be rejected, if $|T_n| \geq t_{\nu,\alpha/2}$, where the critical constant $t_{\nu,\alpha/2}$ is the $100(1-\alpha/2)$th percentile of the central $t$ distribution with $\nu$ degrees of freedom.

To determine the sample size, we need to control the type I error rate $\alpha$, and also to achieve power $1 - \beta$ under the alternative hypothesis. Let $\mathcal{T}(\cdot, c)$ denote the cumulative distribution function of the noncentral $t_\nu(c)$ distribution. Under $H_1$, the power of the two-sample $t$ test is given by

$$1 - \beta = 1 - \mathcal{T}(t_{\nu,\alpha/2}, c) + \mathcal{T}(-t_{\nu,\alpha/2}, c). \tag{6.2}$$

The sample size for the planned study can be solved from (6.2), which, however, does not have a closed form.

If the variance $\sigma^2$ is known, the test statistic becomes

$$T_n = \frac{\bar{Y}_1 - \bar{Y}_2}{\sigma \sqrt{1/n_1 + 1/n_2}},$$

which follows the standard normal distribution under $H_0$, and a normal distribution with a nonzero mean and a variance of one under $H_1$. In a two-sided test, the null hypothesis is rejected at a significance level of $\alpha$ if $|T_n| \geq z_{\alpha/2}$, where $z_{\alpha/2}$ is the $100(1 - \alpha/2)$th percentile of the standard normal distribution. The sample size calculation can be dramatically simplified based on normal distributions, and the sample size formula becomes more explicit.

We specify the treatment difference to be detected as $\theta$ and define

$$Z = \frac{\bar{Y}_1 - \bar{Y}_2 - \theta}{\sigma \sqrt{1/n_1 + 1/n_2}},$$

which is the standard normal random variable. Figure 6.1 shows the type I error rate and power in a two-sided hypothesis test. Under the alternative hypothesis,

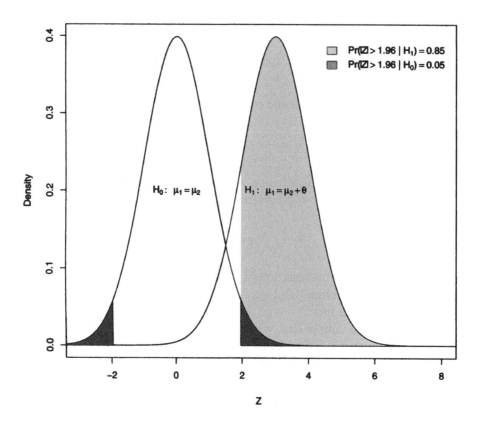

**Figure 6.1** Type I error rate and power under the null and alternative hypotheses based on normal distributions.

the power is given by

$$
\begin{aligned}
1 - \beta &= \Pr\left(\left|\frac{\bar{Y}_1 - \bar{Y}_2}{\sigma\sqrt{1/n_1 + 1/n_2}}\right| \geq z_{\alpha/2}\Big|H_1\right) \\
&= \Pr\left(Z \geq z_{\alpha/2} - \frac{\theta}{\sigma\sqrt{1/n_1 + 1/n_2}}\Big|H_1\right) \\
&\quad + \Pr\left(Z \leq -z_{\alpha/2} - \frac{\theta}{\sigma\sqrt{1/n_1 + 1/n_2}}\Big|H_1\right).
\end{aligned} \tag{6.3}
$$

We now consider the case with positive $\theta$ and that with negative $\theta$, separately. If $\theta > 0$, we can ignore the second term in (6.3) because it is smaller than $\alpha/2$, and then

$$
\beta \approx \Pr\left(Z \leq z_{\alpha/2} - \frac{\theta}{\sigma\sqrt{1/n_1 + 1/n_2}}\Big|H_1\right).
$$

Similarly if $\theta < 0$, we can ignore the first term in (6.3), and then

$$\beta \approx \Pr\left(Z \leq z_{\alpha/2} + \frac{\theta}{\sigma\sqrt{1/n_1 + 1/n_2}}\bigg| H_1\right).$$

By combining the $\theta$ positive and $\theta$ negative cases and ignoring the terms that are smaller than $\alpha/2$, (6.3) is simplified as

$$\beta \approx \Phi\left(z_{\alpha/2} - \frac{|\theta|}{\sigma\sqrt{1/n_1 + 1/n_2}}\right),$$

where $\Phi(\cdot)$ is the cumulative distribution function of the standard normal distribution. Therefore, the sample size is obtained by solving

$$\frac{|\theta|}{\sigma\sqrt{1/n_1 + 1/n_2}} = z_{\alpha/2} + z_\beta.$$

Using an equal allocation of the trial participants with $n_1 = n_2 = n/2$, the total sample size for the trial is

$$n = \frac{4\sigma^2(z_{\alpha/2} + z_\beta)^2}{\theta^2}.$$

Often in practice, relatively more patients are assigned to the new treatment than those to the standard treatment in order to learn more about the experimental drug. If the patient allocation ratio between arm 1 and arm 2 is $r = n_1/n_2$, then

$$n_1 = rn_2 \quad \text{and} \quad n_2 = \frac{(1 + 1/r)\sigma^2(z_{\alpha/2} + z_\beta)^2}{\theta^2}.$$

When using an unbalanced patient allocation, the total sample size needs to be increased in order to maintain the same power as that with a balanced allocation. Figure 6.2 shows that imbalance in the numbers of patients typically leads to some power loss.

**EXAMPLE 6.2**

Suppose that an experimental drug is compared with the standard treatment in terms of lowering a continuous biomarker measurement. The expected treatment difference is $\theta = 1$ and the variance is $\sigma^2 = 4$. If we conduct a two-sided normal $Z$-test at a significance level of $\alpha = 0.05$, the total sample size to achieve a power of 90% is 168, with 84 for each arm. If the assignment ratio between the new and standard treatments is 2:1 (i.e., $r = 2$), then we need 126 subjects in the experimental arm and 63 in the standard arm to achieve the same power 90%.

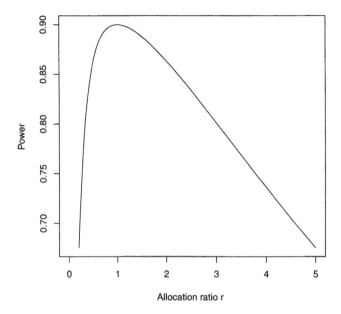

**Figure 6.2**    Power versus the allocation ratio with the total sample size fixed at $n = 168$ and the significance level $\alpha = 0.05$.

### 6.2.2  Superiority Trial

In a superiority trial, one is interested in assessing whether the new treatment is better than the standard treatment. This can be formulated in a one-sided hypothesis test with

$$H_0\colon \theta \leq 0 \quad \text{versus} \quad H_1\colon \theta > 0.$$

Under $H_1$, we choose a clinically meaningful difference $\theta > 0$ and define

$$Z = \frac{\bar{Y}_1 - \bar{Y}_2 - \theta}{\sigma\sqrt{1/n_1 + 1/n_2}},$$

which follows the standard normal distribution. In a one-sided test, the power is given by

$$
\begin{aligned}
1 - \beta &= \Pr\!\left(\frac{\bar{Y}_1 - \bar{Y}_2}{\sigma\sqrt{1/n_1 + 1/n_2}} \geq z_\alpha \middle| H_1\right) \\
&= \Pr\!\left(Z \geq z_\alpha - \frac{\theta}{\sigma\sqrt{1/n_1 + 1/n_2}} \middle| H_1\right),
\end{aligned}
$$

which leads to

$$\frac{\theta}{\sigma\sqrt{1/n_1 + 1/n_2}} = z_\alpha + z_\beta.$$

If the numbers of patients in the two groups are the same with $n_1 = n_2 = n/2$, then the total sample size is

$$n = \frac{4\sigma^2(z_\alpha + z_\beta)^2}{\theta^2},$$

and if the patient allocation is unequal with $n_1 = rn_2$, then

$$n_2 = \frac{(1 + 1/r)\sigma^2(z_\alpha + z_\beta)^2}{\theta^2}.$$

### 6.2.3  Noninferiority Trial

In a noninferiority trial, we are interested in examining whether the new treatment is not worse than the standard treatment by a noninferiority margin, $\delta_N > 0$. The threshold $\delta_N$ specifies the lower bound beyond which the experimental drug is considered unacceptably inferior to the standard drug. In a one-sided hypothesis test with

$$H_0\colon \theta \le -\delta_N \quad \text{versus} \quad H_1\colon \theta > -\delta_N,$$

by rejecting $H_0$, the experimental treatment would be claimed to be noninferior to the standard treatment.

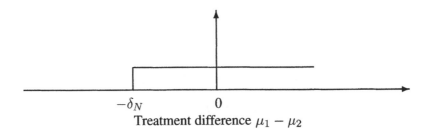

Treatment difference $\mu_1 - \mu_2$

It is critical to choose an appropriate noninferiority margin in such a trial. The noninferiority margin typically should not be larger than the smallest effect size that the standard treatment (active control) would be expected to have in comparison with a placebo. The noninferiority margin $\delta_N$ can be determined based on

- the clinical rationale, for example, $\delta_N$ is specified as the maximum difference that the investigator would tolerate;

- regulatory requirements using the information from previous trials; or

- the statistical "putative placebo" approach, that is to preserve a relevant proportion of the benefit of the active control over the placebo in historical studies.

The sample size for a noninferiority trial is determined as follows. In a one-sided noninferiority test, the null hypothesis is rejected at a significance level of $\alpha$, if

$$\frac{\bar{Y}_1 - \bar{Y}_2 + \delta_N}{\sigma\sqrt{1/n_1 + 1/n_2}} \geq z_\alpha.$$

Define the standard normal variable

$$Z = \frac{\bar{Y}_1 - \bar{Y}_2 - \theta}{\sigma\sqrt{1/n_1 + 1/n_2}},$$

and the power is given by

$$1 - \beta = \Pr\left(\frac{\bar{Y}_1 - \bar{Y}_2 + \delta_N}{\sigma\sqrt{1/n_1 + 1/n_2}} \geq z_\alpha \Big| H_1\right)$$

$$= \Pr\left(Z \geq z_\alpha - \frac{\delta_N + \theta}{\sigma\sqrt{1/n_1 + 1/n_2}} \Big| H_1\right),$$

which leads to

$$\frac{\theta + \delta_N}{\sigma\sqrt{1/n_1 + 1/n_2}} = z_\alpha + z_\beta.$$

If the numbers of patients in the two groups are equal with $n_1 = n_2 = n/2$, then the total sample size is

$$n = \frac{4\sigma^2(z_\alpha + z_\beta)^2}{(\theta + \delta_N)^2}.$$

If the numbers of patients in the two groups are different with $n_1 = rn_2$, then

$$n_2 = \frac{(1 + 1/r)\sigma^2(z_\alpha + z_\beta)^2}{(\theta + \delta_N)^2}.$$

Often in a noninferiority trial, the true mean difference is assumed to be zero (i.e., $\theta = 0$), when estimating the sample size. Because the noninferiority margin $\delta_N$ is typically smaller than the specified treatment difference in a superiority trial, the sample size required for a noninferiority trial is in general much larger than that for a superiority trial.

### 6.2.4  Equivalence Trial

In practice, the therapeutic effects of two treatments cannot be shown to be exactly the same. Equivalence trials aim to demonstrate that the difference between two treatments is less than a prespecified equivalence margin, $\delta_E > 0$. If the therapeutic effects of two treatments differ by more than the equivalence margin along either direction, the equivalence does not hold. Sometimes, a noninferiority trial is also called an equivalence trial because we are only concerned about whether the new treatment is not worse than the standard treatment.

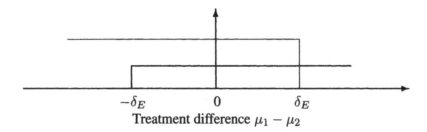

Treatment difference $\mu_1 - \mu_2$

An equivalence trial formulates the null and alternative hypotheses as

$$H_0 \colon |\theta| \geq \delta_E \quad \text{versus} \quad H_1 \colon |\theta| < \delta_E.$$

The null hypothesis $H_0$ would be rejected, leading to the equivalence of two treatments, if

$$\frac{\bar{Y}_1 - \bar{Y}_2 + \delta_E}{\sigma\sqrt{1/n_1 + 1/n_2}} \geq z_\alpha \quad \text{and} \quad \frac{\bar{Y}_1 - \bar{Y}_2 - \delta_E}{\sigma\sqrt{1/n_1 + 1/n_2}} \leq -z_\alpha.$$

The rejection region can be rewritten as

$$z_\alpha - \frac{\delta_E}{\sigma\sqrt{1/n_1 + 1/n_2}} \leq \frac{\bar{Y}_1 - \bar{Y}_2}{\sigma\sqrt{1/n_1 + 1/n_2}} \leq -z_\alpha + \frac{\delta_E}{\sigma\sqrt{1/n_1 + 1/n_2}}.$$

As defined before, let

$$Z = \frac{\bar{Y}_1 - \bar{Y}_2 - \theta}{\sigma\sqrt{1/n_1 + 1/n_2}} \sim \mathrm{N}(0, 1).$$

Under $H_1$, the power is given by

$$1 - \beta = \Pr\left( z_\alpha - \frac{\delta_E + \theta}{\sigma\sqrt{1/n_1 + 1/n_2}} \leq Z \leq -z_\alpha + \frac{\delta_E - \theta}{\sigma\sqrt{1/n_1 + 1/n_2}} \Big| H_1 \right)$$

$$= \Phi\left( -z_\alpha + \frac{\delta_E - \theta}{\sigma\sqrt{1/n_1 + 1/n_2}} \right) - \Phi\left( z_\alpha - \frac{\delta_E + \theta}{\sigma\sqrt{1/n_1 + 1/n_2}} \right).$$

In a conservative derivation with no power inflation, we have that

$$1 - \beta \approx 2\Phi\left( -z_\alpha + \frac{\delta_E - |\theta|}{\sigma\sqrt{1/n_1 + 1/n_2}} \right) - 1,$$

which leads to

$$\frac{\delta_E - |\theta|}{\sigma\sqrt{1/n_1 + 1/n_2}} = z_\alpha + z_{\beta/2}.$$

If the sample sizes of the two groups are the same with $n_1 = n_2 = n/2$, then the total sample size is

$$n = \frac{4\sigma^2(z_\alpha + z_{\beta/2})^2}{(\delta_E - |\theta|)^2}.$$

If the sample sizes of the two groups are different with $n_1 = rn_2$, then

$$n_2 = \frac{(1 + 1/r)\sigma^2(z_\alpha + z_{\beta/2})^2}{(\delta_E - |\theta|)^2},$$

where $\theta$ is often set as zero in practice.

**EXAMPLE 6.3**

Most of the equivalence trials compare a generic drug with the originally approved drug, aiming to establish bioequivalence. The two drugs are generally expected to have similar pharmacokinetic profiles. A bioequivalence trial often uses the 90% rather than the 95% confidence interval. In a clinical trial with cardiovascular disease, both the experimental and the standard therapies target lowering a continuous measurement, such as the blood pressure or cholesterol level. The study is to establish equivalence of the two treatments in terms of therapeutic effects with an equivalence margin $\delta_E = 0.2$. The variance of the medical measurements is estimated as 1 from previous studies. With a type I error rate $\alpha = 0.1$, we need a total sample size of 740 patients in order to achieve a power of 85%.

## 6.3 COMPARING PROPORTIONS FOR BINARY OUTCOMES

### 6.3.1 Testing for Equality

In many clinical trials, the primary endpoint is dichotomous, for example, whether a patient has responded to the treatment, or whether a patient has experienced toxicity. More specifically, consider a two-arm randomized trial with binary outcomes. Let $p_1$ denote the response rate of the experimental drug, $p_2$ as that of the standard drug, and the difference is $\theta = p_1 - p_2$. Let $Y_{ik}$ be the binary outcome for subject $i$ in arm $k$; that is,

$$Y_{ik} = \begin{cases} 1, & \text{with probability } p_k, \\ 0, & \text{with probability } 1 - p_k, \end{cases}$$

for $i = 1, \ldots, n_k$ and $k = 1, 2$. The sum of i.i.d. Bernoulli random variables follows a binomial distribution,

$$\sum_{i=1}^{n_k} Y_{ik} \sim \text{Bin}(n_k, p_k), \quad k = 1, 2.$$

The sample proportion for arm $k$ is

$$\bar{Y}_k = \frac{1}{n_k} \sum_{i=1}^{n_k} Y_{ik}, \quad k = 1, 2,$$

and $\text{E}(\bar{Y}_k) = p_k$ and $\text{Var}(\bar{Y}_k) = p_k(1 - p_k)/n_k$.

To test whether there is any difference between $p_1$ and $p_2$, we formulate a two-sided hypothesis with

$$H_0 \colon \theta = 0 \quad \text{versus} \quad H_1 \colon \theta \neq 0. \tag{6.4}$$

Under the null hypothesis, we may construct a test statistic

$$T_n = \frac{\bar{Y}_1 - \bar{Y}_2}{\sqrt{\bar{Y}(1 - \bar{Y})(1/n_1 + 1/n_2)}},$$

where $\bar{Y}$ is the pooled-sample mean,

$$\bar{Y} = \frac{n_1 \bar{Y}_1}{n_1 + n_2} + \frac{n_2 \bar{Y}_2}{n_1 + n_2}.$$

Noting that $\bar{Y}$ is a consistent estimator of

$$\bar{p} = \frac{n_1 p_1}{n_1 + n_2} + \frac{n_2 p_2}{n_1 + n_2},$$

the test statistic can be approximated by

$$T_n \approx \frac{\bar{Y}_1 - \bar{Y}_2}{\sqrt{\bar{p}(1 - \bar{p})(1/n_1 + 1/n_2)}}. \tag{6.5}$$

Under the null hypothesis, $T_n$ follows the standard normal distribution,

$$T_n | H_0 \sim \text{N}(0, 1),$$

and under the alternative hypothesis,

$$T_n | H_1 \sim \text{N}\left( \frac{\theta}{\sqrt{\bar{p}(1 - \bar{p})(1/n_1 + 1/n_2)}}, \frac{p_1(1 - p_1)/n_1 + p_2(1 - p_2)/n_2}{\bar{p}(1 - \bar{p})(1/n_1 + 1/n_2)} \right).$$

We control the type I error rate at $\alpha$, specify the treatment difference to be detected as $\theta$, and define the standard normal random variable

$$Z = \frac{\bar{Y}_1 - \bar{Y}_2 - \theta}{\sqrt{p_1(1-p_1)/n_1 + p_2(1-p_2)/n_2}}. \tag{6.6}$$

The sample size is computed under $H_1$ to achieve a power of $1 - \beta$,

$$
\begin{aligned}
1 - \beta &= \Pr\left(\left|\frac{\bar{Y}_1 - \bar{Y}_2}{\sqrt{\bar{p}(1-\bar{p})(1/n_1 + 1/n_2)}}\right| \geq z_{\alpha/2}\Big|H_1\right) \\
&= \Pr\left(Z \geq \frac{z_{\alpha/2}\sqrt{\bar{p}(1-\bar{p})(1/n_1 + 1/n_2)} - \theta}{\sqrt{p_1(1-p_1)/n_1 + p_2(1-p_2)/n_2}}\Big|H_1\right) \\
&\quad + \Pr\left(Z \leq \frac{-z_{\alpha/2}\sqrt{\bar{p}(1-\bar{p})(1/n_1 + 1/n_2)} - \theta}{\sqrt{p_1(1-p_1)/n_1 + p_2(1-p_2)/n_2}}\Big|H_1\right).
\end{aligned}
$$

Similar to the case with normally distributed endpoints in (6.3), we simplify the derivation by ignoring the term that is smaller than $\alpha/2$ in the situations with $\theta > 0$ and $\theta < 0$, respectively. So for $\theta > 0$,

$$\beta \approx \Pr\left(Z \leq \frac{z_{\alpha/2}\sqrt{\bar{p}(1-\bar{p})(1/n_1 + 1/n_2)} - \theta}{\sqrt{p_1(1-p_1)/n_1 + p_2(1-p_2)/n_2}}\Big|H_1\right),$$

and for $\theta < 0$,

$$\beta \approx \Pr\left(Z \leq \frac{z_{\alpha/2}\sqrt{\bar{p}(1-\bar{p})(1/n_1 + 1/n_2)} + \theta}{\sqrt{p_1(1-p_1)/n_1 + p_2(1-p_2)/n_2}}\Big|H_1\right).$$

Therefore,

$$\beta \approx \Phi\left(\frac{z_{\alpha/2}\sqrt{\bar{p}(1-\bar{p})(1/n_1 + 1/n_2)} - |\theta|}{\sqrt{p_1(1-p_1)/n_1 + p_2(1-p_2)/n_2}}\right),$$

and the sample size can be obtained by solving

$$|\theta| = z_{\alpha/2}\sqrt{\bar{p}(1-\bar{p})\left(\frac{1}{n_1} + \frac{1}{n_2}\right)} + z_\beta\sqrt{\frac{p_1(1-p_1)}{n_1} + \frac{p_2(1-p_2)}{n_2}}.$$

If $n_1 = n_2 = n/2$, then the total sample size is

$$n = \frac{2}{\theta^2}\left\{z_{\alpha/2}\sqrt{2\bar{p}(1-\bar{p})} + z_\beta\sqrt{p_1(1-p_1) + p_2(1-p_2)}\right\}^2, \tag{6.7}$$

and if $n_1 = rn_2$, then

$$n_2 = \frac{1 + 1/r}{\theta^2}\left\{z_{\alpha/2}\sqrt{\bar{p}(1-\bar{p})} + z_\beta\sqrt{\frac{p_1(1-p_1)/r + p_2(1-p_2)}{1 + 1/r}}\right\}^2.$$

### 6.3.2  Sample Size Formula with Unpooled Variance

In the derivation of the sample size formula (6.7), the samples in the two groups are pooled together under the null hypothesis to estimate the variance. However, if we do not pool the samples, a slightly different but simpler sample size formula can be derived. Under the same two-sided hypothesis as in (6.4), we consider the test statistic

$$T_n = \frac{\bar{Y}_1 - \bar{Y}_2}{\sqrt{\bar{Y}_1(1 - \bar{Y}_1)/n_1 + \bar{Y}_2(1 - \bar{Y}_2)/n_2}},$$

which can be approximated by

$$T_n \approx \frac{\bar{Y}_1 - \bar{Y}_2}{\sqrt{p_1(1 - p_1)/n_1 + p_2(1 - p_2)/n_2}}. \tag{6.8}$$

Under the null hypothesis,

$$T_n | H_0 \sim \mathrm{N}(0, 1),$$

and under the alternative hypothesis,

$$T_n | H_1 \sim \mathrm{N}\left(\frac{\theta}{\sqrt{p_1(1 - p_1)/n_1 + p_2(1 - p_2)/n_2}}, 1\right).$$

Given the specified effect size $\theta$, the power is given by

$$1 - \beta = \Pr\left(\left|\frac{\bar{Y}_1 - \bar{Y}_2}{\sqrt{p_1(1 - p_1)/n_1 + p_2(1 - p_2)/n_2}}\right| \ge z_{\alpha/2}\Big|H_1\right)$$

$$= \Pr\left(Z \ge z_{\alpha/2} - \frac{\theta}{\sqrt{p_1(1 - p_1)/n_1 + p_2(1 - p_2)/n_2}}\Big|H_1\right)$$

$$+ \Pr\left(Z \le -z_{\alpha/2} - \frac{\theta}{\sqrt{p_1(1 - p_1)/n_1 + p_2(1 - p_2)/n_2}}\Big|H_1\right),$$

where $Z$ is defined the same as in (6.6). If we ignore the term that is smaller than $\alpha/2$ when considering $\theta > 0$ and $\theta < 0$, respectively, then

$$\beta \approx \Phi\left(z_{\alpha/2} - \frac{|\theta|}{\sqrt{p_1(1 - p_1)/n_1 + p_2(1 - p_2)/n_2}}\right),$$

and the sample size can be obtained by solving

$$\frac{|\theta|}{\sqrt{p_1(1 - p_1)/n_1 + p_2(1 - p_2)/n_2}} = z_{\alpha/2} + z_\beta.$$

If $n_1 = n_2 = n/2$, then the total sample size is

$$n = \frac{2(z_{\alpha/2} + z_\beta)^2}{\theta^2} \{p_1(1 - p_1) + p_2(1 - p_2)\}, \qquad (6.9)$$

and if $n_1 = rn_2$, then

$$n_2 = \frac{(z_{\alpha/2} + z_\beta)^2}{\theta^2} \{p_1(1 - p_1)/r + p_2(1 - p_2)\}.$$

### EXAMPLE 6.4

Suppose that the standard treatment has a response rate of 30% for metastatic breast cancer patients, and the new treatment is expected to improve the response rate with an increment of 10%. Under this setup, we have that $p_1 = 0.4$, $p_2 = 0.3$, and $\theta = 0.1$. We take a two-sided test with a type I error rate of $\alpha = 0.05$ and a power of 90%. Based on (6.7), the total sample size for this study is 952 patients, with 476 in each arm. Using the alternative sample size formula in (6.9), we need 946 subjects in total, with 473 in each arm.

## 6.3.3 Superiority Trial

Superiority trials are designed to assess whether the new treatment is better than the standard treatment, for which a one-sided hypothesis is formulated as

$$H_0\colon \theta \le 0 \quad \text{versus} \quad H_1\colon \theta > 0.$$

After we specify a clinically meaningful difference $\theta > 0$ under $H_1$, the sample size is determined as follows. The power is given by

$$1 - \beta = \Pr\left( Z \ge \frac{z_\alpha \sqrt{\bar{p}(1 - \bar{p})(1/n_1 + 1/n_2)} - \theta}{\sqrt{p_1(1 - p_1)/n_1 + p_2(1 - p_2)/n_2}} \middle| H_1 \right),$$

where $Z$ is the standard normal variable defined as

$$Z = \frac{\bar{Y}_1 - \bar{Y}_2 - \theta}{\sqrt{p_1(1 - p_1)/n_1 + p_2(1 - p_2)/n_2}}.$$

Therefore, the sample size can be obtained by solving

$$\theta = z_\alpha \sqrt{\bar{p}(1 - \bar{p})\left(\frac{1}{n_1} + \frac{1}{n_2}\right)} + z_\beta \sqrt{\frac{p_1(1 - p_1)}{n_1} + \frac{p_2(1 - p_2)}{n_2}}.$$

If $n_1 = n_2 = n/2$, then the total sample size for the trial is

$$n = \frac{2}{\theta^2} \left\{ z_\alpha \sqrt{2\bar{p}(1 - \bar{p})} + z_\beta \sqrt{p_1(1 - p_1) + p_2(1 - p_2)} \right\}^2,$$

and if $n_1 = rn_2$, then

$$n_2 = \frac{1 + 1/r}{\theta^2} \left\{ z_\alpha \sqrt{\bar{p}(1 - \bar{p})} + z_\beta \sqrt{\frac{p_1(1 - p_1)/r + p_2(1 - p_2)}{1 + 1/r}} \right\}^2.$$

If we use the test statistic in (6.8) without pooling two samples for the variance estimation, the sample size formula for a superiority trial would be slightly different. If $n_1 = n_2 = n/2$, then the total sample size is

$$n = \frac{2(z_\alpha + z_\beta)^2}{\theta^2} \{p_1(1 - p_1) + p_2(1 - p_2)\},$$

and if $n_1 = rn_2$, then

$$n_2 = \frac{(z_\alpha + z_\beta)^2}{\theta^2} \{p_1(1 - p_1)/r + p_2(1 - p_2)\}.$$

**EXAMPLE 6.5**

If the response rate of the standard chemotherapy for prostate cancer is 20%, and we expect that the experimental drug would double the response rate of the standard treatment, so $p_1 = 0.4$ and $p_2 = 0.2$. In a one-sided test, we specify the type I error rate $\alpha = 0.025$ and power 80%. The total sample size required for such a superiority trial is 162 patients. If the allocation ratio between the experimental and the standard arms is 3:1, we need 159 and 53 subjects in the experimental and standard arms, respectively.

### 6.3.4  Noninferiority Trial

Noninferiority trials are conducted to assess whether the new treatment is not worse than the standard treatment by a noninferiority margin, $\delta_N > 0$. The hypothesis test for a noninferiority trial is one-sided, which is formulated as

$$H_0: \theta \leq -\delta_N \quad \text{versus} \quad H_1: \theta > -\delta_N.$$

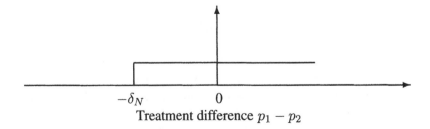
Treatment difference $p_1 - p_2$

The sample size for a noninferiority trial is determined as follows. The null hypothesis is rejected at a significance level of $\alpha$, if

$$\frac{\bar{Y}_1 - \bar{Y}_2 + \delta_N}{\sqrt{\bar{p}(1 - \bar{p})(1/n_1 + 1/n_2)}} \geq z_\alpha.$$

Define the standard normal random variable

$$Z = \frac{\bar{Y}_1 - \bar{Y}_2 - \theta}{\sqrt{p_1(1 - p_1)/n_1 + p_2(1 - p_2)/n_2}},$$

and the power is given by

$$1 - \beta = \Pr\left( Z \geq \frac{z_\alpha\sqrt{\bar{p}(1 - \bar{p})(1/n_1 + 1/n_2)} - (\theta + \delta_N)}{\sqrt{p_1(1 - p_1)/n_1 + p_2(1 - p_2)/n_2}} \Big| H_1 \right).$$

Therefore, the sample size can be obtained by solving

$$\theta + \delta_N = z_\alpha\sqrt{\bar{p}(1 - \bar{p})\left(\frac{1}{n_1} + \frac{1}{n_2}\right)} + z_\beta\sqrt{\frac{p_1(1 - p_1)}{n_1} + \frac{p_2(1 - p_2)}{n_2}}.$$

If $n_1 = n_2 = n/2$, then the total sample size is

$$n = \frac{2}{(\theta + \delta_N)^2}\left\{ z_\alpha\sqrt{2\bar{p}(1 - \bar{p})} + z_\beta\sqrt{p_1(1 - p_1) + p_2(1 - p_2)} \right\}^2,$$

and if $n_1 = rn_2$, then

$$n_2 = \frac{1 + 1/r}{(\theta + \delta_N)^2}\left\{ z_\alpha\sqrt{\bar{p}(1 - \bar{p})} + z_\beta\sqrt{\frac{p_1(1 - p_1)/r + p_2(1 - p_2)}{1 + 1/r}} \right\}^2.$$

If we use the test statistic in (6.8) without pooling two samples for the variance estimation, the sample size formula for a noninferiority trial would be slightly different. If $n_1 = n_2 = n/2$, then the total sample size is

$$n = \frac{2(z_\alpha + z_\beta)^2}{(\theta + \delta_N)^2}\{p_1(1 - p_1) + p_2(1 - p_2)\},$$

and if $n_1 = rn_2$, then

$$n_2 = \frac{(z_\alpha + z_\beta)^2}{(\theta + \delta_N)^2}\{p_1(1 - p_1)/r + p_2(1 - p_2)\}.$$

In practice, we typically take $p_1 = p_2$ for a noninferiority trial; that is, $\theta = 0$. The sample size for a noninferiority trial heavily depends on the choice of the noninferiority margin $\delta_N$. In the following example, we illustrate how to specify $\delta_N$ using the "putative placebo" approach, which preserves a certain proportion of the benefit of the standard treatment versus placebo.

**EXAMPLE 6.6**

We are interested in testing whether a new drug is noninferior to the standard of care, while the new treatment is less toxic and easier to administer. From the statistical perspective, we first estimate the treatment difference between the active control (the standard treatment) and the placebo based on previous studies. Suppose that the estimated difference of the response rates between the active control and placebo is 20%, with a 95% confidence interval of $[0.16, 0.24]$. We may set $\delta_N$ as one half of the minimal estimated difference between the active control and placebo (the lower bound of the 95% confidence interval), that is, $\delta_N = 0.08$. For a one-sided test with $\alpha = 0.025$ and power $= 80\%$, we take $p_1 = p_2 = 0.2$, and thus the sample size required for the trial is 785.

### 6.3.5 Equivalence Trial

Equivalence trials are designed to demonstrate that the difference of the therapeutic effects between two treatments is less than a prespecified equivalence margin, $\delta_E > 0$. For this purpose, a one-sided hypothesis can be formulated as

$$H_0: |\theta| \geq \delta_E \quad \text{versus} \quad H_1: |\theta| < \delta_E.$$

The null hypothesis is rejected at a significance level of $\alpha$, if

$$z_\alpha - \frac{\delta_E}{\sqrt{\bar{p}(1-\bar{p})(1/n_1 + 1/n_2)}} \leq T_n \leq -z_\alpha + \frac{\delta_E}{\sqrt{\bar{p}(1-\bar{p})(1/n_1 + 1/n_2)}},$$

where $T_n$ is defined the same as (6.5).

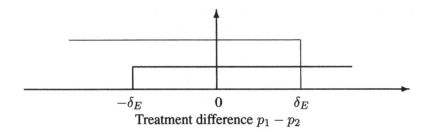

Treatment difference $p_1 - p_2$

Under $H_1$, the power is given by

$$1 - \beta \approx 2\Phi\left(\frac{-z_\alpha\sqrt{\bar{p}(1-\bar{p})(1/n_1 + 1/n_2)} + \delta_E - |\theta|}{\sqrt{p_1(1-p_1)/n_1 + p_2(1-p_2)/n_2}}\right) - 1.$$

Therefore, the sample size can be obtained by solving

$$\delta_E - |\theta| = z_\alpha\sqrt{\bar{p}(1-\bar{p})\left(\frac{1}{n_1} + \frac{1}{n_2}\right)} + z_{\beta/2}\sqrt{\frac{p_1(1-p_1)}{n_1} + \frac{p_2(1-p_2)}{n_2}}.$$

If $n_1 = n_2 = n/2$, then the total sample size is

$$n = \frac{2}{(\delta_E - |\theta|)^2} \left\{ z_\alpha \sqrt{2\bar{p}(1-\bar{p})} + z_{\beta/2} \sqrt{p_1(1-p_1) + p_2(1-p_2)} \right\}^2,$$

and if $n_1 = rn_2$, then

$$n_2 = \frac{1+1/r}{(\delta_E - |\theta|)^2} \left\{ z_\alpha \sqrt{\bar{p}(1-\bar{p})} + z_{\beta/2} \sqrt{\frac{p_1(1-p_1)/r + p_2(1-p_2)}{1+1/r}} \right\}^2.$$

As in Section 6.3.2, if we take the test statistic in (6.8) for an equivalence trial, a different sample size formula can be derived. If $n_1 = n_2 = n/2$, then the total sample size is

$$n = \frac{2(z_\alpha + z_{\beta/2})^2}{(\delta_E - |\theta|)^2} \{ p_1(1-p_1) + p_2(1-p_2) \},$$

and if $n_1 = rn_2$, then

$$n_2 = \frac{(z_\alpha + z_{\beta/2})^2}{(\delta_E - |\theta|)^2} \{ p_1(1-p_1)/r + p_2(1-p_2) \}.$$

## 6.4  SAMPLE SIZE WITH SURVIVAL DATA

### 6.4.1  Comparison of Survival Curves

In clinical trials with continuous or binary endpoints, responses of patients are typically observed immediately or shortly after treatment. However, for cancer and other chronic diseases, it is often of interest to compare the duration of the time from treatment till occurrence of an event (e.g., disease progression or death) between different groups. Phase III trials often collect such time-to-event data to examine whether there are survival differences between treatment groups. As discussed in Section 3.3, survival data are subject to right censoring due to loss of follow-up, interim data monitoring, or the termination of the study.

Consider a two-arm trial, and let $T_{ik}$ denote the failure time of subject $i$ in arm $k$, for $i = 1, \ldots, n_k$ and $k = 1, 2$. Correspondingly, let $C_{ik}$ denote the censoring time, and we observe $X_{ik} = \min(T_{ik}, C_{ik})$ and the censoring indicator $\Delta_{ik} = I(T_{ik} \le C_{ik})$, where $I(\cdot)$ is the indicator function. Under the independent censoring assumption, the survival function for each group, $S_k(t) = P(T_{ik} > t)$, can be estimated using the Kaplan–Meier (1958) estimator. Let $\lambda_k(t)$ be the hazard function for group $k$, and thus $\lambda_k(t) = -\mathrm{d}\log S_k(t)/\mathrm{d}t$.

The null hypothesis states that there is no difference in patients' survival between the two groups,

$$H_0 \colon S_1(t) = S_2(t) \quad \text{or} \quad \lambda_1(t) = \lambda_2(t), \quad \text{for all } t,$$

while the alternative hypothesis claims that $H_1$: $S_1(t) \neq S_2(t)$ for some $t$. The log-rank test is most powerful when the hazards of the two groups are proportional to each other under the alternative hypothesis,

$$H_1: \lambda_1(t) = \lambda_2(t)e^\theta \quad \text{or} \quad \log \lambda_1(t) - \log \lambda_2(t) = \theta.$$

If $\theta > 0$ (i.e., the hazard ratio $e^\theta > 1$), patients in arm 1 are at a higher risk, resulting in worse survival, than those in arm 2; if $\theta = 0$ (i.e., $e^\theta = 1$), there is no survival difference between the two arms, implying that $H_0$ is true; and if $\theta < 0$ (i.e., $e^\theta < 1$), patients in arm 1 have better survival than those in arm 2.

To construct the log-rank test, we first order all the distinct failure times in the pooled samples. Let $m$ denote the total number of distinct failure times. For $i = 1, \ldots, m$, at each of the distinct failure times, we organize the data in a $2 \times 2$ contingency table as follows,

|  | Arm 1 | Arm 2 |  |
|---|---|---|---|
| Number of failures | $D_{1i}$ | $D_{2i}$ | $D_i$ |
| Number of survivors | $R_{1i} - D_{1i}$ | $R_{2i} - D_{2i}$ | $R_i - D_i$ |
| Number of subjects at risk | $R_{1i}$ | $R_{2i}$ | $R_i$ |

As in the Mantel–Haenszel test for multiple $2 \times 2$ tables, $D_{1i}$ follows a hypergeometric distribution conditional on all the marginal counts under $H_0$. After standardization, the log-rank test statistic is given by

$$T_n = \frac{\sum_{i=1}^m (D_{1i} - R_{1i}D_i/R_i)}{\left[ \sum_{i=1}^m R_{1i}R_{2i}D_i(R_i - D_i)/\{R_i^2(R_i - 1)\} \right]^{1/2}}, \qquad (6.10)$$

which asymptotically follows the standard normal distribution under $H_0$.

### 6.4.2  Parametric Approach under Exponential Distribution

In survival analysis, the number of events rather than the number of subjects is more relevant. After entering a trial over a period of accrual time, patients are followed till the occurrence of the event of interest or being censored. If we assume an exponential distribution for the survival time, $T \sim \text{Exp}(\lambda)$, the survival function and the hazard function are given by

$$S(t) = \exp(-\lambda t) \quad \text{and} \quad \lambda(t) = \lambda,$$

respectively. The median survival time is $\lambda^{-1} \log 2$, the mean survival time $\text{E}(T) = 1/\lambda$, and $\text{Var}(T) = 1/\lambda^2$.

Consider a two-arm clinical trial with an equal allocation of the number of patients. Let $\lambda_k(t) = \lambda_k$ be the constant hazard for group $k$, $k = 1, 2$. We are interested in testing a one-sided hypothesis,

$$H_0: \lambda_1 = \lambda_2 \quad \text{versus} \quad H_1: \lambda_1 > \lambda_2,$$

which is equivalent to testing whether the mean or the median survival times are the same across the two groups.

Heuristically speaking, when the number of events is relatively small compared with the number of patients at risk, the variance in (6.10) can be approximated as

$$\sum_{i=1}^{m} \frac{R_{1i} R_{2i} D_i (R_i - D_i)}{R_i^2 (R_i - 1)} \approx \sum_{i=1}^{m} \frac{R_{1i} R_{2i} D_i}{R_i^2}.$$

If the log hazard ratio $\theta$ is small and the accrual rate for each treatment group is similar, then $R_{1i} \approx R_{2i} \approx R_i/2$, and the variance of the log-rank statistic can be further simplified to $\sum_{i=1}^{m} D_i/4 = D/4$, where $D$ is the total number of events, $D = \sum_{i=1}^{m} D_i \approx nP(\Delta = 1)$, and $\Delta$ is the censoring indicator.

Under the null hypothesis, $H_0$: $\lambda_1 = \lambda_2$,

$$T_n | H_0 \sim N(0, 1),$$

and under the alternative hypothesis, $H_1$: $\lambda_1/\lambda_2 = \exp(\theta)$, with $\theta > 0$,

$$T_n | H_1 \sim N(\sqrt{D}\theta/2, 1),$$

where the mean of $T_n$ under $H_1$ can be derived using similar arguments as those in Schoenfeld (1981) and Collett (1994). Therefore, for a one-sided test to maintain a type I error rate of $\alpha$ and achieve a power of $1 - \beta$, the number of events required for a trial is

$$D = \frac{4(z_\alpha + z_\beta)^2}{\theta^2}.$$

In a clinical trial, let $\tau_a$ be the accrual period, and let $\tau_f$ be the follow-up period, then the entire trial duration is $\tau_a + \tau_f$.

If $a(t)$ denotes the accrual rate at calendar time $t$, the total number of subjects to be enrolled in the study is

$$n = \int_0^{\tau_a} a(t)\, dt.$$

If we only consider administrative censoring by the end of the study, the number of expected events is

$$D = \int_0^{\tau_a} a(t) \left[ 1 - \frac{1}{2} \{ S_1(\tau_a + \tau_f - t) + S_2(\tau_a + \tau_f - t) \} \right] dt,$$

where $S_1(\cdot)$ and $S_2(\cdot)$ are the survival functions for the experimental and standard arms, respectively. Furthermore, if the accrual rate is constant, $a(t) = a$, then under the exponential assumption for the survival time,

$$D = a \left[ \tau_a - \frac{\exp(\lambda_1 \tau_a) - 1}{2\lambda_1 \exp\{\lambda_1(\tau_a + \tau_f)\}} - \frac{\exp(\lambda_2 \tau_a) - 1}{2\lambda_2 \exp\{\lambda_2(\tau_a + \tau_f)\}} \right]. \quad (6.11)$$

More discussions on the sample size calculation with survival endpoints are given in Lachin and Foulkes (1986), Lakatos (1988), and Collett (1994).

**EXAMPLE 6.7**

Suppose that the median survival time for patients with brain tumor is 6 months under the standard treatment, and the new treatment is expected to prolong the median survival time to 8 months. Under the exponential model, the hazard for the new treatment is $\lambda_1 = \log(2)/8 \approx 0.0866$ and that for the standard treatment is $\lambda_2 = \log(2)/6 \approx 0.1155$, and thus the log hazard ratio $\theta = \log(\lambda_1/\lambda_2) \approx -0.2877$. If we take a one-sided log-rank test at a significance level of $\alpha = 0.025$ and aim at a power of 80%, the total number of events will be $D = 380$.

The design parameters involved for calculating the total number of subjects include the accrual rate $a$, the length of the accrual period $\tau_a$, and the follow-up time $\tau_f$. Among the three design parameters $(a, \tau_a, \tau_f)$, we can fix any two of them to compute the third based on (6.11). For simplicity, consider a constant accrual rate of $a = 25$ patients per month, and $\tau_f = 24$ months, then we can compute the accrual period $\tau_a = 16$ months and thus the total number of patients is $n = 400$. If we take $a = 20$ and $\tau_f = 12$, then we obtain $\tau_a = 22$ in order to have $D = 380$ events, so we need $n = 440$ subjects. On the other hand, given $\tau_a = 24$ and $\tau_f = 6$ months, we can obtain the accrual rate of $a = 20$ patients per month, which leads to a total sample size of $n = 480$. The shorter the follow-up time, the more subjects are needed to achieve the required number of events. If the number of patients $n$ is fixed, we may extend the follow-up time to reach the target number of events $D$.

### 6.4.3  Nonparametric Approach with Counting Process

The sample size calculation does not necessarily rely upon the exponential distribution for the survival time. To derive the sample size nonparametrically, we introduce the counting process, $N_{ik}(t) = I(X_{ik} \leq t, \Delta_{ik} = 1)$, and the at-risk process, $Y_{ik}(t) = I(X_{ik} \geq t)$, for subject $i$ in group $k$, $i = 1, \ldots, n_k; k = 1, 2$. We can write the martingale as

$$M_{ik}(t) = N_{ik}(t) - \int_0^t Y_{ik}(u) \, d\Lambda_k(u),$$

where $\Lambda_k(t)$ is the cumulative hazard function for group $k$, $\Lambda_k(t) = \int_0^t \lambda_k(u)\,du$. Let $N_k(t) = \sum_{i=1}^{n_k} N_{ik}(t)$, $M_k(t) = \sum_{i=1}^{n_k} M_{ik}(t)$, $Y_k(t) = \sum_{i=1}^{n_k} Y_{ik}(t)$, and $Y(t) = Y_1(t) + Y_2(t)$. The limiting function of $Y_k(t)/n_k$ is denoted by $\pi_k(t) = P(X_{ik} \geq t)$. Let the total sample size be $n = n_1 + n_2$ with an allocation ratio $r = n_1/n_2$, then the limiting function of $Y(t)/n$ is

$$\pi(t) = \frac{r\pi_1(t)}{1+r} + \frac{\pi_2(t)}{1+r}.$$

The Nelson–Aalen estimator of the cumulative hazard function for group $k$ is given by

$$\hat{\Lambda}_k(t) = \int_0^t \frac{dN_k(u)}{Y_k(u)},$$

where $dN_k(u) = N_k((u + du)-) - N_k(u-)$. The usual log-rank statistic (Fleming and Harrington, 1991) can be written as

$$
\begin{aligned}
U_n &= \frac{1}{\sqrt{n}} \int_0^\infty \left\{ \frac{Y_2(t)}{Y(t)} dN_1(t) - \frac{Y_1(t)}{Y(t)} dN_2(t) \right\} \\
&= \frac{1}{\sqrt{n}} \int_0^\infty \left\{ \frac{Y_2(t)}{Y(t)} dM_1(t) - \frac{Y_1(t)}{Y(t)} dM_2(t) \right\} \\
&\quad + \frac{1}{\sqrt{n}} \int_0^\infty \frac{Y_1(t)Y_2(t)}{Y(t)} \{d\Lambda_1(t) - d\Lambda_2(t)\}.
\end{aligned}
$$

Under the null hypothesis, $H_0$: $\Lambda_1(t) = \Lambda_2(t) = \Lambda(t)$, the variance of $U_n$ can be approximated by

$$\hat{\sigma}^2 = \frac{1}{n} \int_0^\infty \frac{Y_1(t)Y_2(t)}{Y(t)} d\hat{\Lambda}(t),$$

which converges in probability to

$$\sigma^2 = \frac{r}{(1+r)^2} \int_0^\infty \frac{\pi_1(t)\pi_2(t)}{\pi(t)} d\Lambda(t). \tag{6.12}$$

Let $G_k(t) = P(C_{ik} \geq t)$ denote the survival function for the censoring time in group $k$, $k = 1, 2$. If the censoring time distributions of the two groups are the same, $G_1(t) = G_2(t) = G(t)$, the variance of $U_n$ can be simplified as follows,

$$
\begin{aligned}
\sigma^2 &= \frac{r}{(1+r)^2} \int_0^\infty \frac{S_1(t)G_1(t)S_2(t)G_2(t)}{S_1(t)G_1(t)r/(1+r) + S_2(t)G_2(t)/(1+r)} d\Lambda(t) \\
&= \frac{r}{(1+r)^2} \int_0^\infty S(t)G(t)\,d\Lambda(t) \\
&= \frac{r}{(1+r)^2} P(\Delta = 1),
\end{aligned}
$$

where $S_1(t) = S_2(t) = S(t)$ under the null hypothesis $H_0$. Therefore, if using an equal allocation for the two arms with $r = 1$, the variance of $U_n$ reduces to

$$\sigma^2 = \frac{1}{4}P(\Delta = 1).$$

To determine the sample size for a clinical trial with a survival endpoint, we consider a one-sided log-rank test with the type I error rate of $\alpha$ and a power of $1 - \beta$. Under the local alternative hypothesis $H_1$: $\lambda_1(t) = \lambda_2(t)e^{\theta}$ where $\theta$ is small, the Taylor series expansion yields $e^{\theta} \approx 1 + \theta$. The log-rank statistic $U_n$ converges in distribution to $N(\mu, \sigma^2)$, where

$$\mu \approx \frac{\sqrt{n}\theta r}{(1 + r)^2} \int_0^{\infty} \frac{\pi_1(t)\pi_2(t)}{\pi(t)} \, d\Lambda(t),$$

and $\sigma^2$ is given in (6.12). Let $\theta$ be the specified log hazard ratio (the effect size) under $H_1$, then the power is given by

$$1 - \beta = \Pr\left(\frac{U_n}{\sigma} \geq z_{\alpha}\Big|H_1\right) = \Pr\left(\frac{U_n - \mu}{\sigma} \geq z_{\alpha} - \frac{\mu}{\sigma}\Big|H_1\right),$$

where $(U_n - \mu)/\sigma$ follows the standard normal distribution. Therefore,

$$z_{\alpha} + z_{\beta} = \frac{\mu}{\sigma} = \sqrt{n}\theta\sigma,$$

which leads to the number of subjects

$$n = \frac{(1 + r)^2(z_{\alpha} + z_{\beta})^2}{rP(\Delta = 1)\theta^2},$$

and the number of events

$$D = nP(\Delta = 1) = \frac{(1 + r)^2(z_{\alpha} + z_{\beta})^2}{r\theta^2}.$$

If $r = 1$, that is an equal allocation with $n_1 = n_2 = n/2$, then the total number of subjects required for the trial is

$$n = \frac{4(z_{\alpha} + z_{\beta})^2}{P(\Delta = 1)\theta^2}.$$

If the numbers of patients assigned to the two treatment groups are different with $n_1 = rn_2$, then

$$n_2 = \frac{(1 + r)(z_{\alpha} + z_{\beta})^2}{rP(\Delta = 1)\theta^2}.$$

## 6.5   SAMPLE SIZE FOR CORRELATED DATA

### 6.5.1   Linear Model with Continuous Data

We have focused on sample size estimation for the i.i.d. data thus far, while correlated data may also arise in clinical trials. In a longitudinal study, the outcome of interest is repeatedly measured over time for each patient, which may induce serial correlations among intra-patient observations. For example, cardiovascular patients may have their systolic and diastolic blood pressures measured once a week to monitor the trend. On the other hand, the data may be naturally or artificially clustered; for example, ophthalmology research often involves paired eyes of each patient, and dental studies may take multiple measurements on several teeth belonging to the same subject. Under such circumstances, correlations are induced among the observed data within each subject/cluster, while the data across different individuals remain independent. Not only does the sample size calculation need to consider all the design parameters pertaining to the independent case (i.e., the effect size and variance), but it also must account for the underlying correlations (Vonesh and Schork, 1986; Rochon, 1991; Liu and Liang, 1997; Liu, Shih, and Gehan, 2002).

Under the generalized estimating equation, Liu and Liang (1997) extend the sample size computation for the generalized linear model (Self and Mauritsen, 1988) to correlated data. For ease of exposition, we consider a two-arm trial, in which each participant has an equal number of measurements; that is, all the cluster sizes are the same, say $K$. Let $Z_i = 0$ if patient $i$ is under the standard treatment, and $Z_i = 1$ if he/she is under the new treatment. Let $Y_{ik}$ denote the observed outcome for the $k$th measurement on the $i$th subject, $i = 1, \ldots, n; k = 1, \ldots, K$. We apply the marginal linear regression model to examine the treatment effect,

$$Y_{ik} = \gamma + \theta Z_i + \epsilon_{ik},$$

where $\gamma$ is the intercept and $\theta$ represents the marginal treatment effect. We assume the error vector $\epsilon_i = (\epsilon_{i1}, \ldots, \epsilon_{iK})^\mathsf{T}$ follows a multivariate normal distribution with mean zero and variance–covariance matrix $\sigma^2 \mathbf{R}$; that is, $\epsilon_i \sim N_K(\mathbf{0}, \sigma^2 \mathbf{R})$, where $\sigma^2$ is the marginal variance and $\mathbf{R}$ is the correlation matrix.

We specify the type I error rate $\alpha$ and power $1 - \beta$, and assume that subjects are equally allocated between the two treatment arms. Under the two-sided hypothesis test with

$$H_0\colon \theta = 0 \quad \text{versus} \quad H_1\colon \theta \neq 0,$$

the total sample size required for the trial is

$$n = \frac{4(z_{\alpha/2} + z_\beta)^2 \sigma^2}{\theta^2 (\mathbf{1}^\mathsf{T} \mathbf{R}^{-1} \mathbf{1})}, \tag{6.13}$$

where $\mathbf{1}$ is a $K$-vector of 1's, and $\theta$ is the specified effect size under $H_1$. If we further assume an exchangeable correlation matrix,

$$
\mathbf{R} = \begin{pmatrix}
1 & \rho & \cdots & \rho \\
\rho & \ddots & & \vdots \\
\vdots & & \ddots & \rho \\
\rho & \cdots & \rho & 1
\end{pmatrix},
$$

where $\rho$ is the correlation coefficient, the sample size formula in (6.13) can be simplified as

$$
n = \frac{4(z_{\alpha/2} + z_\beta)^2 \sigma^2 \{1 + (K-1)\rho\}}{\theta^2 K}.
$$

Therefore, the design parameters $\theta$, $\sigma$, and $\rho$ should all be calibrated from previous studies or expert opinions. Compared with the effective sample size $nK$ for the independent normal data, the total number of observations is inflated by a factor of $1 + (K-1)\rho$ due to correlations. The sample sizes for a superiority trial, a noninferiority trial, and an equivalence trial with correlated data can be derived similarly as those independent cases.

**EXAMPLE 6.8**

To illustrate the influence of correlations on the effective sample size, we consider a longitudinal study with six consecutive measurements; that is, the cluster size is $K = 6$. For simplicity, we assume an exchangeable correlation structure with $\rho = 0.2$, and take $\theta = 0.2$ and $\sigma = 1$. We specify the type I error rate $\alpha = 0.05$ and power 85%. Then the number of clusters required for the trial is $n = 300$, leading to a total number of observations of $nK = 1800$, which doubles the effective sample size of 900 if all of the settings are the same except that the data are assumed to be independent ($\rho = 0$). Certainly, the higher the correlation, the larger the sample size needed to achieve the same power.

### 6.5.2    Logistic Model with Binary Data

Consider a longitudinal study with two treatments; and for simplicity, suppose that each patient has the same number of measurements, $K$. Let $Z_i = 0$ if subject $i$ is treated in the control arm, and otherwise $Z_i = 1$ for the experimental arm. For $i = 1, \ldots, n$ and $k = 1, \ldots, K$, let $Y_{ik}$ denote a binary outcome for the $k$th measurement of the $i$th subject, which takes a value of 1 with probability $p_{ik}$, and 0 with probability $1 - p_{ik}$. The observations for the $i$th subject, $Y_{i1}, \ldots, Y_{iK}$, are correlated due to repeated measurements. We apply a logistic regression model to examine the marginal treatment effect,

$$
\mathrm{logit}(p_{ik}) = \gamma + \theta Z_i.
$$

We are interested in testing whether there is a difference in the response rates between the treatment and control groups; that is,

$$H_0: \theta = 0 \quad \text{versus} \quad H_1: \theta \neq 0. \tag{6.14}$$

Following the logistic model, the probabilities of response for the control and treatment are given by

$$p_0 = \frac{\exp(\gamma)}{1 + \exp(\gamma)} \quad \text{and} \quad p_1 = \frac{\exp(\gamma + \theta)}{1 + \exp(\gamma + \theta)},$$

respectively. Hence, the hypothesis testing in (6.14) is equivalent to

$$H_0: p_0 = p_1 \quad \text{versus} \quad H_1: p_0 \neq p_1.$$

With an equal allocation between the two arms, the total number of patients needed is

$$n = \frac{2(z_{\alpha/2} + z_\beta)^2 \{p_0(1 - p_0) + p_1(1 - p_1)\}}{\theta^2 (\mathbf{1}^\mathsf{T} \mathbf{R}^{-1} \mathbf{1})},$$

where $\mathbf{R}$ is the $K \times K$ correlation matrix. If we further assume an exchangeable correlation matrix with correlation coefficient $\rho$, the sample size is simplified to

$$n = \frac{2(z_{\alpha/2} + z_\beta)^2 \{p_0(1 - p_0) + p_1(1 - p_1)\}\{1 + (K - 1)\rho\}}{\theta^2 K}.$$

Compared with the sample size formula for the i.i.d. binary data in (6.9), the inflation factor $1 + (K - 1)\rho$ indicates that the higher is the correlation, the more observations are needed.

## 6.6   GROUP SEQUENTIAL METHODS

Conventional clinical trial designs typically determine the total sample size in advance and only perform one final analysis after all the data are collected according to the planned sample size. These methods are known as fixed-sample designs, which are easy to plan and implement, but lacks flexibility. In addition, the trial conduct is rigid, strictly complying with the prefixed sample size, regardless of unexpected interim results, such as better-than-expected superiority or futility. By contrast, group sequential methods are much more flexible, which regularly examine the efficacy data over administratively convenient intervals, and also monitor possible futility stopping along the course of the study (Jennison and Turnbull, 2000). If the experimental treatment shows an overwhelmingly strong beneficial effect at the interim analyses, it would be desirable to stop the trial early to allow patients on the inferior arms to receive the more effective treatment and, more importantly, to move the drug developmental process rapidly such as to benefit more patients in the general population (Pocock, 1977; O'Brien and Fleming, 1979; Lan and DeMets, 1983).

Continuous data monitoring refers to a fully sequential analysis of the accumulating data after observing every single outcome, which, however, may be practically infeasible. Group sequential methods offer a compromise between trial flexibility and practicality. In particular, Pocock (1977) and O'Brien and Fleming (1979) describe two-arm group sequential tests with different stopping boundaries for the significance region: The former takes equal testing boundaries throughout the trial, while the later allocates more stringent levels of significance at the beginning of the study and alleviates the significance levels towards the end of the trial. Based on a more general boundary specification, Wang and Tsiatis (1987) develop a class of group sequential tests, which includes Pocock's design and O'Brien and Fleming's design as special cases. Classical sequential designs aim for early termination of a trial when interim data demonstrate notable treatment differences. Modified one-sided group sequential designs may also allow trials to terminate early for a lack of treatment effects (DeMets and Ware, 1980; 1982; Gould and Pecore, 1982; Whitehead and Stratton, 1983).

### 6.6.1 Multiple Testing

Multiplicity may arise when several hypotheses are tested simultaneously or the same hypothesis is tested sequentially over time as in the group sequential trial design. As a consequence, the $p$-value needs to be adjusted in order to control the familywise type I error rate. To be more specific, let $\theta$ denote the parameter of interest, and there are $K$ hypotheses to be tested, denoted as $\{H_{01}, \ldots, H_{0K}\}$. Define the parameter space of $\theta$ under the null hypothesis,

$$\Theta = \left\{ \theta : \bigcap_{k=1}^{K} H_{0k} \text{ is true} \right\}.$$

The familywise error rate is controlled at level $\alpha$, if

$$\sup_{\theta \in \Theta} \Pr(\text{reject at least one } H_{0k}, k = 1, \ldots, K) \leq \alpha.$$

Suppose that we perform $K$ hypothesis tests. If each test is conducted at a significance level of $\alpha = 0.05$, then the overall type I error rate will be inflated, which deteriorates as the number of tests $K$ increases. For $K$ from 1 to 10, we list the overall type I error rate below:

| Number of Tests ($K$) | 1 | 2 | 5 | 10 |
|---|---|---|---|---|
| Type I Error Rate | 0.05 | 0.083 | 0.142 | 0.193 |

We first introduce the closed testing principle to maintain the overall type I error rate at $\alpha$ (Marcus, Peritz, and Gabriel, 1976). Based on $\{H_{01}, \ldots, H_{0K}\}$, we may reject any one of the hypotheses, say $H_{0k}$, if all possible intersection hypotheses involving $H_{0k}$ can be rejected by using level-$\alpha$ tests. This would control the familywise error rate for all the $K$ hypotheses at the significance level of $\alpha$. As an example, if there are three hypotheses $\{H_{01}, H_{02}, H_{03}\}$ under consideration, and the overall type I error rate is 0.05, then $H_{01}$ can be rejected at a significance level of 0.05 if $H_{01}$, $H_{01} \cap H_{02}$, $H_{01} \cap H_{03}$ and $H_{01} \cap H_{02} \cap H_{03}$ can all be rejected using statistical tests at $\alpha = 0.05$.

Controlling the familywise type I error rate is an effective way to prevent the occurrence of false positives, which is of paramount importance in the new drug development. The easiest way to preserve the overall type I error rate is to use the Bonferroni correction by splitting $\alpha$ over all the tests. Suppose that there are $K$ hypotheses to be tested, and as usual we test one hypothesis at a statistical significance level of $\alpha$. The familywise error rate will be preserved if each individual hypothesis is tested at a significance level of $\alpha/K$. Despite its simplicity, Bonferroni's correction is the most stringent and conservative way to control false positives. The split of $\alpha$ over the $K$ hypothesis tests may not necessarily be even. The familywise type I error rate is maintained as long as $\alpha_1 + \cdots + \alpha_K = \alpha$, where $\alpha_k$ is the significance level of test $k$, for $k = 1, \ldots, K$.

Compared with Bonferroni's correction, Holm's step-down method (Holm, 1979) is less conservative and thus yields higher power, which is described as follows:

(1) Order all the $p$-values from the $K$ tests,

$$p_{(1)} \leq p_{(2)} \leq \cdots \leq p_{(K-1)} \leq p_{(K)},$$

and denote the corresponding hypotheses as $\{H_{0(1)}, \ldots, H_{0(K)}\}$. Compare the smallest $p$-value $p_{(1)}$ to $\alpha/K$. If $p_{(1)} < \alpha/K$, then reject $H_{0(1)}$ and go to step (2); otherwise stop.

(2) Compare the second smallest $p$-value $p_{(2)}$ to $\alpha/(K-1)$. If $p_{(2)} < \alpha/(K-1)$, then reject $H_{0(2)}$ and go to step (3); otherwise stop.

$$\vdots$$

(K) Compare the largest $p$-value $p_{(K)}$ to $\alpha$. If $p_{(K)} < \alpha$, then reject the corresponding hypothesis $H_{0(K)}$ and stop.

Holm's procedure sequentially compares the $p$-values from the smallest to the largest with a sequence of significance levels $\{\alpha/K, \alpha/(K-1), \ldots, \alpha\}$, until the first hypothesis cannot be rejected. At that point, stop and accept the hypothesis that was not rejected and all the remaining hypotheses that have not been tested. Based on the Bonferroni inequality, Holm's method is valid regardless of the joint distribution of the test statistics.

On the other hand, Hochberg's step-up method (Hochberg, 1988) proceeds in a reversed order, which is described as follows:

(1) Order all the $p$-values from the $K$ tests,

$$p_{(1)} \le p_{(2)} \le \cdots \le p_{(K-1)} \le p_{(K)},$$

and denote the corresponding hypotheses as $\{H_{0(1)}, \ldots, H_{0(K)}\}$. Compare the largest $p$-value $p_{(K)}$ to $\alpha$. If $p_{(K)} < \alpha$, then reject all the hypotheses $\{H_{0(1)}, \ldots, H_{0(K)}\}$ and stop; otherwise go to step (2).

(2) Compare the second largest $p$-value $p_{(K-1)}$ to $\alpha/2$. If $p_{(K-1)} < \alpha/2$, then reject the hypotheses $\{H_{0(1)}, \ldots, H_{0(K-1)}\}$ and stop; otherwise go to step (3).

$$\vdots$$

($K$) Compare the smallest $p$-value $p_{(1)}$ to $\alpha/K$. If $p_{(1)} < \alpha/K$, then reject the hypothesis $H_{0(1)}$ and stop.

In general, Hochberg's step-up procedure is relatively more powerful than Holm's step-down procedure, while more restrictions are required for Hochberg's test statistics—for example, independence or having distributions with multivariate total positivity of order two or a scale mixture thereof (Sarkar, 1998; Huang and Hsu, 2007). Clearly, both Holm's and Hochberg's methods are not applicable in group sequential designs for which the tests are sequentially conducted on the data that accrue over time.

### 6.6.2  Pocock's Design

If multiple tests are conducted during the interim monitoring of a trial, spurious treatment effects may arise due to chance or random fluctuations of the efficacy data. As a consequence, the type I and type II error rates would be inflated. Controlling the type I error rate would prevent an undesirably large number of false-positive findings into the drug development. In the group sequential design, stopping boundaries are developed for sequential tests along the trial to maintain the overall type I error rate. Toward this goal, Pocock (1977) proposes conducting repeated significance tests at a constant nominal level during the course of a trial.

In a two-arm trial, suppose that the outcomes are i.i.d. normal with a known variance $\sigma^2$; that is, $Y_{1i} \sim N(\mu_1, \sigma^2)$ for subject $i$ in the experimental arm, and $Y_{2i} \sim N(\mu_2, \sigma^2)$ for that in the standard arm. The treatment difference is $\theta = \mu_1 - \mu_2$, and we are interested in testing the hypotheses,

$$H_0: \theta = 0 \quad \text{versus} \quad H_1: \theta \ne 0.$$

For simplicity, patients are divided into $K$ equal-size groups according to their enrollment dates. For each sequentially accrued group, an equal number of patients are allocated to each treatment. Let $N_k$ denote the cumulative sample

**Table 6.1    Critical Constants $c_{\mathrm{Po}}(K, \alpha)$ under Pocock's Design, with $K$ Two-Sided Sequential Tests and the Type I Error Rate $\alpha$**

| $K$ | $\alpha = 0.01$ | $\alpha = 0.05$ | $\alpha = 0.1$ |
|---|---|---|---|
| 1 | 2.576 | 1.960 | 1.645 |
| 2 | 2.772 | 2.178 | 1.875 |
| 3 | 2.873 | 2.289 | 1.992 |
| 4 | 2.939 | 2.361 | 2.067 |
| 5 | 2.986 | 2.413 | 2.122 |
| 6 | 3.023 | 2.453 | 2.164 |
| 7 | 3.053 | 2.485 | 2.197 |
| 8 | 3.078 | 2.512 | 2.225 |
| 9 | 3.099 | 2.535 | 2.249 |
| 10 | 3.117 | 2.555 | 2.270 |

size up to group $k$, and a total of $N_K$ subjects are needed in such a group sequential study. After enrolling $k$ groups, we observe the accumulated data $\{(Y_{1i}, Y_{2i}), i = 1, \ldots, N_k/2\}$, and the standardized test statistic for the $k$th interim analysis is

$$Z_k = \frac{1}{\sqrt{N_k}\sigma} \sum_{i=1}^{N_k/2} (Y_{1i} - Y_{2i}), \quad k = 1, \ldots, K.$$

Based on a two-sided test, if $|Z_k|$ is large enough to exceed the critical boundary, we stop the trial with a rejection of the null hypothesis. However, due to multiple testing with $K > 1$, the familywise or overall type I error rate is inflated, such that we cannot use the usual significance level $\alpha = 0.05$ for each of the $K$ tests.

To preserve the overall type I error rate at $\alpha = 0.05$, Pocock (1977) computes the critical constant $c_{\mathrm{Po}}(K, \alpha)$ such that

$$\Pr(|Z_k| \geq c_{\mathrm{Po}}(K, \alpha) \text{ at any } k \text{ in a sequential order} \mid H_0) = \alpha.$$

The critical value $c_{\mathrm{Po}}(K, \alpha)$ is a constant across all the $K$ tests, which are given in Table 6.1 for different $K$'s under each specified significance level $\alpha$. More specifically, Pocock's design is carried out as follows.

- *Interim analysis*:
  After observing the accumulated data up to group $k$, $k = 1, \ldots, K - 1$, if $|Z_k| \geq c_{\mathrm{Po}}(K, \alpha)$, stop the trial with a rejection of $H_0$; otherwise, continue to enroll group $k + 1$.

- *Final analysis*:
  After observing all the data from the planned $K$ groups, if $|Z_K| \geq c_{\mathrm{Po}}(K, \alpha)$, reject $H_0$; otherwise, accept $H_0$.

**Table 6.2**   **Critical Constants $c_{\mathrm{OF}}(K, \alpha)$ under O'Brien and Fleming's Design, with $K$ Two-Sided Sequential Tests and the Type I Error Rate $\alpha$**

| $K$ | $\alpha = 0.01$ | $\alpha = 0.05$ | $\alpha = 0.1$ |
|---|---|---|---|
| 1 | 2.576 | 1.960 | 1.645 |
| 2 | 2.580 | 1.977 | 1.678 |
| 3 | 2.595 | 2.004 | 1.710 |
| 4 | 2.609 | 2.024 | 1.733 |
| 5 | 2.621 | 2.040 | 1.751 |
| 6 | 2.631 | 2.053 | 1.765 |
| 7 | 2.640 | 2.063 | 1.776 |
| 8 | 2.648 | 2.072 | 1.786 |
| 9 | 2.654 | 2.080 | 1.794 |
| 10 | 2.660 | 2.087 | 1.801 |

In principle, the type I error rate $\alpha$ is split among the $K$ analyses such that the overall test size of $\alpha$ is maintained at the desired level. In the general sequential setting, the critical constants for the $K$ tests, $c_{(1,\alpha)}, \ldots, c_{(K,\alpha)}$, may not necessarily be all the same, as long as they are chosen to yield the overall type I error rate of $\alpha$. We can solve for $c_{(k,\alpha)}$ from the following equations iteratively,

$$\Pr\{|Z_1| \geq c_{(1,\alpha)}|H_0\} = \alpha_1,$$

and for $k = 2, \ldots, K$,

$$\alpha_{k-1} + \Pr\{|Z_1| < c_{(1,\alpha)}, \ldots, |Z_{k-1}| < c_{(k-1,\alpha)}, |Z_k| \geq c_{(k,\alpha)}|H_0\} = \alpha_k,$$

with $\alpha_K \equiv \alpha$.

### 6.6.3   O'Brien and Fleming's Design

Intuitively, a more stringent threshold should be exceeded if a trial is to be terminated earlier. Thus, instead of using a constant nominal level for all the $K$ tests, O'Brien and Fleming (1979) propose making the rejection of $H_0$ much more difficult at the earlier interim analyses, and alleviating the test boundaries as the trial proceeds. In other words, the trial would only be terminated for superiority if an extreme treatment difference could be shown earlier. Still, the overall type I error rate should be preserved. O'Brien and Fleming's design is described as follows.

- *Interim analysis*:
  After observing the accumulated data up to group $k$, $k = 1, \ldots, K - 1$, if $|Z_k| \geq c_{\mathrm{OF}}(K, \alpha)\sqrt{K/k}$, stop the trial with a rejection of $H_0$; otherwise, continue to enroll group $k + 1$.

**Table 6.3** **Critical Constants $c_{WT}(K, \alpha = 0.05, \gamma)$ under Wang and Tsiatis's Design, with $K$ Two-Sided Sequential Tests and Different Values of the Transformation Parameter $\gamma$, while Fixing the Type I Error Rate $\alpha = 0.05$**

| $K$ | $\gamma = 0.1$ | $\gamma = 0.25$ | $\gamma = 0.4$ |
|---|---|---|---|
| 1 | 1.960 | 1.960 | 1.960 |
| 2 | 1.994 | 2.038 | 2.111 |
| 3 | 2.026 | 2.083 | 2.186 |
| 4 | 2.050 | 2.113 | 2.233 |
| 5 | 2.068 | 2.136 | 2.267 |
| 6 | 2.083 | 2.154 | 2.292 |
| 7 | 2.094 | 2.168 | 2.313 |
| 8 | 2.104 | 2.180 | 2.329 |
| 9 | 2.113 | 2.190 | 2.343 |
| 10 | 2.120 | 2.199 | 2.355 |

- *Final analysis*:
  After observing all the data from the planned $K$ groups, if $|Z_K| \geq c_{OF}(K, \alpha)$, reject $H_0$; otherwise, accept $H_0$.

Table 6.2 presents the critical constants at different significance levels for the final stage $K$, and thus the rest of the critical constants along the sequential tests can be computed as $c_{OF}(k, \alpha) = c_{OF}(K, \alpha)\sqrt{K/k}$, for $k = 1, \ldots, K$. Clearly, as $k$ increases, the critical values become smaller and the critical intervals become narrower, which makes it easier to cross (i.e., to reject the null).

More generally, Wang and Tsiatis (1987) propose a family of sequential tests indexed by a power transformation parameter $\gamma$, which includes Pocock's and O'Brien and Fleming's designs as special cases. For a fixed value of $\gamma$, the critical constant at stage $k$ is $c_{WT}(k, \alpha, \gamma) = c_{WT}(K, \alpha, \gamma)(k/K)^{\gamma-1/2}$, $k = 1, \ldots, K$. Table 6.3 gives $c_{WT}(K, \alpha, \gamma)$, the critical constant at the $K$th stage for $\alpha = 0.05$ and a particular value of $\gamma$. Obviously, Wang and Tsiatis's design reduces to Pocock's design if $\gamma = 1/2$, and to O'Brien and Fleming's design if $\gamma = 0$. Other values of $\gamma$ between 0 and 1/2 produce some encompassing shapes of critical boundaries. The trial design using Wang and Tsiatis's stopping boundaries proceeds as follows.

- *Interim analysis*:
  After observing the accumulated data up to group $k$, $k = 1, \ldots, K - 1$, if $|Z_k| \geq c_{WT}(K, \alpha, \gamma)(k/K)^{\gamma-1/2}$, stop the trial with a rejection of $H_0$; otherwise, continue to enroll group $k + 1$.

- *Final analysis*:
  After observing all the data from the planned $K$ groups, if $|Z_K| \geq c_{WT}(K, \alpha, \gamma)$, reject $H_0$; otherwise, accept $H_0$.

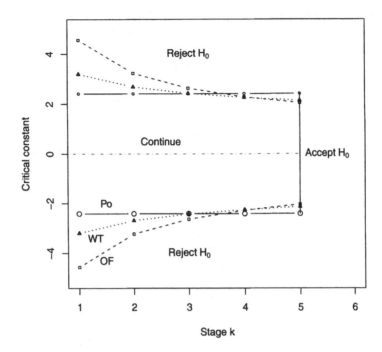

**Figure 6.3**    Critical constants under two-sided group sequential tests with $K = 5$ groups: Pocock's design (Po), O'Brien and Fleming's design (OF) and Wang and Tsiatis's design (WT) with $\gamma = 0.25$.

To illustrate different shapes of stopping boundaries, we take $K = 5$ and $\alpha = 0.05$. Figure 6.3 shows the three stopping boundaries: Pocock's stopping boundaries are constant and parallel to the horizontal axis; those of O'Brien and Fleming's test are wider (more stringent) at the early interim analyses, and become narrower (more relaxed) toward the end of the trial; and Wang and Tsiatis's boundaries with $\gamma = 0.25$ lie in the between.

### 6.6.4   Information and Asymptotic Distribution

In a group sequential design, suppose that we monitor the trial at the prespecified calendar times, $\tau_1, \ldots, \tau_K$. Let $\theta$ be the treatment difference that is of clinical interest, for example, $\theta = \mu_1 - \mu_2$ for the difference of normal means with continuous endpoints; $\theta = p_1 - p_2, p_1/p_2$, or $\{p_1/(1-p_1)\}/\{p_2/(1-p_2)\}$ for the difference, ratio, or odds ratio of response rates with binary outcomes; and $\theta = \log(\lambda_1/\lambda_2)$ for the logarithm of the hazard ratios with time-to-event data.

During the trial, as more subjects are accrued and longer follow-ups are taken, more information would be accumulated in the study. If the primary endpoint is normal or binary, the accumulating number of subjects $N_k$ by calendar time $\tau_k$ characterizes the trial information $\mathcal{I}_k$, while for time-to-event endpoints, the accumulating number of events or failures $D_k$ up to $\tau_k$ determines $\mathcal{I}_k$. In general, the information increases as the trial proceeds because more subjects are enrolled and more events are expected to occur with a longer follow-up. The information at $\tau_k$ can be characterized by the usual Fisher information, $\mathcal{I}_k = \{\mathrm{Var}(\hat{\theta}_k)\}^{-1}$, where $\hat{\theta}_k$ is the maximum likelihood estimator (MLE) of $\theta$ based on the data accumulated up to $\tau_k$. If a total of $K$ tests are planned for a trial that includes $K-1$ interim analyses and the $K$th final analysis, then the maximum information $\mathcal{I}_K$ is characterized by the maximum sample size, $N_K$, or the total number of events by time $\tau_K$, $D_K$. We take the accumulated information from $\tau_1$ up to $\tau_K$ as some fraction of the maximum information $\mathcal{I}_K$, and define

$$t_k = \begin{cases} N_k/N_K, & \text{for normal or binary endpoints,} \\ D_k/D_K, & \text{for survival endpoints,} \\ \mathcal{I}_k/\mathcal{I}_K, & \text{for general cases,} \end{cases}$$

where $\mathcal{I}_k/\mathcal{I}_K = \mathrm{Var}(\hat{\theta}_K)/\mathrm{Var}(\hat{\theta}_k)$. Note that $t_k$ increases from 0 to 1 as $k$ approaches $K$, which can be viewed as a standardized internal time of a trial. At the internal time $t_K \equiv 1$, the trial stops and attains the maximum information of $\mathcal{I}_K$.

At the internal monitoring time $t_k$, we obtain the MLE $\hat{\theta}_k$ and its variance based on all the data accumulated up to $t_k$. The Wald test statistic is given by

$$Z(t_k) = \frac{\hat{\theta}_k}{\{\mathrm{Var}(\hat{\theta}_k)\}^{1/2}} = \hat{\theta}_k\sqrt{\mathcal{I}_k}, \quad k = 1, \ldots, K.$$

Across all the internal monitoring times $t_1, \ldots, t_K$, the sequential test statistics $Z(t_1), \ldots, Z(t_K)$ jointly follow a multivariate normal distribution (Scharfstein, Tsiatis, and Robins, 1997; Jennison and Turnbull, 1997). The marginal distribution of $Z(t_k)$ is

$$Z(t_k) \sim \mathrm{N}(\theta\sqrt{\mathcal{I}_k}, 1), \quad k = 1, \ldots, K,$$

and the covariance function between $Z(t_j)$ and $Z(t_k)$ for $0 < t_j \le t_k < 1$ is

$$\mathrm{Cov}\{Z(t_j), Z(t_k)\} = \sqrt{\mathcal{I}_j/\mathcal{I}_k}.$$

**EXAMPLE 6.9**

As an illustration, we consider a two-arm randomized trial with normal endpoints. Given a common known variance $\sigma^2$, $Y_{1i} \sim \mathrm{N}(\mu_1, \sigma^2)$ for subject $i$ in arm 1 (the experimental treatment), and $Y_{2i} \sim N(\mu_2, \sigma^2)$ for that in arm 2 (the standard treatment). For $k = 1, \ldots, K$, let $N_k$ be the cumulative sample size up to group $k$, and $N_k/2$ patients are allocated to each arm. Let $\bar{Y}_1^{(k)}$ and $\bar{Y}_2^{(k)}$ denote the sample means of arm 1 and arm 2 up to stage $k$, respectively. The treatment difference $\theta = \mu_1 - \mu_2$ can then be estimated by

$$\hat{\theta}_k = \bar{Y}_1^{(k)} - \bar{Y}_2^{(k)} = \frac{2}{N_k} \sum_{i=1}^{N_k/2} (Y_{1i} - Y_{2i}).$$

At the internal time $t_k$, the standardized test statistic for the $k$th interim analysis is

$$Z(t_k) = \frac{\sqrt{N_k}}{2\sigma}(\bar{Y}_1^{(k)} - \bar{Y}_2^{(k)}) = (\bar{Y}_1^{(k)} - \bar{Y}_2^{(k)})\sqrt{\mathcal{I}_k}.$$

The test statistics $Z(t_1), \ldots, Z(t_K)$ jointly follow a multivariate normal distribution, since marginally each $Z(t_k)$ is a linear combination of normal random variables, and

$$Z(t_k) \sim N(\theta\sqrt{\mathcal{I}_k}, 1), \quad k = 1, \ldots, K.$$

The covariance function between $Z(t_j)$ and $Z(t_k)$ for $0 < t_j \leq t_k < 1$ is given by

$$\begin{aligned}
\text{Cov}\{Z(t_j), Z(t_k)\} &= \text{Cov}\left\{(\bar{Y}_1^{(j)} - \bar{Y}_2^{(j)})\sqrt{\mathcal{I}_j},\ (\bar{Y}_1^{(k)} - \bar{Y}_2^{(k)})\sqrt{\mathcal{I}_k}\right\} \\
&= \left(\frac{2}{N_j} \times \frac{2}{N_k} \times \frac{N_j}{2}\sigma^2 + \frac{2}{N_j} \times \frac{2}{N_k} \times \frac{N_j}{2}\sigma^2\right)\sqrt{\mathcal{I}_j\mathcal{I}_k} \\
&= \sqrt{\mathcal{I}_j/\mathcal{I}_k}.
\end{aligned}$$

If we denote the drift parameter $\eta = \theta\sqrt{\mathcal{I}_K}$, then

$$Z(t_k) \sim N(\eta\sqrt{t_k}, 1), \quad k = 1, \ldots, K.$$

Under the null hypothesis, $H_0$: $\theta = 0$, the drift term $\eta = 0$. We can derive a simplified version of the Gaussian process with independent increments,

$$W(t_k) = \sqrt{t_k} Z(t_k), \quad k = 1, \ldots, K,$$

such that the joint distribution of $W(t_1), \ldots, W(t_K)$ is also multivariate normal. For each $k$, the marginal distribution of $W(t_k)$ is

$$W(t_k) \sim N(\eta t_k, t_k),$$

and the covariance function between $W(t_j)$ and $W(t_k)$ for $0 < t_j \leq t_k < 1$ is

$$\mathrm{Cov}\{W(t_j), W(t_k)\} = t_j,$$

which implies that $W(t_j)$ and $W(t_k) - W(t_j)$ are independent. Based on the independent increment property of the process $W(t_k)$, the stopping boundaries of a group sequential design can be computed efficiently through recursive integration, as will be discussed in the next section.

### 6.6.5  Stopping Boundary Computation

We outline the basic steps for calculating the stopping boundaries in a group sequential design with a total of $K$ analyses. The vector of the standard test statistics $(Z(t_1), \ldots, Z(t_K))^{\mathsf{T}}$ follows a multivariate normal distribution:

- $\mathrm{E}\{Z(t_k)\} = \theta\sqrt{\mathcal{I}_k}$,

- $\mathrm{Cov}\{Z(t_j), Z(t_k)\} = \sqrt{\mathcal{I}_j/\mathcal{I}_k}, \quad 1 \leq j \leq k \leq K$,

- $Z(t_1) \sim \mathrm{N}(\theta\sqrt{\mathcal{I}_1}, 1)$, and the increment

$$Z(t_k)\sqrt{\mathcal{I}_k} - Z(t_{k-1})\sqrt{\mathcal{I}_{k-1}} \sim \mathrm{N}(\theta(\mathcal{I}_k - \mathcal{I}_{k-1}), \ \mathcal{I}_k - \mathcal{I}_{k-1}),$$

which is independent of all the previous test statistics $Z(t_1), \ldots, Z(t_{k-1})$.

Let $c_1, \ldots, c_K$ be the stopping boundaries corresponding to the interim monitoring times $t_1, \ldots, t_K$. We stop the trial with a rejection of $H_0$ at the first $t_k$ that satisfies

$$|Z(t_1)| < c_1, \ldots, |Z(t_{k-1})| < c_{k-1}, \text{ and } |Z(t_k)| \geq c_k.$$

To preserve the type I error rate at the conventional significance level of $\alpha$, the $c_k$'s need to be chosen such that

$$\mathrm{Pr}\left\{ \bigcap_{k=1}^{K} (|Z(t_k)| < c_k) \middle| H_0 \right\} = 1 - \alpha,$$

which, however, by itself cannot uniquely determine the values of $c_k$. Based on the concept of the $\alpha$-spending function (Lan and DeMets, 1983), we can specify a monotone increasing function $\alpha(t)$, such as

$$\alpha(t) = \alpha \log\{1 + (e - 1)t\}, \quad t \in [0, 1],$$

which corresponds to the stopping boundaries of Pocock (1977). To generate the stopping boundaries of O'Brien and Fleming (1979), the $\alpha$-spending function takes the form of

$$\alpha(t) = 4 - 4\Phi\left(\frac{z_{\alpha/4}}{\sqrt{t}}\right).$$

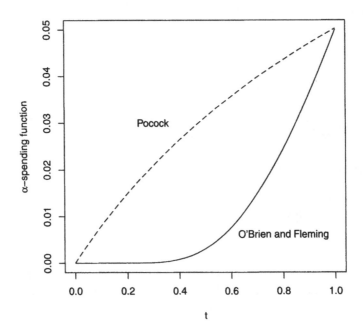

**Figure 6.4** The $\alpha$-spending functions corresponding to Pocock (1977) and O'Brien and Fleming (1979) group sequential designs, respectively.

Figure 6.4 exhibits the shapes of the $\alpha$-spending functions for these two designs, while other $\alpha$-spending functions may also work in group sequential designs. No matter which $\alpha$-spending function is used, it must be specified in advance before any data are collected.

Based on the predetermined $\alpha$-spending function, we can construct the following set of equations,

$$\alpha(t_1) = \Pr(|Z(t_1)| \geq c_1)|H_0),$$
$$\alpha(t_2) = \alpha(t_1) + \Pr(|Z(t_1)| < c_1, |Z(t_2)| \geq c_2)|H_0),$$
$$\vdots$$
$$\alpha(t_K) = \alpha(t_{K-1})$$
$$\qquad + \Pr(|Z(t_1)| < c_1, \ldots, |Z(t_{K-1})| < c_{K-1}, |Z(t_K)| \geq c_K)|H_0).$$

By recursively solving these $K$ equations, we can obtain the stopping boundaries $c_1, \ldots, c_K$. During the entire trial conduct, the probability of ever crossing the efficacy boundary under $H_0$ is

$$\Pr(|Z(t_1)| \geq c_1|H_0) + \Pr(|Z(t_1)| < c_1, |Z(t_2)| \geq c_2|H_0) + \cdots$$
$$+ \Pr(|Z(t_1)| < c_1, \ldots, |Z(t_{K-1})| < c_{K-1}, |Z(t_K)| \geq c_K|H_0),$$

which simplifies to

$$\alpha(t_1) + \{\alpha(t_2) - \alpha(t_1)\} + \cdots + \{\alpha(t_K) - \alpha(t_{K-1})\} = \alpha(t_K) \equiv \alpha.$$

Therefore, group sequential designs continuously spend $\alpha$ over each interim test until the overall type I error rate $\alpha$ is exhausted.

### 6.6.6   Sample Size and Inflation Factor

With the drift parameter $\eta = \theta\sqrt{\mathcal{I}_K}$, the marginal distribution of the test statistic at the $k$th interim analysis is

$$Z(t_k) \sim \mathrm{N}(\eta\sqrt{t_k}, 1), \quad k = 1, \ldots, K.$$

To determine the sample size for a group sequential trial, we first compute the drift term $\eta$ such that the trial is able to detect the treatment difference $\theta$ with power $1 - \beta$. Under the alternative hypothesis, the type II error rate is given by

$$\Pr\left\{\bigcap_{k=1}^{K}(|Z(t_k)| < c_k)\Big|H_1\right\} = \beta, \tag{6.15}$$

from which we can obtain $\eta$. Thus, the amount of information needed to achieve power $1 - \beta$ is $\mathcal{I}_K = (\eta/\theta)^2$. The total information by the end of the trial is $\mathcal{I}_K = \{\mathrm{Var}(\hat{\theta}_K)\}^{-1}$, where $\hat{\theta}_K$ is the MLE based on all $K$ groups of data. Intuitively, we should keep enrolling patients into the trial until the reciprocal of the variance of $\hat{\theta}_K$ is equal to $\mathcal{I}_K$.

More specifically, consider a two-arm trial with normal endpoints sharing a common known variance $\sigma^2$; that is, $Y_{1i} \sim \mathrm{N}(\mu_1, \sigma^2)$ and $Y_{2i} \sim \mathrm{N}(\mu_2, \sigma^2)$. The goal is to calculate an adequate sample size in order to detect the treatment difference $\theta = \mu_1 - \mu_2$. Let $\bar{Y}_1$ and $\bar{Y}_2$ denote the sample means of arm 1 and arm 2 after all the $K$ groups of patients are enrolled, respectively. The difference of the sample means between the two arms, $\hat{\theta}_K = \bar{Y}_1 - \bar{Y}_2$, can be used to estimate $\theta$. Let $N_K$ denote the total sample size, and each arm is allocated $N_K/2$ subjects, then

$$\mathrm{Var}(\hat{\theta}_K) = \frac{4\sigma^2}{N_K}.$$

Therefore, the maximum sample size for the group sequential trial is $N_K = 4\sigma^2\mathcal{I}_K$.

If we consider a two-arm trial with binary endpoints, let $p_1$ be the response rate of the experimental treatment, and let $p_2$ be that of the standard treatment.

**Table 6.4    Sample Size Inflation Factors of Group Sequential Designs Relative to Fixed-Sample Designs for Two-Sided Tests with $\alpha = 0.05$**

| $\alpha$-Spending Function | $K$ | Power $= 1 - \beta$ | | |
| | | 0.80 | 0.90 | 0.95 |
| --- | --- | --- | --- | --- |
| Pocock | 2 | 1.11 | 1.10 | 1.09 |
| | 3 | 1.17 | 1.15 | 1.14 |
| | 4 | 1.20 | 1.18 | 1.17 |
| | 5 | 1.23 | 1.21 | 1.19 |
| O'Brien and Fleming | 2 | 1.01 | 1.01 | 1.01 |
| | 3 | 1.02 | 1.02 | 1.02 |
| | 4 | 1.02 | 1.02 | 1.02 |
| | 5 | 1.03 | 1.03 | 1.02 |

The dichotomous outcomes are $Y_{1i} \sim \text{Bernoulli}(p_1)$ and $Y_{2i} \sim \text{Bernoulli}(p_2)$, and the difference of the response rates is $\theta = p_1 - p_2$. The estimate for $\theta$ is $\hat{\theta}_K = \bar{Y}_1 - \bar{Y}_2$, and the corresponding variance is given by

$$\text{Var}(\hat{\theta}_K) = \frac{2\{p_1(1 - p_1) + p_2(1 - p_2)\}}{N_K},$$

which yields the maximum sample size $N_K = 2\{p_1(1 - p_1) + p_2(1 - p_2)\}\mathcal{I}_K$.

When designing a group sequential trial, besides the specification of the type I and type II error rates (i.e., $\alpha$ and $\beta$), we also need to determine the number of planned analyses, $K$, and the $\alpha$-spending function. We can then compute the drift parameter $\eta$ from (6.15) through recursive integration, and we can also obtain $\mathcal{I}_K = (\eta/\theta)^2$ and eventually the total sample size $N_K$. It is more convenient to express the maximum information as

$$\mathcal{I}_K = \left(\frac{z_{\alpha/2} + z_\beta}{\theta}\right)^2 \times \text{IF},$$

where the inflation factor (IF) is defined as

$$\text{IF} = \left(\frac{\eta}{z_{\alpha/2} + z_\beta}\right)^2.$$

Therefore, for a group sequential trial with continuous outcomes, the total sample size needed is

$$N_K = 4\sigma^2 \mathcal{I}_K = \frac{4\sigma^2 (z_{\alpha/2} + z_\beta)^2}{\theta^2} \times \text{IF},$$

and for a group sequential trial with binary outcomes,

$$N_K = \frac{2(z_{\alpha/2} + z_\beta)^2}{\theta^2}\{p_1(1 - p_1) + p_2(1 - p_2)\} \times \text{IF}.$$

The sample size required for a group sequential trial is enlarged by the inflation factor compared with that of the corresponding fixed-sample design. For convenience of sample size calculation, Table 6.4 provides the inflation factors under the commonly encountered configurations of the Pocock and O'Brien and Fleming designs, respectively.

**EXAMPLE 6.10**

We illustrate group sequential methods with a two-arm clinical trial design. The endpoint is a continuous measurement, which is assumed to be normally distributed. The treatment difference between the new and standard drugs is specified as $\theta = 1$, and the variance is $\sigma^2 = 4$. Under a two-sided test with $\alpha = 0.05$ and $\beta = 0.1$, the fixed-sample design needs a total sample size of $n = 168$. If we use Pocock's stopping boundaries with $K = 3$ groups, the required sample size is $N_{\text{Po}} = 168 \times 1.15 = 194$, with approximately 64 subjects in each group. During the trial conduct, we perform one hypothesis test of $H_0: \theta = 0$, after enrolling every 64 patients in a sequential order, and each test statistic is compared with the same critical constant 2.289. The trial will be stopped when for the first time one of the three tests crosses the critical boundary, and then we claim that there is a significant difference between the two treatments. Otherwise, we continue to enroll the next group of patients till the end of the trial.

On the other hand, if we use O'Brien and Fleming's stopping boundaries with $K = 5$, then the total sample size is $N_{\text{OF}} = 168 \times 1.03 = 174$ with approximately 36 subjects in each group. In a sequential order, the five critical constants are 4.562, 3.226, 2.634, 2.281, and 2.040, computed by $2.040 \times \sqrt{5/k}$, for $k = 1, \ldots, 5$. The trial proceeds until one of the five tests along the sequential order first crosses the corresponding boundary, and then we reject the null hypothesis; otherwise we continue to enroll the next group till the end of the trial. If the trial runs to the last group, the final test statistic will be compared with the critical constant 2.040.

### 6.6.7   Futility Stopping Boundary

During the interim monitoring, if the observed effect size is too small to warrant continuation, we may stop the trial early. Such futility stopping boundaries can be derived in parallel to the aforementioned efficacy stopping boundaries. The probability of ever crossing the futility boundaries under $H_1$ is the type II error rate $\beta$, which leads to the $\beta$-spending function to generate the futility boundaries. We force the stopping boundaries for efficacy and futility to meet at the final analysis by choosing an appropriate drift parameter $\eta$. Therefore, at the end of the trial, a definitive conclusion must be drawn: Either the null hypothesis is rejected (for superiority), or the null hypothesis is accepted (for futility).

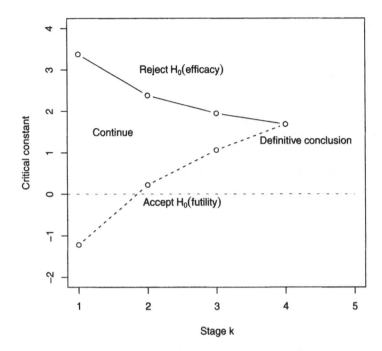

**Figure 6.5** Critical constants under one-sided group sequential tests with superiority and futility stopping boundaries and $K = 4$.

To determine the efficacy and futility boundaries and the drift parameter $\eta$, we need to spend both the type I and type II error rates, $\alpha$ and $\beta$, simultaneously, based on the following iterative procedure:

(1) Initiate a value for $\eta$.

(2) Find the paired values of $(l_1, u_1)$ satisfying

$$\alpha(t_1) = \Pr\{Z(t_1) \geq u_1 | H_0\},$$

and

$$\beta(t_1) = \Pr\{Z(t_1) \leq l_1 | H_1\},$$

where the upper bound $u_1$ is for efficacy stopping and the lower bound $l_1$ is for futility stopping.

(3) For $k = 2, \ldots, K$, solve recursively for $(l_k, u_k)$, such that

$$\alpha(t_k) = \alpha(t_{k-1})$$
$$+ \Pr\{l_1 < Z(t_1) < u_1, \ldots, l_{k-1} < Z(t_{k-1}) < u_{k-1}, Z(t_k) \geq u_k | H_0\}$$

and

$$\beta(t_k) = \beta(t_{k-1})$$
$$+ \Pr\{l_1 < Z(t_1) < u_1, \ldots, l_{k-1} < Z(t_{k-1}) < u_{k-1}, Z(t_k) \le l_k | H_1\},$$

with $\alpha(t_K) = \alpha$ and $\beta(t_K) = \beta$.

(4) Repeat steps (1)–(3) by fixing $\eta$ at different values until we find the value of $\eta$ such that $l_K = u_K$.

This guarantees that the upper and lower stopping boundaries meet at the end of the trial (stage $K$), as shown in Figure 6.5.

### 6.6.8   Repeated Confidence Intervals

In a group sequential trial, repeated confidence intervals may be constructed along the sequential tests (Jennison and Turnbull, 1989). For $k = 1, \ldots, K$, the usual Wald test statistic is given by

$$Z(t_k) = \hat{\theta}_k \sqrt{\mathcal{I}_k},$$

where $\hat{\theta}_k$ is the MLE of the parameter $\theta$ at the $k$th interim analysis. Let $c_k$ be the stopping boundary for stage $k$. Under $H_0$: $\theta = 0$, $Z(t_k) \sim \mathrm{N}(0, 1)$, and

$$\Pr\left\{ \bigcap_{k=1}^{K} (|Z(t_k)| < c_k) \Big| H_0 \right\} = 1 - \alpha.$$

Under $H_1$: $\theta \neq 0$,

$$Z(t_k) - \theta\sqrt{\mathcal{I}_k} \sim \mathrm{N}(0, 1), \quad k = 1, \ldots, K,$$

while the covariance structure is still the same as that under $H_0$. The $k$th confidence interval for $\theta$ is given by

$$\left( \hat{\theta}_k - \frac{c_k}{\sqrt{\mathcal{I}_k}}, \ \hat{\theta}_k + \frac{c_k}{\sqrt{\mathcal{I}_k}} \right), \quad k = 1, \ldots, K,$$

and the probability that all the $K$ repeated confidence intervals simultaneously cover $\theta$ is $1 - \alpha$,

$$\Pr\left( \hat{\theta}_k - \frac{c_k}{\sqrt{\mathcal{I}_k}} < \theta < \hat{\theta}_k + \frac{c_k}{\sqrt{\mathcal{I}_k}}, \text{ for } k = 1, \ldots, K \right) = 1 - \alpha.$$

## 6.7   ADAPTIVE DESIGNS

### 6.7.1   Motivation

In a phase III clinical trial, patients are randomized to different treatment arms for comparing their therapeutic effects. In the planning stage, we need to specify the type I error rate and power, and determine the effect size and variance for the treatment. Classical fixed-sample designs require precise information on these design parameters to produce an accurate sample size. The effect size and variance are typically elicited from expert experience or estimated from historical data, such as previous phase II trials. However, due to different study conditions and patient populations, as well as small sample sizes in early-phase trials, the estimates of the effect size and variance may not be reliable for the current phase III trial design. Consequently, the sample size for the phase III trial may be overestimated and thus wasting resources, or underestimated and leading to a low power. Imagine a situation in which a $p$-value lies between 0.05 and 0.1; that is, the $p$-value barely misses the conventional significance level of $\alpha = 0.05$. Clearly, in this case there is considerable evidence showing the treatment to be effective, but it is still not strong enough to reach the nominal level. As a result, the trial may fail to detect a clinically meaningful difference due to inadequacy of the sample size. If we extend the patient enrollment to collect a few more samples in order to reach the statistical significance, the type I error rate is generally inflated if the original fixed-sample test is used. On the other hand, if we abandon the current study to redesign and rerun such a large pivotal trial, it would certainly be expensive and time-consuming. Therefore, it is desirable to develop more flexible designs that are capable of extending a trial based on the cumulated data while still controlling the type I error rate. Otherwise, the trial may use a sample size that is not large enough to detect an important clinical difference, due to either an overestimation of the actual treatment difference or an underestimation of the standard error.

Group sequential methods may terminate a trial early for some extreme interim findings, such as markable treatment effects of a particular arm, a lack of beneficial effects of a certain treatment, or severe adverse events in a subgroup. Whether to call a trial design adaptive or nonadaptive is relative; some designs could be more adaptive than others. Compared with fixed-sample designs, group sequential methods are clearly more flexible, which, however, still require fixing the total number of subjects, or the maximum number of tests with prespecified group sizes in advance. In other words, group sequential methods do not allow the maximum sample size to be modified in the middle of the trial for achieving a desired power.

Adaptive designs have been developed to offer the possibility of re-estimating the sample size based on the observed data in the course of a trial (Wassmer, 1998; Gould, 2001; Shun et al., 2001; Shih, 2001). These "real" adaptive methods are more flexible because they update the initial design parameters using the ongoing trial data and re-estimate the sample size at the interim stages to ensure an adequate testing power. Colton and McPherson (1976), Elashoff and Reedy (1984), and Proschan and Hunsberger (1995) propose various two-stage designs to re-estimate the sample size using the data in the first stage, while constraining the significance level at each stage to preserve the overall type I error rate. Gould (1992) and Shih (1992) re-estimate variances at the interim analyses without unblinding the trial. Fisher (1998), Shen and Fisher (1999), and Yin and Shen (2005a, 2005b) propose self-designing trials, in which the variance or the weight function is sequentially spent to modify the sample size to achieve the desired power. Bauer and Köhne (1994), Cui, Hung, and Wang (1999), Liu and Chi (2001), Lehmacher and Wassmer (1999), Posch and Bauer (2000), and Müller and Schäfer (2001) develop various adaptive methods with similar motivations by modifying a design based on interim data.

### 6.7.2  Fisher's Combination Criterion

Consider a randomized trial to compare an experimental treatment and a control. The null hypothesis is that there is no difference between the two treatments, and the alternative is that there is a difference. In the notion of sample size re-estimation, Bauer and Köhne (1994) propose a two-stage trial design, in which the sample size in stage 2 may depend on the data observed in stage 1. In the middle of a trial, there is an adaptation point that switches the design from stage 1 to stage 2. This switching point partitions the entire trial data into two nonoverlapping samples, and each sample is used to test the same null hypothesis. At the end of the trial, the error probabilities are combined from the two disjoint samples to control the overall type I error rate.

We examine the data observed before and after the adaptation takes place separately. By formulating the null hypotheses $H_{01}$ and $H_{02}$ corresponding to stage 1 and stage 2, the trial aims to test their intersection:

$$H_0: H_{01} \cap H_{02} \text{ (there is no treatment difference)}.$$

Let $p_1$ be the $p$-value from the test of $H_{01}$ for the data collected prior to the sample size re-estimation (the adaptation point), and let $p_2$ be that of $H_{02}$ for the sample accrued after the adaptation. At the end of the trial, based on Fisher's combination criterion, the null hypothesis $H_0$ would be rejected, if

$$p_1 p_2 \leq c_\alpha \equiv \exp(-\chi^2_{4,\alpha}/2), \tag{6.16}$$

where $\chi^2_{4,\alpha}$ is the $100(1 - \alpha)$th percentile of the chi-squared distribution with 4 degrees of freedom. We can derive (6.16) based on the fact that $p_1$ and $p_2$ are independent and uniformly distributed under $H_0$.

Suppose that $n_1$ subjects are recruited in stage 1, and the corresponding $p$-value, $p_1$, is obtained. Let $\alpha_0$ and $\alpha_1$ denote probability cutoffs, with $\alpha_0 < \alpha_1$. The trial proceeds in the following two sequential stages, in which futility stopping may also be incorporated for trial early termination.

- If $p_1 \leq \alpha_0$, stop the trial and reject $H_0$.

- If $p_1 \geq \alpha_1$, stop the trial and accept $H_0$.

- If $\alpha_0 < p_1 < \alpha_1$, continue the trial to stage 2 and enroll additional $n_2$ subjects, where $n_2$ may depend on the data observed in stage 1.

- After the trial is completed with a total of $n_1 + n_2$ subjects, if $p_1 p_2 \leq c_\alpha$, reject $H_0$; otherwise accept $H_0$.

To preserve an overall significance level of $\alpha$, for a given value of $\alpha_1$ the value of $\alpha_0$ can be solved from

$$\alpha_0 + \int_{\alpha_0}^{\alpha_1} \frac{c_\alpha}{p_1} dp_1 = \alpha_0 + c_\alpha(\log \alpha_1 - \log \alpha_0) = \alpha.$$

At the conventional significance level $\alpha = 0.05$, the critical constant $c_{0.05} = \exp(-\chi^2_{4,0.05}/2) = 0.0087$; thus given different values of $\alpha_1$ for futility stopping, we can obtain the corresponding values of $\alpha_0$ as follows:

| $\alpha_1$ | 0.1 | 0.2 | 0.3 | 0.4 | 0.5 | 0.6 |
|---|---|---|---|---|---|---|
| $\alpha_0$ | 0.0426 | 0.0348 | 0.0299 | 0.0263 | 0.0233 | 0.0207 |

### 6.7.3 Conditional Power

Fisher's combination test lays out the framework of combining the two $p$-values in a two-stage adaptive design. However, it does not demonstrate how to re-estimate the sample size in stage 2 based on the data observed in stage 1. Towards this goal, Proschan and Hunsberger (1995) propose using the conditional power to re-estimate the sample size in a two-stage sequential procedure.

For ease of exposition, consider a two-arm clinical trial with normally distributed outcomes. For subject $i$ in arm 1, $Y_{1i} \sim N(\mu_1, \sigma^2)$, and for that in arm 2, $Y_{2i} \sim N(\mu_2, \sigma^2)$, where the common variance $\sigma^2$ is assumed to be known. Let $\theta = \mu_1 - \mu_2$ denote the difference in the treatment effect between the experimental and standard arms. We are interested in testing a one-sided hypothesis of

$$H_0: \theta = 0 \quad \text{versus} \quad H_1: \theta > 0.$$

In stage 1, $n_1$ patients are enrolled, and for simplicity suppose that $n_1/2$ subjects are allocated to each arm. Using the standardized sample means, we can construct a test statistic as

$$Z_1 = \frac{\sqrt{n_1}(\bar{Y}_1 - \bar{Y}_2)}{2\sigma}.$$

In stage 2, we plan to recruit $n_2$ subjects and denote the sample means of those subjects in the experimental and standard arms as $\bar{X}_1$ and $\bar{X}_2$, respectively. Let $\text{CP}_\theta(n_2, c|Z_1)$ denote the conditional power, which is the probability that the final test statistic based on $n_1 + n_2$ observations exceeds the critical constant

$c$ (the value of $c$ is to be determined) given $Z_1$ and the treatment difference $\theta$. In a one-sided test,

$$
\begin{aligned}
&\mathrm{CP}_\theta(n_2, c|Z_1) \\
&= \Pr\left\{ \frac{n_1(\bar{Y}_1 - \bar{Y}_2) + n_2(\bar{X}_1 - \bar{X}_2)}{2\sigma\sqrt{n_1 + n_2}} \geq c \Big| Z_1 \right\} \\
&= \Pr\left\{ \frac{\sqrt{n_2}(\bar{X}_1 - \bar{X}_2 - \theta)}{2\sigma} \geq \frac{\sqrt{n_1 + n_2}c - \sqrt{n_1}Z_1}{\sqrt{n_2}} - \frac{\sqrt{n_2}\theta}{2\sigma} \Big| Z_1 \right\}.
\end{aligned}
$$

Noting that $\sqrt{n_2}(\bar{X}_1 - \bar{X}_2 - \theta)/(2\sigma)$ follows the standard normal distribution, this leads to

$$
\mathrm{CP}_\theta(n_2, c|Z_1) = 1 - \Phi\left( \frac{\sqrt{n_1 + n_2}c - \sqrt{n_1}Z_1}{\sqrt{n_2}} - \frac{\sqrt{n_2}\theta}{2\sigma} \right).
$$

Both the critical value $c \equiv c(n_2, Z_1)$ and the conditional power depend on $n_2$. Let $\phi(\cdot)$ denote the density function of the standard normal distribution, that is, $\phi(z) = \mathrm{d}\Phi(z)/\mathrm{d}z$, then the type I error rate in the two-stage design is

$$
\int \mathrm{CP}_{\theta=0}(n_2, c|Z_1)\phi(Z_1)\,\mathrm{d}Z_1.
$$

To compute $n_2$ and the critical constant $c(n_2, Z_1)$, we first specify a conditional error function $F(\cdot)$, which is an increasing function over $[0, 1]$ and satisfies

$$
\int F(Z_1)\phi(Z_1)\,\mathrm{d}Z_1 = \alpha.
$$

Given the test statistic $Z_1$ of stage 1, $F(Z_1)$ characterizes how much of the conditional type I error is allowed at the end of the trial. After collecting $n_1$ observations in stage 1, we can determine $n_2$ and the critical constant $c(n_2, Z_1)$ such as to obtain an exact $\alpha$-level test. To preserve the type I error rate, let

$$
\mathrm{CP}_{\theta=0}(n_2, c|Z_1) = F(Z_1),
$$

from which we can obtain the critical value

$$
c(n_2, Z_1) = \frac{\sqrt{n_1}Z_1 + \sqrt{n_2}z_{F(Z_1)}}{\sqrt{n_1 + n_2}}.
$$

Following this procedure, an exact $\alpha$-level test is guaranteed no matter how the future sample size $n_2$ is chosen. Naturally, we can compute $n_2$ to achieve the conditional power of $1 - \beta$,

$$
\mathrm{CP}_\theta(n_2, c|Z_1) = 1 - \Phi\left( z_{F(Z_1)} - \frac{\sqrt{n_2}\theta}{2\sigma} \right) = 1 - \beta.
$$

Therefore, we have

$$n_2 = \frac{4\sigma^2 (z_{F(Z_1)} + z_\beta)^2}{\theta^2}$$

and

$$c(n_2, Z_1) = \frac{\sqrt{n_1} Z_1 \theta + 2\sigma(z_{F(Z_1)} + z_\beta) z_{F(Z_1)}}{\sqrt{n_1 \theta^2 + 4\sigma^2 (z_{F(Z_1)} + z_\beta)^2}}.$$

If we replace $\theta$ by its MLE $\hat{\theta}$ based on the data in stage 1, then

$$n_2 = \frac{(z_{F(Z_1)} + z_\beta)^2}{Z_1^2} n_1$$

and

$$c(n_2, Z_1) = \frac{Z_1^2 + z_{F(Z_1)}(z_{F(Z_1)} + z_\beta)}{\sqrt{Z_1^2 + (z_{F(Z_1)} + z_\beta)^2}}.$$

### 6.7.4  Adaptive Group Sequential Method

Group sequential methods and adaptive designs are developed extensively in parallel. In general, classical group sequential methods require data-independent group sizes and a fixed number of interim looks. In other words, the group sizes and the number of tests are typically fixed in the planning stage. It may also happen that the interim analyses are performed at specific calendar times rather than after accruing a specified number of subjects or observing a fixed number of events, so the group sizes may be different and unknown in advance. However, the group sizes in the subsequent stages must not depend on the data observed in the previous groups. Whereas adaptive designs allow the sample sizes or the group sizes in the future stages to depend on the data observed previously. Certainly, a flexible design that is capable of updating the sample size, as well as terminating the trial early for strong efficacy, is desirable, since it would balance both power requirements and ethical concerns at the same time. Lehmacher and Wassmer (1999) propose an adaptive inferential strategy within the classical group sequential framework, which, however, does not provide a sample size updating procedure to achieve the desired power. Cui, Hung, and Wang (1999) apply a combination principle with prefixed weights within a group sequential trial. Müller and Schäfer (2001) integrate the adaptive interim analyses into the classical group sequential testing. These "more" adaptive methods fix the maximum number of group sequential tests, while allowing the group sizes to change during the trial. Tsiatis and Mehta (2003) compare group sequential designs with certain two-stage adaptive designs, and conclude the former to be more efficient.

Lehmacher and Wassmer (1999) compare the average of the test statistics with the classical stopping boundaries and conclude that the adaptively varied group sizes will not affect group sequential tests as long as the test statistics are conditionally independent and follow the standard normal distribution. More specifically, consider a two-arm group sequential trial with normally distributed outcomes with a common and known variance $\sigma^2$; that is, $Y_{1i} \sim \mathrm{N}(\mu_1, \sigma^2)$ and $Y_{2i} \sim \mathrm{N}(\mu_2, \sigma^2)$ for the $i$th patient in arm 1 and arm 2, respectively. We are interested in testing whether there is a significant difference between the two treatments. Suppose that a total of $K$ analyses are planned in advance, with group sizes of $n_1, \ldots, n_K$. Let $N_k = \sum_{j=1}^{k} n_j$ denote the cumulative sample size up to group $k$. Using an equal allocation for each group, $n_k/2$ subjects are assigned to each arm for $k = 1, \ldots, K$. Under $H_0$, the test statistic based on the data in the $k$th group is given by

$$Z_k = \frac{\sqrt{n_k}(\bar{Y}_{1k} - \bar{Y}_{2k})}{2\sigma} \sim \mathrm{N}(0, 1),$$

where $\bar{Y}_{1k}$ and $\bar{Y}_{2k}$ are sample means corresponding to arm 1 and arm 2 in group $k$. The cumulative test statistic up to group $k$ also follows the standard normal distribution; that is,

$$T_k = \frac{1}{\sqrt{N_k}} \sum_{j=1}^{k} \sqrt{n_j} Z_j \sim \mathrm{N}(0, 1).$$

If the group sizes $n_1, \ldots, n_K$ are all equal, at stage $k$ we may use

$$T_k = \frac{1}{\sqrt{k}} \sum_{j=1}^{k} Z_j \tag{6.17}$$

as the test statistic, which is compared with the critical boundaries in the classical group sequential test.

In an adaptive design, $n_k$ may depend on the information available prior to stage $k$. That is, group sizes are allowed to be data-dependent and adaptively changing throughout the trial. Note that $Z_1, \ldots, Z_K$ are independent, and each follows the standard normal distribution irrespective of how the group sizes are chosen. If we use (6.17) as the test statistic and the classical group sequential boundaries, the type I error rate $\alpha$ will still be preserved. The test statistic in (6.17) can be rewritten as

$$T_k = \frac{1}{\sqrt{k}} \sum_{j=1}^{k} \Phi^{-1}(1 - p_j),$$

where $p_j$ is the $p$-value corresponding to $Z_j$ and $\Phi^{-1}(\cdot)$ is the inverse cumulative distribution function of the standard normal distribution.

### 6.7.5 Self-Designing Strategy

The goal of the adaptive designs discussed thus far is to re-estimate the total sample size based on the cumulated data in the trial so as to achieve the specified power. From a slightly different perspective, the self-designing scheme fixes the group sizes while allowing the total number of groups to change during the trial (Fisher, 1998; Shen and Fisher, 1999; Yin and Shen, 2005a; 2005b). The design automatically decides whether to stop the trial for futility or extend patient accrual to achieve the desired power, and also preserves the overall type I error rate.

Consider a two-arm trial with normally distributed outcomes sharing a common and known variance $\sigma^2$,

$$Y_{1i} \sim \mathrm{N}(\mu_1, \sigma^2) \quad \text{and} \quad Y_{2i} \sim \mathrm{N}(\mu_2, \sigma^2),$$

for the $i$th patient in arm 1 and that in arm 2, respectively. Let $\theta = \mu_1 - \mu_2$ denote the treatment difference, and we are interested in testing a one-sided hypothesis,

$$H_0\colon \theta = 0 \quad \text{versus} \quad H_1\colon \theta > 0.$$

The data are partitioned into groups of fixed sizes $n_1, \ldots, n_K$, while the total number of groups, $K$, is not determined in advance. Thus, the total sample size $\sum_{k=1}^{K} n_k$ is not prefixed but may be adaptively updated during the trial conduct. With an equal allocation between the two arms, $n_k/2$ subjects are assigned to each arm for the $k$th group. Accordingly, the difference in the sample means is given by

$$\bar{Y}_{1k} - \bar{Y}_{2k} \sim \mathrm{N}\left(\theta, \frac{4\sigma^2}{n_k}\right),$$

and after standardization we have

$$S_k = \frac{\sqrt{n_k}(\bar{Y}_{1k} - \bar{Y}_{2k})}{2\sigma} \sim \mathrm{N}\left(\frac{\sqrt{n_k}\theta}{2\sigma}, 1\right).$$

Once the trial is completed with a total of $K$ groups, the final test statistic is constructed as a weighted sum of the standardized sample means,

$$T_K = \sum_{k=1}^{K} w_k S_k,$$

where the weights $w_k$ satisfy $\sum_{k=1}^{K} w_k^2 = 1$. Under $H_0$, $T_K \sim \mathrm{N}(0, 1)$, and thus we can reject $H_0$ if $T_K \geq z_\alpha$.

The weight function plays a key role in extending or stopping the trial. Suppose that there are $k - 1$ groups in the trial thus far. We compute the future sample size $N_k^*$ to achieve power $1 - \beta$ as if the next group $k$ would be the last group to enroll. Based on the sample means of the future data, $\bar{X}_{1k}$ and $\bar{X}_{2k}$, the standardized test statistic is given by

$$S_k^* = \frac{\sqrt{N_k^*}(\bar{X}_{1k} - \bar{X}_{2k})}{2\sigma}.$$

Then the conditional power can be computed as

$$1 - \beta = \Pr\left(\sum_{j=1}^{k-1} w_j S_j + w_k S_k^* \geq z_\alpha \Big| D_{k-1}\right)$$

$$= \Pr\left(S_k^* - \frac{\sqrt{N_k^*}\hat{\theta}_{k-1}}{2\sigma} \geq \frac{z_\alpha - \sum_{j=1}^{k-1} w_j S_j}{w_k} - \frac{\sqrt{N_k^*}\hat{\theta}_{k-1}}{2\sigma}\Big| D_{k-1}\right),$$

where $\hat{\theta}_{k-1}$ is the MLE of $\theta$ based on the data accumulated up to group $k-1$, $D_{k-1}$, and $w_k^2 = 1 - \sum_{j=1}^{k-1} w_j^2$. Since the conditional distribution of $S_k^*$ given $D_{k-1}$ is normal, the sample size of the next group (assumed to be the last group) is given by

$$N_k^* = \frac{4\sigma^2}{\hat{\theta}_{k-1}^2}\left\{\frac{z_\alpha - \sum_{j=1}^{k-1} w_j S_j}{(1 - \sum_{j=1}^{k-1} w_j^2)^{1/2}} + z_\beta\right\}^2.$$

Clearly, the larger the observed treatment effect $\hat{\theta}_{k-1}$, the smaller the conditional sample size needed to achieve the desired power $1 - \beta$.

Instead of directly enrolling $N_k^*$ subjects, we translate the information in the conditional sample size into the weight function while keeping the group size $n_k$ fixed *a priori*. Intuitively, the weight should be inversely proportional to the conditional sample size. For a larger value of $N_k^*$, a smaller weight should be assigned to the next group. The weight for the first group may not be too small because the trial needs an adequate amount of data before adaptation takes place. For group $k$, the weight $w_k$ is given by

$$w_k = \left\{\frac{n_k}{N_k^*}\left(1 - \sum_{j=1}^{k-1} w_j^2\right)\right\}^{1/2}.$$

During the trial, the self-designing strategy assesses the data periodically after enrolling every group of subjects. Based on the interim data, if the new treatment is ineffective compared with the standard therapy, the trial will be terminated for futility (Demets and Ware, 1980). After the $(k-1)$th group is enrolled, we first compute $N_k^*$ and $w_k$. If $\sum_{j=1}^{k} w_j^2 < 1$, the trial, if not stopped for futility, will enroll the next group because more data are needed to draw a conclusion. If $\sum_{j=1}^{k} w_j^2 > 1$, the $k$th group would be the last group whose weight will be reassigned as $(1 - \sum_{j=1}^{k-1} w_j^2)^{1/2}$. The diagram of the self-designing trial is given below.

| Weight Function | Decision Making after $k - 1$ Groups |
|---|---|
| $\displaystyle\sum_{j=1}^{k} w_j^2 < 1$ | $\left\{ \begin{array}{l} \text{If futility stopped, accept } H_0. \\ \text{Otherwise, enroll the next group.} \end{array} \right.$ |
| $\displaystyle\sum_{j=1}^{K-1} w_j^2 < 1 \text{ and } \sum_{j=1}^{K} w_j^2 = 1$ | $\left\{ \begin{array}{l} \text{If } T_K \geq z_\alpha, \text{ reject } H_0. \\ \text{Otherwise, accept } H_0. \end{array} \right.$ |

When the treatment is truly effective but the effect size is overestimated or the variance is underestimated, the trial would not be able to achieve the desired power if using the originally planned sample size in the fixed-sample design. Suppose that the targeted power of a two-arm randomized trial is 90%. Depending on how badly the effect size and variance are specified, the fixed-sample design may only lead to a power of 70% to 80%. By contrast, the self-designing trial has the capability of gaining more power, by extending the enrollment based on the cumulative data.

There is no single definition for adaptive designs; adaptations may involve early-stopping due to efficacy, futility, or toxicity, and sample size re-estimation. It is also possible to seamlessly bridge phase II and phase III trials through jointly modeling their respective endpoints (Inoue, Thall, and Berry, 2002; Liu and Pledger, 2005). No matter how adaptive a clinical trial is, the key issue is always to maintain the type I error rate. Indeed, adaptive designs are more flexible in terms of sample size adjustment, more efficient to achieve the desired power, and more ethical for their early-stopping provisions. Nevertheless, such adaptive trials often involve enormous logistical planning and complicated information tracking and updating, which make them much more challenging to design and implement in practice.

## 6.8 CAUSALITY AND NONCOMPLIANCE

### 6.8.1 Causal Inference and Counterfactuals

The goal of randomization in a clinical trial is to balance patients in each treatment arm, so that patients in different groups are "alike" on average. Ideally, the only difference between comparative groups should be the treatment and thus a "clean" comparison can be made. However, if certain characteristics of the patient groups are confounded with treatments, the difference in the responses between different treatments may be attributed to those unbalanced confounding effects rather than the treatment effects.

Randomization allows us to make causal inference regarding the treatment effects. Consider a two-arm randomized controlled trial with treatment 1 (the experimental drug) and treatment 0 (the active control or placebo). Let $\tilde{Y}_1$ and $\tilde{Y}_0$ be the "imaginary" response if a subject were assigned to arm 1 or arm 0, respectively. In reality, it is impossible to observe both outcomes on any given individual, because the subject is assigned to either treatment 1 or 0, but not both (except for the crossover study which is not considered here). The variables $\tilde{Y}_1$ and $\tilde{Y}_0$ are called counterfactuals because they are contrary to the fact of observing both $\tilde{Y}_1$ and $\tilde{Y}_0$ on the same subject. If we had known which treatment works better on a patient, the decision would simply be to assign that patient whichever treatment works better on him/her. However, this information is unobtainable for any individual subject. At the population level, the population mean causal effect is defined as

$$\theta = E(\tilde{Y}_1) - E(\tilde{Y}_0).$$

If $\theta > 0$, we say that on average treatment 1 would lead to a better response than treatment 0. Although this does not necessarily guarantee that any specific individual will benefit more from treatment 1, the population as a whole will do better under treatment 1. If we can estimate the average causal effect at the population level, then in the absence of any additional knowledge that would distinguish one individual from the other, the best treatment choice for any patient in the general population is treatment 1 (given that $\theta > 0$).

The data from a clinical trial may be summarized as $\{(Y_i, A_i), i = 1, \dots, n\}$, where $A_i = 0$ or 1 indicates the treatment assignment for subject $i$, $Y_i$ denotes the actual response, and $n$ is the total number of patients. If all patients comply with their treatment assignments, we would observe

$$Y_i = \tilde{Y}_{1i} I(A_i = 1) + \tilde{Y}_{0i} I(A_i = 0),$$

where $I(\cdot)$ is the indicator function. Due to randomization, the treatment assignment $A_i$ is independent of $(\tilde{Y}_{1i}, \tilde{Y}_{0i})$, so the potential response of an individual has no effect on which treatment this subject will receive. We are interested in estimating the true population treatment effect,

$$\theta = E(Y_i | A_i = 1) - E(Y_i | A_i = 0).$$

In a randomized clinical trial, we can estimate $\theta$ using the difference between the treatment-specific sample averages,

$$\hat{\theta} = \frac{\sum_{i=1}^n Y_i I(A_i = 1)}{\sum_{i=1}^n I(A_i = 1)} - \frac{\sum_{i=1}^n Y_i I(A_i = 0)}{\sum_{i=1}^n I(A_i = 0)}.$$

### 6.8.2  Noncompliance and Intent-to-Treat Analysis

In practice, there is almost always some kind of noncompliance or deviation from the intended treatment regimen in a randomized clinical trial. For example, noncompliance may be caused by patients' failure to understand and follow the detailed instructions. Sometimes, patients may refuse to start the assigned treatment because they believe that the other treatment would work better, or they may discontinue the assigned treatment due to intolerable side effects. In certain situations, physicians may have to switch patients to a salvage therapy when a front-line therapy fails, or allow patients to change to a different treatment due to severe adverse events, disease progression, or deterioration of patients' health. Under all of these circumstances, noncompliance issues arise, which make treatment comparison and inference much more difficult.

When analyzing the data from a randomized clinical trial, there are in general three major analysis populations in accommodation with noncompliance, which correspond to intent-to-treat, as-treated, and per-protocol analyses, respectively. Trials' conclusions and inferences may change under different analysis populations. In principle, one needs to ensure that exclusion of any patient from the analysis should not cause bias in the treatment effects. Thus, excluding patients based on post-randomization considerations, such as noncompliance, is generally not allowed for the primary analysis.

Intent-to-treat (ITT) analysis, also called as-randomized analysis, includes all of the randomized patients in the treatment groups to which they were originally assigned. The data would be analyzed as the patients were randomized regardless of their compliance with the entry criteria, the treatment they actually received, and subsequent withdrawal from treatment or deviation from the protocol. ITT analysis ignores noncompliance, and thus patients who have dropped out of the trial should also be included in the analysis. Generally speaking, ITT analysis examines the treatment effects as well as accounting for difficulties in drug administration and noncompliance issues. On the other hand, per-protocol (PP) analysis compares only the patients who have fully complied with their assigned treatment regimen while excluding those noncompliers from the analysis. Hence, PP analysis evaluates the maximum beneficial effect from a treatment given perfect compliance. Finally, as-treated (AT) analysis takes a middle ground between the ITT and PP analyses, which compares patients based on the actual treatment they received, not the treatment they were originally assigned to.

Compliers and noncompliers are often prognostically different. For example, if patients with refractory or more serious problems tend to drop out (i.e., sicker or nonresponding patients are more likely to quit the treatment), then an ineffective treatment may appear to be beneficial if one merely compares those who finished the treatment with the control. ITT analysis tries to avoid such misleading artifacts that may arise during the intervention. It takes everyone who begins the treatment as belonging to that treatment group, whether they finish the entire treatment or not. Hence, ITT analysis preserves the integrity of randomization. Moreover, when some patients do not comply with the intended treatment, ITT analysis is a more conservative approach because it would diminish the treatment effect towards the null in a superiority trial. On the other hand, both PP and

AT analyses may result in bias because the prognostic effect of noncompliance cannot be separated out from that of treatment.

### 6.8.3 Instrumental Variable Approach

Let $A$ be the indicator for the treatment assignment with $A = 1$ if a patient is assigned to the experimental arm and $A = 0$ if he/she is assigned to the control arm. Let $Z$ denote the treatment actually received by the patient; that is, $Z = 1$ if the patient received the experimental treatment, and $Z = 0$ if the patient received the control. Each patient in the population may be called a

- complier, if $(A = 1, Z = 1)$ or $(A = 0, Z = 0)$;

- never-taker, if $(A = 1, Z = 0)$ or $(A = 0, Z = 0)$;

- always-taker, if $(A = 0, Z = 1)$ or $(A = 1, Z = 1)$; or

- defier, if $(A = 1, Z = 0)$ or $(A = 0, Z = 1)$.

Using the counterfactual notation $(\tilde{Y}_0, \tilde{Y}_1)$, let $\mu_0 = \mathrm{E}(\tilde{Y}_0)$, $\mu_1 = \mathrm{E}(\tilde{Y}_1)$, $\tilde{y}_0 = \tilde{Y}_0 - \mu_0$, and $\tilde{y}_1 = \tilde{Y}_1 - \mu_1$; then the observed outcome is

$$Y = \tilde{Y}_0(1 - Z) + \tilde{Y}_1 Z$$
$$= \mu_0 + (\mu_1 - \mu_0)Z + \tilde{y}_0 + (\tilde{y}_1 - \tilde{y}_0)Z.$$

If we define $\epsilon = \tilde{y}_0 + (\tilde{y}_1 - \tilde{y}_0)Z$ and $\theta = \mu_1 - \mu_0$, then

$$Y = \mu_0 + \theta Z + \epsilon.$$

The indicator for treatment assignment $A$ can be viewed as a binary instrumental variable (IV), because $\mathrm{Cov}(A, Z) \neq 0$ and $\mathrm{Cov}(A, \epsilon) = 0$; that is, $A$ is associated with $Z$ but not associated with $\epsilon$ and any effect of $A$ on $Y$ must be through an effect of $A$ on $Z$. Conditional on the IV,

$$\mathrm{E}(Y|A = 1) - \mathrm{E}(Y|A = 0)$$
$$= \theta\{\mathrm{E}(Z|A = 1) - \mathrm{E}(Z|A = 0)\} + \mathrm{E}(\epsilon|A = 1) - \mathrm{E}(\epsilon|A = 0),$$

and by noting $\mathrm{E}(\epsilon|A = 1) - \mathrm{E}(\epsilon|A = 0) = 0$, we have

$$\theta = \frac{\mathrm{E}(Y|A = 1) - \mathrm{E}(Y|A = 0)}{\mathrm{E}(Z|A = 1) - \mathrm{E}(Z|A = 0)}.$$

For a better understanding of the differences between the IV, ITT, PP and AT estimators, we consider a study comparing two treatments (Angrist, Imbens, and Rubin, 1996; Bang and Davis, 2007). Let $A_i$ be the treatment indicator for patient $i$, and let $\tilde{Y}_{1i}$ and $\tilde{Y}_{0i}$ denote the counterfactuals, for $i = 1, \ldots, n$. We assume that there are counterfactual doses under each treatment, denoted by $\tilde{Z}_{1i}$

and $\tilde{Z}_{0i}$, which also take a value of 0 or 1. In reality, we only observe the actually received dose $Z_i$ and the induced response $Y_i$, which are given by

$$Z_i = (1 - A_i)\tilde{Z}_{0i} + A_i\tilde{Z}_{1i},$$
$$Y_i = (1 - Z_i)\tilde{Y}_{0i} + Z_i\tilde{Y}_{1i}.$$

The ITT estimator of the treatment effect is defined as

$$\hat{\theta}_{\text{ITT}} = \frac{\sum_{i=1}^{n} Y_i I(A_i = 1)}{\sum_{i=1}^{n} I(A_i = 1)} - \frac{\sum_{i=1}^{n} Y_i I(A_i = 0)}{\sum_{i=1}^{n} I(A_i = 0)},$$

which ignores post-randomization compliant status and compares the treatment groups formed by virtue of randomization. Under noncompliance, the ITT estimator is generally attenuated toward the null in a superiority trial, and toward the alternative in a noninferiority or an equivalence trial. The IV estimator is the ratio of the ITT effect of $A_i$ on $Y_i$ and that of $A_i$ on $Z_i$; that is,

$$\hat{\theta}_{\text{IV}} = \frac{\dfrac{\sum_{i=1}^{n} Y_i I(A_i = 1)}{\sum_{i=1}^{n} I(A_i = 1)} - \dfrac{\sum_{i=1}^{n} Y_i I(A_i = 0)}{\sum_{i=1}^{n} I(A_i = 0)}}{\dfrac{\sum_{i=1}^{n} Z_i I(A_i = 1)}{\sum_{i=1}^{n} I(A_i = 1)} - \dfrac{\sum_{i=1}^{n} Z_i I(A_i = 0)}{\sum_{i=1}^{n} I(A_i = 0)}}.$$

The AT estimator examines the difference between actual recipients and nonrecipients of the treatment, defined as

$$\hat{\theta}_{\text{AT}} = \frac{\sum_{i=1}^{n} Y_i I(Z_i = 1)}{\sum_{i=1}^{n} I(Z_i = 1)} - \frac{\sum_{i=1}^{n} Y_i I(Z_i = 0)}{\sum_{i=1}^{n} I(Z_i = 0)}.$$

The PP estimator compares the subjects who have strictly followed the protocol and fully complied with their assigned treatments, which is given by

$$\hat{\theta}_{\text{PP}} = \frac{\sum_{i=1}^{n} Y_i I(A_i = 1, Z_i = 1)}{\sum_{i=1}^{n} I(A_i = 1, Z_i = 1)} - \frac{\sum_{i=1}^{n} Y_i I(A_i = 0, Z_i = 0)}{\sum_{i=1}^{n} I(A_i = 0, Z_i = 0)}.$$

Although the AT and PP estimators are generally not recommended to be used alone, they can serve as complementary estimates to the ITT or IV analysis.

In summary, the ITT analysis includes all the randomized patients in the groups to which they were randomly assigned, regardless of their adherence with the entry criteria, the treatment they actually received, subsequent withdrawal from treatment, or any deviation from the protocol (Fisher et al., 1990). The ITT estimator compares treatment effects as randomized, which preserves the initial randomization and the baseline comparability among treatment groups. It also minimizes bias and prevents conscious or unconscious attempts to influence the study findings by excluding certain patients. The ITT analysis typically yields conservative estimates for treatment differences in superiority trials and thus is particularly preferred for comparisons of multiple treatments.

## 6.9   POST-APPROVAL TRIAL—PHASE IV

### 6.9.1   Limitations of Phase I–III Trials

If an experimental drug is shown to be effective in phase I–III trials, it will be filed to the FDA for approval. However, constrained by both the scopes and sizes, phase I, II, and III clinical trials have a number of limitations:

- more homogeneous and selective patient populations due to eligibility criteria,

- small sample sizes and less representative of the entire population,

- relatively short follow-ups,

- the use of surrogate endpoints, and

- a lack of generality of routine clinical practice.

In a phase IV trial, a larger number of patients with more diverse conditions are exposed to the approved drug, such that the "real-world" information on the drug's efficacy and safety can be obtained (Glasser, Salas, and Delzell, 2007; Kelly, Spielberg, and McAuliffe, 2008). The general population is much more heterogeneous than the patients studied in randomized controlled clinical trials due to the strict and specific enrollment criteria. In addition, the ways that patients are treated in routine clinical practice are very different from those in the "gold standard" phase III trials: The former may require patients taking multiple prescriptions or medications to manage both chronic and acute conditions, while the latter generally involves more intensive and well-controlled medical care with more frequent clinic visits and extra medical examinations.

Phase IV trials may be initiated as

- conditions required by the FDA or post-marketing commitments following the drug's approval,

- further investigations to support various drug development aspects sponsored by the pharmaceutical company,

- scientifically rigorous studies similar to randomized controlled phase III trials, or

- observational studies by investigators.

### 6.9.2   Drug Withdrawal

Phase IV trials aim to delineate more information on the drug's risks and benefits, so as to achieve its optimal use. In particular, phase IV trials may study different doses/schedules and routes of administration from those approved, treat patients with less stringent medical conditions or other stages of the disease in general clinical practice, demonstrate the drug's superiority over other competing agents, attain approval of new indications or label changes, and establish safety and efficacy in different patient populations.

As post-marketing studies, phase IV trials keep drug safety under close surveillance. To detect any rare or long-term adverse effects, a much larger patient population needs to be followed for a much longer period of time, which is typically not feasible in phase I–III clinical trials. Based on the nature and frequency of unintended adverse effects and thorough comparisons with alternative therapies, the FDA can add new risks to the warning label on the medication and, in a more serious occasion, the approved drug may be taken off the market. Withdrawal of a drug may be caused by rare and unpredictable adverse effects that have not been observed in previous studies. Prior to the FDA approval, a new drug is usually tested among 3,000 to 10,000 patients through phase I–III trials. As an example, if some severe drug-induced liver dysfunction or kidney failure only occurs at a rate of 1 in 5,000 to 10,000 exposures or less, these rare events will only surface when the drug is used in the general public. Some drugs may also be taken off the market because they are more toxic than expected, they interact with other prescription drugs or those over-the-counter resulting in "dangerous" drug combinations, or safer alternatives are developed and become available. After the approval, approximately 50% of drugs have label changes due to major safety concerns; 20% are issued new black box warnings; and 3% to 4% are ultimately withdrawn for severe safety reasons (Strom, 2006).

Compared with a phase III clinical trial, a phase IV trial enrolls a much larger number of heterogeneous samples with more diverse conditions. As usual, we can determine the sample size based on the effect size of the intervention and the nature of comparisons to be made with other standards of care. Nevertheless, phase IV trials often enroll patients attending different clinics, treated in different settings, or seen by different doctors. Because the data are often nested within clusters (e.g., doctors or clinics), intra-cluster correlations among the primary outcomes should be taken into consideration for power and sample size calculation; see Section 6.5.

In summary, interventions that have been shown to be effective in well-controlled clinical trials should be further evaluated under diverse "real-world" conditions. This is particularly important for the drugs that have been given accelerated approval, such as some HIV/AIDS drugs. To fulfill these purposes, phase IV trials should contain scientifically sound objectives. The design and implementation of these studies must allow us to reach firm conclusions on the impact and risks/benefits of new drugs through the widespread use in clinical practice.

## EXERCISES

**6.1**   In a superiority trial, suppose that the response rate of the standard treatment is 25%, and we expect that of the experimental treatment to be 40%. With the type I error rate $\alpha = 0.025$ and a power of 80%, what is the total sample size if the ratio of allocation between the experimental and standard arms is 2:1? Compare the sample size estimation based on the two different formulae (depending on whether to pool data together under the null hypothesis). How about the sample size using an allocation ratio of 1:1?

**6.2**   In a noninferiority trial, suppose that the noninferiority margin $\delta_N = 0.05$, and we take the response rates of both the standard and experimental treatments to be 30%. For a type I error rate of $\alpha = 0.05$ and a power of 90%, what is the total sample size of the trial with an allocation ratio of 1:1?

**6.3**   Consider the parametric approach to calculating the sample size for a clinical trial with survival endpoints. Assume exponential models with constant hazards $\lambda_1$ and $\lambda_2$ in groups 1 and 2, respectively. Under the alternative hypothesis $H_1$: $\lambda_1/\lambda_2 = \exp(\theta)$, with $\theta > 0$, show that

$$T_n|H_1 \sim \mathrm{N}(\sqrt{D}\theta/2, 1),$$

where $T_n$ is the log-rank statistic and $D$ is the total number of events.

**6.4**   Due to multiple testing, the overall type I error rate may be inflated. Given that each test is conducted at a significance level of $\alpha = 0.05$, verify that the overall type I error rate is 0.083 when two tests are conducted. How about the overall type I error rate with three tests?

**6.5**   In the group sequential designs, there are many other families of $\alpha$-spending functions, such as

$$\alpha(t) = \alpha \times \left( \frac{1 - e^{-\gamma t}}{1 - e^{-\gamma}} \right), \quad \gamma \neq 0,$$

or

$$\alpha(t) = \alpha t^{\gamma}.$$

Plot these two $\alpha$-spending functions under different values of $\gamma$. For what values of $\gamma$, Pocock's and O'Brien and Fleming's stopping boundaries can be generated, respectively?

**6.6**   In a two-arm group sequential trial with normal endpoints, show that the covariance function between the two test statistics $Z(t_j)$ and $Z(t_k)$ is

$$\mathrm{Cov}\{Z(t_j), Z(t_k)\} = \sqrt{\mathcal{I}_j/\mathcal{I}_k}, \quad 0 < t_j \leq t_k < 1,$$

where $\mathcal{I}_k$ is the information up to group $k$, and also show that

$$Z(t_k)\sqrt{\mathcal{I}_k} - Z(t_{k-1})\sqrt{\mathcal{I}_{k-1}} \sim \mathrm{N}(\theta(\mathcal{I}_k - \mathcal{I}_{k-1}), \mathcal{I}_k - \mathcal{I}_{k-1}).$$

Furthermore, prove that $Z(t_{k-1})$ and $Z(t_k)\sqrt{\mathcal{I}_k} - Z(t_{k-1})\sqrt{\mathcal{I}_{k-1}}$ are independent.

**6.7**   In the adaptive design with Fisher's combination test, show that the null hypothesis $H_0$ would be rejected if the $p$-values from the two stages satisfy

$$p_1 p_2 \le c_\alpha \equiv \exp(-\chi^2_{4,\alpha}/2).$$

# CHAPTER 7

# ADAPTIVE RANDOMIZATION

## 7.1 INTRODUCTION

The general goals of randomized clinical trials are to

- treat patients effectively, and

- differentiate treatment effects efficiently,

albeit the inherent conflict between the two due to individual versus collective ethics. On one hand, a clinical trial tries to discriminate the effects of different treatments quickly, so that more patients outside of the trial would benefit from the more efficacious treatment sooner. For this purpose, patients' allocation should be (nearly) balanced across the comparative arms. On the other hand, each trial participant should be treated the most effectively, and patients themselves also hope that they would be assigned to the arm that performs better. This often leads to an unbalanced allocation through adaptive randomization by equipping a better arm with a higher allocation probability. Therefore, randomized clinical trials need to strike a balance between individual and collective ethics.

To ensure an objective comparison of different treatments, patients' allocation should be random (or unpredictable) so that different groups are balanced with

*Clinical Trial Design.* By Guosheng Yin
Copyright © 2012 John Wiley & Sons, Inc.

respect to all known and unknown prognostic factors that may affect the response. In practice, investigators might consciously or unconsciously assign patients under certain conditions to a specific treatment—for example, always giving healthier patients the treatment that is believed to work better. Such potential selection bias can be prevented if using randomization in conjunction with a double-blind scheme.

Not only can randomization effectively reduce bias and confounding effects, but it also forms the fundamental basis for statistical analysis. Although post-adjustment procedures, such as analysis of covariance or regression models, may account for a lack of comparability between treatment groups, clinical trials with well-balanced prognostic variables are more credible and efficient. In general, randomization can be classified as follows:

- *Simple randomization* is the most straightforward way for patient allocation, which fixes randomization probabilities but may lead to unbalanced groups.

- *Permuted block randomization* guarantees the number of subjects in each group to be the same during the trial.

- *Stratified randomization* first stratifies participants by certain important prognostic factors, and then allocates them within each stratum. Thus at least, the numbers of patients for those stratification factors can be balanced.

- *Adaptive randomization* allows the allocation probability for each arm to change as the trial progresses. It can be covariate-adaptive to balance the baseline prognostic factors or outcome-adaptive to assign more patients to better treatment arms.

The first three randomization procedures have fixed allocation probabilities. The use of block and stratification in randomization helps to balance different groups and also to control unwanted variations. By contrast, adaptive randomization allows the randomization probabilities to change throughout the trial. Covariate-adaptive randomization intends to make patients in different groups more alike, while response- or outcome-adaptive randomization aims to treat more patients with better treatments.

Response or outcome-based adaptive randomization, simply abbreviated as AR from now on, is the main focus of this chapter. Under such an AR scheme, the responses of the currently treated patients in the trial are used to determine the treatment allocation for future participants. The purpose is to increase the number of patients assigned to the superior arm, so that more patients will benefit from the better treatment based upon the evidence accumulated from the data.

Historically, equal randomization is the standard for treatment assignment due to its ease of implementation and the state of equipoise (genuine uncertainty about which treatment is more beneficial). In general, equal randomization leans toward collective ethics, because if a trial can demonstrate the effectiveness of an experimental treatment earlier (due to higher power), more patients outside of the trial would benefit from it sooner. By contrast, AR is more concerned with individual ethics; that is to treat patients in the current trial more effectively using the better treatment. While it appears to be more ethical and appealing to each individual patient, AR may lead to imbalanced numbers of patients among different arms and thus result in loss of efficiency for the study. Moreover, real-time AR requires patients' outcomes to be ascertainable immediately or shortly after treatment; otherwise, new participants may have to wait for treatment assignment until the responses of all the previous patients are obtained. However, it is neither sensible nor ethical to withhold treatment from patients due to others' delayed responses.

The history of AR can be traced back to the pioneering work of Thompson (1933) and Robbins (1952). Zelen (1969) introduces the play-the-winner rule for a two-arm trial: The next patient is assigned to the same treatment if the previous patient responded, or to the other treatment if the previous patient did not respond. Wei and Durham (1978) extend the deterministic allocation in the play-the-winner rule to a randomized version. Efron (1971) studies the biased coin design to balance the patient allocation based on the extent of imbalance among different arms. Eisele (1994) develops a doubly adaptive biased coin design to target a certain allocation proportion. Berry and Eick (1995) make a through comparison of several AR procedures, including a two-arm bandit and a robust Bayesian method. Thall and Wathen (2007) take AR as a compromise between equal randomization and treatment assignment based on physicians' preference. Although AR is useful to mitigate ethical issues, it may cause imbalance of the prognostic factors among different groups. To bridge response-adaptive and covariate-adjusted randomization, the allocation probability may be skewed to more effective treatments, while at the same time the distributions of the covariates are adjusted toward balance (Ning and Huang, 2010; Yuan, Huang, and Liu, 2011). For comprehensive coverage on various randomization methods, see Rosenberger and Lachin (2002) and Hu and Rosenberger (2006).

## 7.2  SIMPLE RANDOMIZATION

In simple randomization, the probability that a patient is assigned to each treatment arm is fixed throughout the trial with no regard to the history of patient allocations. If equal randomization is used in a trial with $K$ treatments, each participant is simply assigned with probability $1/K$ to one of the $K$ groups. For a two-arm trial as shown in Figure 7.1, equal randomization can be achieved by tossing a fair coin. In some circumstances, it may be desirable to allocate more subjects to a certain treatment, because that treatment is believed to work

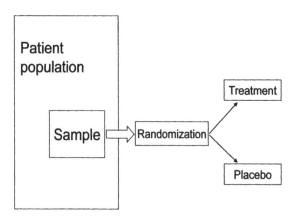

**Figure 7.1**   Simple randomization in a two-arm trial.

better or investigators are interested in learning more about a specific drug. If the allocation ratio to the new therapy versus the standard therapy is 2:1, then more information can be gained on the new treatment.

The allocation unit can be either individual-based or group/cluster-based. For individual-based randomization, patients are randomized on a one-by-one basis. For group-based randomization, a group of subjects belonging to the same family, clinic, or community is randomized together to a particular intervention group. Simple randomization is straightforward and unpredictable, while it may cause imbalance among different groups.

## 7.3   PERMUTED BLOCK RANDOMIZATION

To achieve perfect balance across different groups, we may use the so-called permuted block randomization. By permuting the patient allocation within each block, the method guarantees an equal number of patients assigned to each treatment during the course of the trial (Simon, 1979). For illustration, suppose that we want to compare three treatments, say A, B, and C, in a randomized trial. If the permuted block randomization uses a block size of three, then the possible permutation sequences are

$$\{ABC, \ ACB, \ BAC, \ BCA, \ CAB, \ CBA\}.$$

At the randomization, a block is randomly chosen first, say BAC; that means, the first patient in the block will receive treatment B, the second will receive treatment A, and the third will receive treatment C. This ensures that exactly one

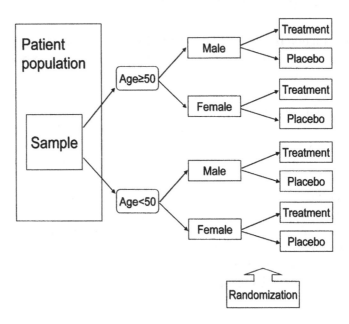

**Figure 7.2**    Stratified randomization by the age of 50 years and patient sex in a two-arm trial.

patient is assigned to each treatment within the block. As another example, we consider a randomized two-arm trial with treatments A and B. If we use a block size of four, then two patients in each block will be assigned to treatment A and the other two will receive treatment B. As a result, the permutation sequences can be written as

$$\{AABB, \ ABAB, \ ABBA, \ BBAA, \ BABA, \ BAAB\}.$$

Obviously, such permuted block randomization guarantees the number of patients allocated to each treatment arm to be the same.

However, there is a potential for selection bias if the practitioner is aware of the block size. By the end of each block, the treatment assigned to the last participant in the block will always be known as long as the previous treatment assignments have been kept track of. A natural remedy to prevent such selection bias is to make the block size unpredictable as well. For example, in a clinical trial with three treatments, the block size may be randomly chosen from $\{3, 6, 9\}$; in a study with two treatments, the block size may be randomly selected from $\{2, 4, 6, 8\}$. This additional randomness in the block size makes the permuted block randomization unpredictable.

## 7.4  STRATIFIED RANDOMIZATION

Simple randomization and permuted block randomization may not be able to balance certain prognostic factors of particular interest. To balance over some particular covariates of importance, randomization may be stratified by them. Subjects entering the trial are first classified into mutually exclusive strata, and then within each stratum separately, patients are randomly allocated to each treatment. Figure 7.2 displays that patients are stratified by the age of 50 years and sex, before randomization takes place. However, the number of strata increases multiplicatively with the number of stratification factors. If the number of strata is relatively large in comparison to the number of subjects, some strata may have few or even no patients assigned. This, in turn, may yield considerable imbalance among treatment groups (Therneau, 1993).

In a small study, a few strata for the most important risk factors may be identified in advance to assure appropriate balance for those factors at least. In a large multi-center trial, the center is often used as one of the stratification factors, which may limit the number of additional prognostic factors for stratification.

## 7.5  COVARIATE-ADAPTIVE ALLOCATION BY MINIMIZATION

When there is a large number of prognostic factors in a trial, it becomes difficult to achieve overall balance across all of the covariates. Taves (1974) and Pocock and Simon (1975) propose the minimization method (also known as dynamic allocation, covariate-adaptive, or -adjusted randomization) for sequential treatment assignment. During the randomization process, the allocation of each subject is determined by the current overall balance among the treatment groups. Hence, the randomization probability to each treatment arm is not fixed, but keeps changing as the trial proceeds. The minimization method determines treatment assignment based on the distributions of covariates in order to achieve desirable balancing properties.

All of the important prognostic factors should be identified prior to the initiation of the trial. Continuous prognostic factors need to be categorized into meaningful ordinal levels. The dynamic allocation (minimization) procedure works toward minimizing the total imbalance of all the prognostic variables, which is mainly characterized by

- the amount of variation or imbalance across different arms for each factor level marginally,

- the measure of the total imbalance across all the treatment groups, and

- the prespecified assignment probabilities for the $K$ groups, $p_{(1)} > \cdots > p_{(K)}$, where $p_{(1)}$ is the probability of assignment to the treatment that would lead to the least total imbalance, $p_{(2)}$ is the second in reducing the total imbalance, $p_{(3)}$ is the third, and so on.

More specifically, let $I$ denote the total number of prognostic factors under consideration. In a two-arm trial with $K = 2$, let $n_{i1}$ be the number of subjects assigned to treatment 1 and $n_{i2}$ be that assigned to treatment 2, then the difference for factor $i$ is given by

$$g_i = |n_{i1} - n_{i2}|, \quad i = 1, \ldots, I. \tag{7.1}$$

For a multi-arm trial with $K > 2$, define

$$g_i = \max_{j,k=1,\ldots,K} |n_{ij} - n_{ik}|, \quad i = 1, \ldots, I,$$

which measures the most imbalance in any pair of treatment groups for the $i$th factor.

The total imbalance is measured by summing over the marginal imbalance for each factor, $G = \sum_{i=1}^{I} g_i$. If some prognostic factors are considered more important than others—for example, tumor stage is clinically more relevant in oncology than patients' sex and age—it is more sensible to use a weighted sum,

$$G = \sum_{i=1}^{I} w_i g_i,$$

where $w_i$ is the prefixed weight characterizing the importance of the $i$th factor. If the total imbalance $G$ is the same regardless of which treatment is assigned to the new patient, the treatment allocation would be purely at random; otherwise, the next patient is more likely to receive the treatment that would lead to the least overall imbalance.

**Table 7.1    Illustration of the Minimization Method, with the First 40 Patients Distributed across the Three Prognostic Factors of Sex, Race, and Tumor Stage**

| Prognostic Factor | Level | Treatment A | Treatment B | Imbalance |
|---|---|---|---|---|
| Sex | Male | 10 | 8 | 2 |
|  | Female | 9 | 13 | 4 |
| Race | Caucasian | 11 | 12 | 1 |
|  | Hispanic | 8 | 9 | 1 |
| Tumor stage | I | 7 | 6 | 1 |
|  | II | 9 | 12 | 3 |
|  | III | 3 | 3 | 0 |

We present an example in Table 7.1 to demonstrate how to achieve overall balance on three prognostic factors: sex, race, and tumor stage. For any given factor level, the measure of imbalance between treatment groups A and B is based upon the absolute difference $g_i$ in (7.1). The total imbalance $G$ is measured by a sum of the $g_i$'s (with equal weights $w_1 = w_2 = w_3 = 1$ for sex, race, and tumor stage). The largest assignment probability is prespecified as $p_{(1)} = 0.75$, with which the subject will be allocated to the treatment group that would yield the least overall imbalance, and thus $p_{(2)} = 0.25$. The values of $p_{(1)}$ and $p_{(2)}$ are specified arbitrarily, as long as each new patient will have a higher probability to be assigned to an arm that tends to reduce the total imbalance.

As shown in Table 7.1, 40 subjects have been enrolled in the trial thus far. Suppose that the next subject entering the trial is a male Hispanic patient with tumor stage II. To determine which treatment this patient will be assigned, we consider the following two hypothetical situations:

- If this subject receives treatment A, the updated table of imbalance would be

| Prognostic Factor | Level | Treatment A | Treatment B | Imbalance |
| --- | --- | --- | --- | --- |
| Sex | Male | 11 | 8 | 3 |
| Race | Hispanic | 9 | 9 | 0 |
| Tumor stage | II | 10 | 12 | 2 |

which leads to the total imbalance of $G = 3 + 0 + 2 = 5$.

- If this subject receives treatment B, the updated table of imbalance would be

| Prognostic Factor | Level | Treatment A | Treatment B | Imbalance |
| --- | --- | --- | --- | --- |
| Sex | Male | 10 | 9 | 1 |
| Race | Hispanic | 8 | 10 | 2 |
| Tumor stage | II | 9 | 13 | 4 |

which leads to the total imbalance of $G = 1 + 2 + 4 = 7$.

The total imbalance between the two treatment groups would be minimized if this patient were assigned to treatment A. Therefore, this subject will be assigned to arm A with probability $p_{(1)} = 0.75$ and to arm B with probability $p_{(2)} = 0.25$.

Following covariate-adaptive randomization, the usual two-sample $t$ test without adjusting for any covariate is conservative. Shao, Yu, and Zhong (2010) provide a valid statistical test by using the correct model between outcomes and covariates, and they also develop a two-sample $t$ test based on the bootstrap procedure.

## 7.6  BIASED COIN DESIGN

In a two-arm randomized study, the biased coin design (BCD) can be used to sequentially allocate patients between the two treatments (Blackwell and Hodges, 1957; Efron, 1971). The BCD specifies the sequential randomization rule by the means of hypothetically tossing a biased coin which has a probability of $p$ $(p > 1/2)$ landing on the head. For illustration, let $n_1$ and $n_2$ denote the numbers of subjects assigned to arm 1 and arm 2, respectively. Let $p$ be the randomization probability for arm 1, and thus $1 - p$ is that for arm 2. As the trial proceeds, a new patient will be allocated to arm 1 with a probability of

$$\text{Pr(assigned to arm 1)} = \begin{cases} p, & \text{if } n_1 < n_2, \\ 1/2, & \text{if } n_1 = n_2, \\ 1 - p, & \text{if } n_1 > n_2. \end{cases}$$

For example, if $p = 2/3$, then each randomization step favors the treatment that has been underrepresented thus far.

Sometimes, simply using the difference in the number of subjects may not be sufficient to characterize how unbalanced the two groups are. For example, an allocation with $n_1 = 100$ versus $n_2 = 95$ is not considered as unbalanced as that with $n_1 = 10$ versus $n_2 = 5$, although the actual differences are the same. In this case, the relative difference $\Delta/n$ is more relevant, where $\Delta = n_1 - n_2$ and $n = n_1 + n_2$ is the total sample size. Let $g(\cdot)$ be a known decreasing function with $g(0) = 1/2$. To put more weight on the relative imbalance, Wei (1978) recommends the allocation probability to arm 1 as

$$p \equiv g\left(\frac{\Delta}{n}\right) = \frac{1}{2}\left(1 - \frac{\Delta}{n}\right).$$

Nevertheless, using the relative difference to characterize the imbalance may also cause ambiguity. For example, the case with $n_1 = 3$ and $n_2 = 2$ (i.e., $\Delta/n = 1/5$) and that with $n_1 = 12$ and $n_2 = 8$ (i.e., $\Delta/n = 4/20$) are indistinguishable based on the relative difference, while the former is as balanced as it can be but the later is clearly unbalanced.

Antognini and Giovagnoli (2004) propose an adjustable BCD—the more imbalanced the two groups, the more strength will be imposed to pull the samples back to balance. Let $g(x)$ be a function that maps from an integer to a probability, which satisfies that $g(x)$ is decreasing and $g(-x) = 1 - g(x)$. Among a variety of allocation probability functions, the one of particular interest is given by

$$g_\gamma(\Delta) = \begin{cases} |\Delta|^\gamma/(|\Delta|^\gamma + 1), & \text{if } \Delta \leq -1, \\ 1/2, & \text{if } \Delta = 0, \\ 1/(|\Delta|^\gamma + 1), & \text{if } \Delta \geq 1, \end{cases}$$

where the power parameter $\gamma \geq 0$ adjusts how much strength is exerted to pull the unbalanced sample sizes toward balance.

**Table 7.2** **Play-the-Winner Rule with Dichotomous Outcomes—Treatment Success (S) or Failure (F)**

| Order of Participants | 1 | 2 | 3 | 4 | 5 | 6 | 7 | 8 | 9 | 10 |
|---|---|---|---|---|---|---|---|---|---|---|
| Treatment A | S | S | F | – | – | – | – | S | F | – |
| Treatment B | – | – | – | S | S | S | F | – | – | F |

## 7.7 PLAY-THE-WINNER RULE

### 7.7.1 Deterministic Scheme

The play-the-winner rule (Zelen, 1969) is a simple response-adaptive design as described below. In a study comparing two treatments A and B, suppose that patients' responses are dichotomous: success or failure. The first patient is randomized to either treatment A or B with an equal probability. If the previous patient's response is a success, the next patient will be assigned the same treatment as the previous one. If the previous patient's response is a failure, the next patient will receive the other treatment. Therefore, once the outcome of the previous patient is obtained, the treatment assignment for the next patient is completely determined; that is to stay with the winner until a failure occurs and then switch to the alternative treatment.

As illustrated in Table 7.2, the first participant is randomized to treatment A or B with a probability of 0.5. Suppose that by chance, this subject received treatment A. Because the response of the first patient was a success, the second patient was assigned to arm A as well, and the response was again a success. Then, the third participant continued to receive treatment A, but a failure was observed, which triggered a switch of the treatment. Therefore, the fourth subject changed to treatment B; and because a subsequent success was observed, the fifth participant stayed on treatment B. Such a process continues until the total sample size is exhausted. The ratio of the numbers of subjects assigned to treatment A and treatment B tends to $(1 - p_B)/(1 - p_A)$ as the number of patients in the trial goes to infinity, where $p_A$ and $p_B$ denote the response rates of treatments A and B, respectively.

### 7.7.2 Randomized Scheme

The original play-the-winner rule lacks randomness because each treatment assignment is fully and only determined by the outcome of the previous patient, regardless of the outcomes of other patients. By contrast, the randomized play-the-winner rule gives a higher probability to change to the other treatment for the next patient if a failure is observed from the previous patient, instead of a definitive switch of treatment (Wei and Durham, 1978).

The randomized play-the-winner rule can be described with an urn model. Suppose that in an urn, there are two types of balls, marked as A or B. Starting with $n$ balls of each type, we randomly draw a ball with replacement to determine which treatment will be assigned to a new patient. If the ball is of type A, the subject is assigned to arm A. If the subsequent response of this subject is a success, additional $\alpha$ balls of type A and $\beta$ balls of type B are added to the urn, with $\alpha \geq \beta \geq 0$. Therefore, the next subject would have a higher probability of

$$\Pr(\text{next drawn ball is A}) = \frac{\alpha + n}{\alpha + \beta + 2n} \geq 0.5,$$

to be assigned to arm A. On the other hand, if the response of this subject is a failure, additional $\beta$ balls of type A and $\alpha$ balls of type B are added to the urn, so that the next subject would have a lower probability of

$$\Pr(\text{next drawn ball is A}) = \frac{\beta + n}{\alpha + \beta + 2n} \leq 0.5,$$

to be assigned to arm A. In practice, it may happen that when a new patient enters the trial, the response of the previous subject is still not available (i.e., delayed response). In this circumstance, we may immediately draw a ball from the urn of current status for this new participant. We will update the balls' composition in the urn whenever the response of that previously treated patient is obtained.

If the urn starts as empty with $n = 0$, a patient would be randomized with an equal probability of 0.5 to each treatment. Whenever an outcome is observed, the allocation probability will be skewed in favor of the better-performing treatment thus far. If $\alpha = 1$ and $\beta = 0$, and every time before a ball is drawn we reset the urn to be empty with $n = 0$, then the randomized play-the-winner rule reduces to the original design with deterministic treatment allocation.

## 7.8  DROP-THE-LOSER RULE

Similar to the play-the-winner rule, the drop-the-loser rule also assigns more patients to a better treatment. The two designs target the same allocation proportion; that is $(1 - p_B)/(1 - p_A)$ between treatment A and treatment B, where $p_A$ and $p_B$ are the corresponding response rates. The drop-the-loser rule may produce a less variable proportion during patients' allocation to treatment groups (Ivanova, 2003; Zhang et al., 2007). The reduction in the allocation variability often leads to improvement in the statistical power.

In a two-arm trial with treatments A and B, we describe the drop-the-loser rule with an urn model. Suppose that an urn contains three types of balls: Balls of types A and B represent treatments, and balls of type 0 are called immigration balls whose function is to avoid extinction of those treatment balls. The urn starts with $n_A$, $n_B$, and $n_0$ balls of types A, B, and 0, respectively. Upon a patient's arrival, one ball is drawn at random. If a treatment ball is selected, either A or B, the corresponding treatment is given to the subject. If the patient's response to the treatment is a failure, the ball will not be replaced back to the urn (i.e., the "loser" is dropped); and if the response is a success, the ball will be replaced and consequently the composition of the urn remains unchanged. If an immigration ball of type 0 is selected, no treatment is assigned to the patient and the ball will be replaced back to the urn together with one ball of type A and one ball of type B; and then we draw another ball for this patient.

## 7.9 OPTIMAL ADAPTIVE RANDOMIZATION

### 7.9.1 Dichotomous Outcome

Adaptive randomization may be optimized with respect to a certain criterion, for example, to minimize the variance (equivalently, to maximize power) or to minimize the number of nonresponders in a trial (Rosenberger et al., 2001). Such a randomization procedure targets a specific allocation proportion, which turns into a constrained optimization problem. In general, a trial may be evaluated by the target allocation proportion, and the bias and variability of randomization procedure (Melfi, Page, and Geraldes, 2001; Hu and Rosenberger, 2003).

To avoid unnecessary complications, we consider a randomized two-arm trial with dichotomous and immediately known responses. Let $p_1$ be the response rate of treatment 1, and let $p_2$ be that of treatment 2. We are interested in testing whether there is a difference between the two treatments,

$$H_0: p_1 = p_2 \quad \text{versus} \quad H_1: p_1 \neq p_2.$$

Suppose that at a certain point of trial conduct, $y_1$ patients have responded among the $n_1$ patients in arm 1 and $y_2$ have responded among the $n_2$ patients in arm 2. If we denote the allocation ratio $r = n_1/n_2$ and the total sample size $n = n_1 + n_2$, then

$$n_1 = \frac{nr}{1+r} \quad \text{and} \quad n_2 = \frac{n}{1+r}.$$

The consistent estimators for $p_1$ and $p_2$ are the corresponding sample proportions, $\hat{p}_1 = y_1/n_1$ and $\hat{p}_2 = y_2/n_2$, and the variance of the response difference is

$$
\begin{aligned}
V &\equiv \text{Var}(\hat{p}_1 - \hat{p}_2) \\
&= \frac{p_1(1-p_1)}{n_1} + \frac{p_2(1-p_2)}{n_2} \\
&= \frac{p_1(1-p_1)}{n}\left(1+\frac{1}{r}\right) + \frac{p_2(1-p_2)}{n}(1+r).
\end{aligned} \tag{7.2}
$$

The so-called Neyman allocation is obtained by minimizing the variance, which leads to the allocation ratio between arm 1 and arm 2 as

$$r_{\text{Neyman}} = \frac{\sqrt{p_1(1-p_1)}}{\sqrt{p_2(1-p_2)}}.$$

In other words, the optimal allocation (to maximize power while fixing the total sample size) is to assign patients proportional to the squared root of the variance of the parameter estimate. Neyman's allocation can also be interpreted as minimizing the total sample size while fixing the variance. However, Neyman's allocation may not be ethical because it may assign more patients to an inferior treatment when $p_1 + p_2 > 1$, say, $p_1 = 0.5$ and $p_2 = 0.6$. A simple remedy to Neyman's allocation is to take equal randomization whenever the assignment probability to the inferior arm is higher than that to the superior arm.

From an ethical perspective, Rosenberger et al. (2001) propose an optimal allocation scheme that minimizes the expected number of nonresponders while fixing the variance of the test statistic. Following this route, we can minimize

$$n_1(1-p_1) + n_2(1-p_2) = \frac{nr}{1+r}(1-p_1) + \frac{n}{1+r}(1-p_2), \qquad (7.3)$$

subject to fixing the variance of $\hat{p}_1 - \hat{p}_2$ in (7.2) as a constant. Thus after plugging in

$$n = \frac{1}{V}\left\{ p_1(1-p_1)\left(1+\frac{1}{r}\right) + p_2(1-p_2)(1+r) \right\},$$

we take the first derivative of (7.3) with respect to $r$, which leads to an optimal allocation ratio of

$$r_{\text{opt}} = \frac{\sqrt{p_1}}{\sqrt{p_2}}.$$

In the application of adaptive randomization, $p_1$ and $p_2$ are unknown; we can continuously replace them by the sample proportions $\hat{p}_1$ and $\hat{p}_2$.

### 7.9.2 Continuous Outcome

Although dichotomous outcomes are intuitive and widely used to characterize patients' responses after treatment, continuous outcomes may also arise as the primary endpoint in clinical trials (Zhang and Rosenberger, 2006). For example, the reduction in the diastolic blood pressure may be used to evaluate antihypertensive efficacy of losartan and amlodipine (Wilson, Lacourcière, and Barnes, 1998), and the Hamilton depression rating scale is often measured on patients with depressive disorder treatments (Vieta et al., 2002). To avoid cumbersome calculations, we assume that continuous outcomes are normally distributed, $Y_1 \sim \text{N}(\mu_1, \sigma_1^2)$ and $Y_2 \sim \text{N}(\mu_2, \sigma_2^2)$ for treatment 1 and treatment 2, respectively. We are interested in testing whether there is a difference between the two treatments; that is,

$$H_0: \mu_1 = \mu_2 \quad \text{versus} \quad H_1: \mu_1 \neq \mu_2.$$

Based on the consistent estimators $\hat{\mu}_1$, $\hat{\mu}_2$, $\hat{\sigma}_1^2$, and $\hat{\sigma}_2^2$, we can construct a $Z$-test statistic

$$Z = \frac{\hat{\mu}_1 - \hat{\mu}_2}{\sqrt{\hat{\sigma}_1^2/n_1 + \hat{\sigma}_2^2/n_2}},$$

which follows the standard normal distribution asymptotically. By minimizing the variance

$$\begin{aligned} \text{Var}(\hat{\mu}_1 - \hat{\mu}_2) &= \frac{\sigma_1^2}{n_1} + \frac{\sigma_2^2}{n_2} \\ &= \frac{\sigma_1^2}{n}\left(1 + \frac{1}{r}\right) + \frac{\sigma_2^2}{n}(1 + r) \end{aligned} \tag{7.4}$$

with respect to $r$, we obtain Neyman's allocation ratio,

$$r_{\text{Neyman}} = \frac{\sigma_1}{\sigma_2}.$$

On the other hand, we may minimize the total expected response from all patients if a smaller response is preferred (e.g., lowering the blood pressure). Hence, we minimize

$$n_1 \mu_1 + n_2 \mu_2$$

subject to fixing the variance as a constant $V \equiv \text{Var}(\hat{\mu}_1 - \hat{\mu}_2)$ given in (7.4). This leads to an allocation ratio of

$$r_{\text{opt}} = \frac{\sigma_1 \sqrt{\mu_2}}{\sigma_2 \sqrt{\mu_1}}.$$

However, it may happen that more patients are allocated to the inferior treatment with certain values of $\mu_1$, $\mu_2$, $\sigma_1$, and $\sigma_2$; for example, $\mu_1 = 0.1$, $\mu_2 = 0.2$, and $\sigma_1 = \sigma_2 = 1$. Whenever such an inappropriate allocation is observed, we should take equal randomization, so that the assignment probability to a better treatment group is guaranteed to be at least $1/2$. If a larger response is preferred in a trial, we may minimize

$$\frac{n_1}{\mu_1} + \frac{n_2}{\mu_2}$$

subject to the same variance constraint in (7.4), which results in an allocation ratio of

$$r_{\text{opt}} = \frac{\sigma_1 \sqrt{\mu_1}}{\sigma_2 \sqrt{\mu_2}}.$$

Biswas and Mandal (2004) propose an alternative optimal criterion based on a probit transformation. Let $\Phi(\cdot)$ denote the cumulative distribution function of the standard normal distribution, and let $c$ be a constant beyond which the response is considered undesirable. We can minimize

$$n_1 \Phi \left( \frac{\mu_1 - c}{\sigma_1} \right) + n_2 \Phi \left( \frac{\mu_2 - c}{\sigma_2} \right),$$

which is equivalent to minimizing the number of patients with responses greater than $c$. The resulting allocation ratio is

$$r_{\mathrm{opt}} = \frac{\sigma_1 \sqrt{\Phi\{(\mu_2 - c)/\sigma_2\}}}{\sigma_2 \sqrt{\Phi\{(\mu_1 - c)/\sigma_1\}}}.$$

### 7.9.3   Time-to-Event Outcome

For time-to-event endpoints, Zhang and Rosenberger (2007) develop an optimal allocation while assuming parametric survival models. Let $T$ denote the failure time with an exponential density function,

$$f(t) = \lambda \exp(-\lambda t),$$

and a survival function,

$$S(t) = \exp(-\lambda t),$$

where $\lambda$ is the constant hazard rate.

Due to independent right censoring, we actually observe i.i.d. replicates of $X_i = \min(T_i, C_i)$ and $\Delta_i = I(T_i \leq C_i)$, where $C_i$ is the censoring time, for $i = 1, \ldots, n$. Under the exponential model, the likelihood function is given by

$$L(\lambda) = \prod_{i=1}^{n} \{\lambda \exp(-\lambda X_i)\}^{\Delta_i} \{\exp(-\lambda X_i)\}^{1-\Delta_i}.$$

We take the first derivative of the log-likelihood function with respect to $\lambda$, which leads to the score function

$$\frac{\mathrm{d} \log L(\lambda)}{\mathrm{d}\lambda} = \frac{1}{\lambda} \sum_{i=1}^{n} \Delta_i - \sum_{i=1}^{n} X_i,$$

and thus the maximum likelihood estimator (MLE) of $\lambda$ is

$$\hat{\lambda} = \frac{\sum_{i=1}^{n} \Delta_i}{\sum_{i=1}^{n} X_i}.$$

By taking the second derivative of $-\log L(\lambda)$, the observed information for $\lambda$ is given by

$$I_n(\lambda) = \frac{\sum_{i=1}^{n} \Delta_i}{\lambda^2},$$

and the expected information for $\lambda$ is

$$\mathcal{I}(\lambda) = \frac{n\delta}{\lambda^2},$$

where $\delta = \mathrm{E}(\Delta_i) = \mathrm{Pr}(\Delta_i = 1)$. The estimate for the variance of $\hat{\lambda}$ is $I_n^{-1}(\hat{\lambda})$.

If we compare two exponential survival distributions with respective hazard rates $\lambda_1$ and $\lambda_2$ for treatment group 1 and group 2, the hypothesis testing formulates

$$H_0\colon \lambda_1 = \lambda_2 \quad \text{versus} \quad H_1\colon \lambda_1 \neq \lambda_2.$$

The total sample size is $n = n_1 + n_2$ and the allocation ratio between arm 1 and arm 2 is $r = n_1/n_2$. We can construct a Wald test statistic,

$$Z = \frac{\hat{\lambda}_1 - \hat{\lambda}_2}{\sqrt{\hat{\lambda}_1^2/\sum_{i=1}^{n_1}\Delta_{1i} + \hat{\lambda}_2^2/\sum_{i=1}^{n_2}\Delta_{2i}}},$$

where $\Delta_{1i}$ and $\Delta_{2i}$ are the censoring indicators in group 1 and group 2, respectively. Let $\delta_1 = \mathrm{E}(\Delta_{1i})$ and $\delta_2 = \mathrm{E}(\Delta_{2i})$. By minimizing the variance

$$\begin{aligned}
\mathrm{Var}(\hat{\lambda}_1 - \hat{\lambda}_2) &= \frac{\lambda_1^2}{n_1\delta_1} + \frac{\lambda_2^2}{n_2\delta_2} \\
&= \frac{\lambda_1^2}{n\delta_1}\left(1 + \frac{1}{r}\right) + \frac{\lambda_2^2}{n\delta_2}(1 + r)
\end{aligned} \tag{7.5}$$

with respect to $r$, we obtain Neyman's allocation ratio,

$$r_{\mathrm{Neyman}} = \frac{\lambda_1\sqrt{\delta_2}}{\lambda_2\sqrt{\delta_1}}.$$

To derive the optimal allocation that minimizes the total expected hazard, we minimize

$$n_1\lambda_1 + n_2\lambda_2$$

subject to fixing the variance in (7.5) at a constant. The optimal allocation ratio is given by

$$r_{\mathrm{opt}} = \frac{\sqrt{\lambda_1\delta_2}}{\sqrt{\lambda_2\delta_1}}.$$

Alternatively, we may use a more meaningful optimal criterion; for example, to maximize the total number of patients who have survived beyond a constant time $c$, $n_1 S_1(c) + n_2 S_2(c)$, where $S_1(t)$ and $S_2(t)$ are the survival functions for group 1 and group 2, respectively. However, such a maximum does not exist. By contrast, we may minimize the total number of patients who have experienced the event (failure or death) by time $c$,

$$n_1\{1 - S_1(c)\} + n_2\{1 - S_2(c)\},$$

subject to fixing the variance in (7.5) at a constant. As a result, the optimal allocation ratio is

$$r_{\text{opt}} = \frac{\lambda_1 \sqrt{\delta_2 \{1 - \exp(-\lambda_2 c)\}}}{\lambda_2 \sqrt{\delta_1 \{1 - \exp(-\lambda_1 c)\}}}.$$

## 7.10  DOUBLY ADAPTIVE BIASED COIN DESIGN

When the randomization probability adaptively changes in the course of a trial, there is often a target allocation ratio between the two arms. The doubly adaptive biased coin design allows the randomization probability to explicitly depend on both the observed allocation proportion and the estimated target allocation ratio (Eisele, 1994; Eisele and Woodroofe, 1995; Hu and Zhang, 2004). It simultaneously takes into consideration both the future goal and the current situation by using an allocation function $g(x, \rho)$ to balance the current allocation proportion $x$ and the target allocation probability $\rho$:

$$g(x, \rho) = \begin{cases} \dfrac{\rho(\rho/x)^\gamma}{\rho(\rho/x)^\gamma + (1 - \rho)\{(1 - \rho)/(1 - x)\}^\gamma}, & \text{if } 0 < x < 1, \\ 1 - x, & \text{if } x = 0 \text{ or } 1. \end{cases}$$

The power parameter $\gamma > 0$ controls the degree of randomness of the procedure.

The target allocation probability $\rho$ may be obtained by using the optimal adaptive randomization methods discussed in the previous section. For example, to minimize the number of nonresponders, the target allocation probability to arm 1 is $\rho = \sqrt{p_1}/(\sqrt{p_1} + \sqrt{p_2})$. Suppose that $y_k$ patients have responded among $n_k$ patients who were enrolled in treatment arm $k$. We can estimate the response rates by $\hat{p}_k = y_k/n_k$, for $k = 1, 2$. Since the current allocation proportion in arm 1 is $x = n_1/(n_1 + n_2)$, the probability that the next patient will be assigned to treatment 1 is $g(x, \hat{\rho})$, where

$$\hat{\rho} = \frac{\sqrt{\hat{p}_1}}{\sqrt{\hat{p}_1} + \sqrt{\hat{p}_2}}.$$

## 7.11  BAYESIAN ADAPTIVE RANDOMIZATION

### 7.11.1  Two-Arm Comparison

Using the "learn as we go" approach, AR assigns more patients to better treatment arms based on the outcomes of previous patients in the on-going trial. There is typically a prephase of equal randomization (ER) at the beginning of a trial, due

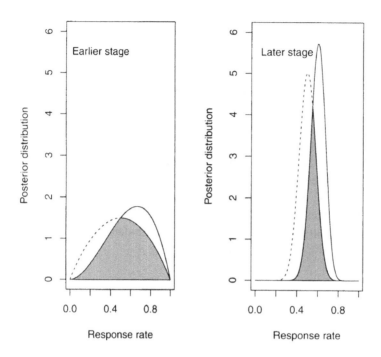

**Figure 7.3**   Posterior distributions of the response rates in a two-arm randomized trial with a small amount of data at the earlier stage of a trial (left panel), and more observed data at the later stage (right panel).

to a lack of information on the treatments. The study design needs to compromise between power and the trial ethics: ER yields nearly the highest power, while AR benefits more trial participants at the sacrifice of power.

For ease of exposition, we consider a two-arm randomized trial. Let $p_1$ and $p_2$ denote the probabilities of response for treatments 1 and 2, respectively. For the implementation of AR, a common practice is to take the assignment probability proportional to the estimated response rate of each treatment. In fact, AR is not uniquely attached to Bayesian or frequentist methods; either approach can assign a new patient to arm $k$ with a probability of $\hat{p}_k/(\hat{p}_1 + \hat{p}_2)$ for $k = 1, 2$, where $\hat{p}_k$ is the posterior mean or the MLE of $p_k$. Nevertheless, such an AR scheme solely depends on the point estimates of the response rates and does not account for their variabilities. From the Bayesian point of view, Figure 7.3 illustrates that based on a small amount of data observed at the early stage of a trial, the posterior distributions of $p_1$ and $p_2$ are widely spread and largely overlapped. In this situation, the point estimates of the response rates of arms 1 and 2, say, $\hat{p}_1 = 0.6$ and $\hat{p}_2 = 0.5$, should not play a dominant role in patient assignment, because more data are needed to confirm that treatment 1 is indeed superior to treatment 2. As more data are accumulated at the later stage of the trial, if we still observe $\hat{p}_1 = 0.6$ and $\hat{p}_2 = 0.5$, the posterior distributions of $p_1$ and $p_2$ would be much separated as shown in Figure 7.3. At that time, we could be more confident in assigning more patients to arm 1, because its superiority would then be much more strongly supported. Therefore, in addition to the point estimates of the $p_k$'s, their variance estimates are also essential in determining the randomization probabilities.

However, it is not straightforward to incorporate the estimation variability in the frequentist AR procedure. In the Bayesian approach, we may naturally assign patients to treatment 1 with a probability of

$$\lambda = \Pr(p_1 > p_2 | D), \tag{7.6}$$

where $D$ represents the accumulated data in the trial. By comparing the posterior distributions $p_1$ and $p_2$, (7.6) automatically accounts for both the point and variance estimates of the treatment response rates. We may explore a more flexible class of randomization probabilities through a power transformation,

$$\pi(\lambda, \gamma) = \frac{\lambda^\gamma}{\lambda^\gamma + (1 - \lambda)^\gamma}, \tag{7.7}$$

where $0 \le \gamma \le 1$. If $\gamma = 0$, the randomization scheme reduces to ER with an equal assigning probability of 0.5 regardless of the value of $\lambda$; and if $\gamma = 1$, $\pi(\lambda, \gamma) = \lambda$. On the other hand, if $\lambda = 0.5$ (the therapeutic effects of the two treatments are the same), (7.7) reduces to ER with $\pi(\lambda, \gamma) = 0.5$, no matter what value $\gamma$ takes. If $\lambda > 0.5$ (treatment 1 is more effective than treatment 2), then a larger value of $\gamma$ would skew more toward the assigning probability to arm 1, i.e., $\pi(\lambda, \gamma) > \lambda$ with $\gamma > 1$. Therefore, the family of randomization probabilities is much enriched by incorporating the extra power parameter $\gamma$ in (7.7).

More interestingly, the power parameter may be allowed to depend on the accumulating sample size $n$,

$$\gamma_n = \frac{n}{2N},$$

where $N$ is the total sample size planned for the trial (Thall and Wathen, 2007). At the beginning of a trial, very few subjects are treated, so $\gamma_n$ is close to zero, which would down-weigh $\lambda$ and virtually lead to ER. As more data are collected during the trial, $\lambda$ starts playing a more dominant role in determining the randomization probabilities. At the completion of the trial with $n = N$, $\gamma_n$ attains the maximum value of 0.5.

### 7.11.2   Fixed-Reference Adaptive Randomization

In a multi-arm randomized trial, let $p_k$ denote the probability of response for treatment $k$, $k = 1, \ldots, K$. To construct the randomization probabilities, we may compare each $p_k$ to a fixed reference, say, a constant $p_0$ between 0 and 1. We take the assignment probability for arm $k$ proportional to the posterior probability

$$\lambda_k = \Pr(p_k > p_0 | D), \quad k = 1, \ldots, K,$$

such that a patient would be assigned to treatment $k$ with probability

$$\pi_k(\gamma) = \frac{\lambda_k^\gamma}{\sum_{j=1}^K \lambda_j^\gamma}, \quad k = 1, \ldots, K, \tag{7.8}$$

where $\gamma$ is the same transformation parameter as in (7.7). However, if two or more $p_k$'s are much smaller or much larger than $p_0$, the corresponding posterior probabilities $\lambda_k$ would be either close to 0 or 1, and thus it would be difficult to distinguish which treatment is better. Therefore, the AR procedure with a fixed reference may not work well if $p_0$ is not chosen properly.

In general, all the treatments in a study are comparable, and one may simply take an arbitrary treatment as the reference, say, the first arm with the probability of response $p_1$. The randomization probabilities are then based on

$$\lambda_k = \Pr(p_k > p_1 | D), \quad k = 2, \ldots, K, \tag{7.9}$$

and $\lambda_1 = 0.5$. However, if $p_1$ is much smaller than other $p_k$'s, it would be difficult to distinguish those treatments. Suppose that in a three-arm trial with $p_1 = 0.1$, $p_2 = 0.4$, and $p_3 = 0.6$, the probabilities of assigning a patient to arm 2 and to arm 3 may be very similar because both $\lambda_2$ and $\lambda_3$ are close to 1. In addition, because $\lambda_1 = 0.5$, no matter how "bad" treatment 1 is, it always has an assignment probability of at least $1/5$. This reveals a serious limitation of the fixed-reference AR. In the case of a two-arm trial with $p_1 = 0.1$ and $p_2 = 0.6$, arm 1 has an assignment probability of at least $1/3$. In the extreme, if $p_1 = 0$ and $p_2 = 1$, there is still a probability of $1/3$ that a patient will be assigned to arm 1.

Instead of using an arbitrary treatment as the reference, we may compare all treatments with the most effective one. We first identify the best treatment, $p_{\max} = \max\{p_1, \ldots, p_K\}$, and then we compute $\lambda_k = \Pr(p_k > p_{\max} | D)$ to form the randomization probabilities as in (7.8). However, if two treatments, say, with $p_1$ and $p_2$, are far inferior to the best treatment, it would be difficult to make a distinction between them since $\Pr(p_1 > p_{\max} | D) \approx \Pr(p_2 > p_{\max} | D) \approx 0$.

### 7.11.3   Moving-Reference Adaptive Randomization

The fixed-reference AR procedures as discussed previously compare each treatment with the same baseline to determine the randomization probability. By

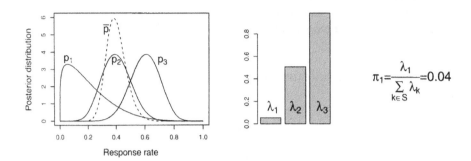

Remove arm 1 from the comparison set S

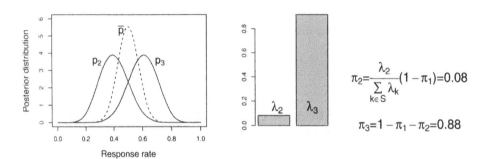

**Figure 7.4** Diagram of the Bayesian moving-reference adaptive randomization for a three-arm trial. Based on the posterior distributions of $p_1, p_2, p_3$, and $\bar{p}$, we calculate $\lambda_k = \Pr(p_k > \bar{p}|D)$ for $k = 1, 2, 3$; and assign the arm with the smallest value of $\lambda_k$ (arm 1 in this case) a randomization probability $\pi_1$. After spending $\pi_1$, we remove arm 1 from the comparison set $S$ and distribute the remaining randomization probability to the other two arms in a similar way.

contrast, the moving-reference AR takes the reference to be the average of the response rates of the treatments in the comparison set. The randomization probability to each treatment arm is computed on a one-by-one basis. Once an arm is assigned a randomization probability, it will be removed from the comparison set, such that we are able to zoom in and accomplish a higher resolution to differentiate treatments.

For illustration, we exhibit the diagram of the Bayesian moving-reference AR in Figure 7.4 using a three-arm randomized trial. In a more general setting with $K$ treatments, we describe the AR procedure based on the posterior samples of $p_1, \ldots, p_K$ as follows:

(1) Let $\mathcal{S}$ denote the set of treatments that needs to be assigned randomization probabilities, and let $\mathcal{S}^c$ denote the set that has been given randomization probabilities. We start with a full set of $\mathcal{S} = \{1, \ldots, K\}$ and an empty set $\mathcal{S}^c$.

(2) Obtain the posterior distribution of the average response rate for the treatments belonging to $\mathcal{S}$,

$$\bar{p} = \frac{\sum_{k \in \mathcal{S}} p_k}{|\mathcal{S}|},$$

where $|\mathcal{S}|$ represents the number of treatments in $\mathcal{S}$.

(3) Taking $\bar{p}$ as the reference, compute $\lambda_k = \Pr(p_k > \bar{p}|D)$ for $k \in \mathcal{S}$, and identify the arm that has the smallest value of $\lambda_k$, denoted as arm $\ell$ with $\lambda_\ell = \min_{k \in \mathcal{S}} \lambda_k$.

(4) Assign arm $\ell$ a randomization probability of

$$\pi_\ell = \frac{\lambda_\ell}{\sum_{k \in \mathcal{S}} \lambda_k} \left(1 - \sum_{j \in \mathcal{S}^c} \pi_j\right),$$

and then remove arm $\ell$ from $\mathcal{S}$ to $\mathcal{S}^c$. Because the assignment probability $\sum_{j \in \mathcal{S}^c} \pi_j$ has been "spent" previously, $\pi_\ell$ is a fraction of the remaining probability $1 - \sum_{j \in \mathcal{S}^c} \pi_j$.

(5) Continue to spend the remaining probability until all of the arms are assigned randomization probabilities, $\pi_1, \ldots, \pi_K$.

**Table 7.3    Comparison of the Number of Patients Randomized to Each Treatment Arm Using the Fixed-Reference and Moving-Reference Adaptive Randomization**

|     | Response Rate | | | Fixed-Reference AR | | | Moving-Reference AR | | |
|-----|------|------|------|-------|-------|-------|-------|-------|-------|
| Sc. | $p_1$ | $p_2$ | $p_3$ | Arm 1 | Arm 2 | Arm 3 | Arm 1 | Arm 2 | Arm 3 |
| 1 | 0.1 | 0.2 | **0.3** | 27.7 | 31.8 | **40.6** | 12.5 | 29.0 | **58.5** |
| 2 | 0.2 | 0.1 | **0.3** | 40.5 | 17.2 | **42.4** | 27.3 | 13.0 | **59.7** |
| 3 | **0.3** | 0.1 | 0.2 | **61.1** | 13.7 | 25.2 | **58.4** | 13.1 | 28.5 |
| 4 | 0.1 | 0.3 | **0.6** | 23.3 | 33.8 | **42.9** | 5.5 | 13.3 | **81.3** |
| 5 | 0.3 | **0.6** | 0.1 | 34.4 | **54.6** | 11.0 | 13.9 | **80.5** | 5.5 |
| 6 | **0.6** | 0.3 | 0.1 | **82.2** | 12.5 | 5.3 | **81.8** | 12.8 | 5.3 |
| 7 | 0.01 | 0.4 | **0.6** | 21.0 | 38.7 | **40.3** | 3.7 | 20.6 | **75.7** |
| 8 | 0.01 | 0.01 | **0.5** | 25.8 | 25.1 | **49.1** | 5.3 | 5.3 | **89.4** |

Note: Sc. stands for Scenario.

To compare the performance of the moving-reference AR and the fixed-reference AR in (7.9), we consider a three-arm trial with a sample size of 100. Based the binomial likelihood, if we take a noninformative beta prior distribution for each $p_k$, $k = 1, 2, 3$, the posterior of $p_k$ is also a beta distribution. Table 7.3 presents the number of subjects allocated to each arm averaged over 1,000 simulated trials under eight scenarios. Scenarios 1 to 3 simulate cases in which the first arm has the lowest, intermediate and highest efficacy, respectively. Scenarios 4 to 6 have a similar pattern, but with much larger differences in the response rates. There are one or two futile arms in scenarios 7 and 8. Clearly, patients could be allocated more efficiently using the moving-reference AR as more patients received the best treatment. In scenarios 4 through 6, the number of patients assigned to the best treatment (the one with a response rate of 0.6)

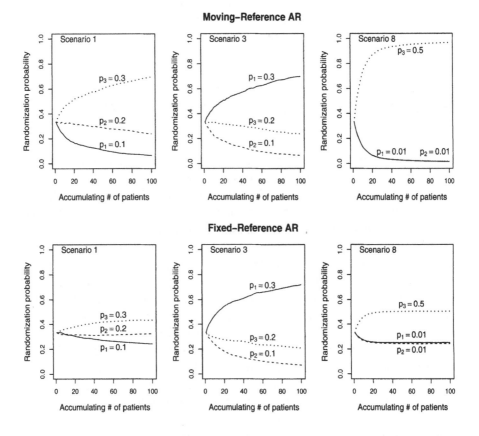

**Figure 7.5**    Randomization probabilities of the moving-reference adaptive randomization and fixed-reference adaptive randomization with accumulating numbers of patients under scenarios 1, 3, and 8, respectively.

using the fixed-reference AR changed dramatically from 42.9 to 82.2, while that using the moving-reference AR stayed approximately the same around 81 subjects. This phenomenon demonstrates the invariance of the moving-reference AR to treatment label switching, while the fixed-reference AR is sensitive to the choice of the reference arm. In scenarios 7 and 8, there is a lower bound of 20% for the assignment probability to arm 1 if using the fixed-reference AR.

For scenarios 1, 3, and 8, Figure 7.5 shows the randomization probabilities for the three arms with respect to the cumulative number of patients using the moving- and fixed-reference AR, respectively. The moving-reference AR exhibits a much higher resolution to distinguish these treatments by separating their curves much faster than the fixed-reference AR. In scenario 1, the curves spread out after approximately 20 patients under the moving-reference AR, but are still not well-separated after 40 patients under the fixed-reference AR. Furthermore, scenarios 1 and 3 are in fact the same except that the treatment labels were switched. The randomization probability curves based on the moving-reference AR are very similar in these two scenarios, while those under the fixed-reference AR unfortunately depend on treatment labeling.

## 7.12 ADAPTIVE RANDOMIZATION WITH EFFICACY AND TOXICITY TRADE-OFFS

In conventional settings, AR is often characterized by a binary efficacy endpoint, such as partial or complete clinical response. However, it may take a long period of time to evaluate such efficacy events after treatment. The potential delay in observing patients' responses makes the real-time implementation of AR very challenging. When a new cohort arrives, estimation using the currently observed data while ignoring the missing data may cause bias, and it is also impractical and unethical to withhold treatment from trial participants. Therefore, binary-endpoint AR may not be the best strategy if the outcomes are not immediately ascertainable. A natural remedy is to model efficacy as time-to-event data so that the unobserved efficacy events become censored. Along this direction, Louis (1977) compares treatments with respect to survival by assuming an exponential distribution. Eick (1988) introduces a general two-arm bandit model with delayed responses assuming geometric lifetimes. Zhang and Rosenberger (2007) study optimized AR procedures under the exponential and Weibull survival models, respectively. Besides efficacy, treatments may induce various levels of toxicity or adverse events. The trend of jointly modeling efficacy and toxicity has grown because neglecting either endpoint is a waste of the information. Rosenberger (1996) combines efficacy and toxicity into a trichotomous outcome, and develops an urn model-based AR procedure. Ji and Bekele (2009) study an AR scheme based on joint efficacy and toxicity outcomes, while Lei, Yuan, and Yin

(2011) model efficacy as time-to-event data and toxicity as dichotomous data through random effects.

### 7.12.1  Survival Model for Efficacy

Let $T_i$ denote the time to disease progression for the $i$th patient, and let $C_i$ denote the censoring time due to decision making for AR. The observed data consist of $X_i = \min(T_i, C_i)$, the censoring indicator $\Delta_i = I(T_i \leq C_i)$, and covariates $\mathbf{Z}_i$ that may include treatments and other important prognostic factors, for $i = 1, \ldots, n$.

Under the proportional hazards model (Cox, 1972), the hazard function for patient $i$ is

$$\lambda(t|\mathbf{Z}_i, b_i) = \lambda_0(t) \exp(\boldsymbol{\beta}^{\mathsf{T}} \mathbf{Z}_i + b_i),$$

where $\lambda_0(t)$ is the baseline hazard function, and $b_i$ is an unobservable frailty or random effect, $b_i \sim \mathrm{N}(0, \sigma^2)$. Under a Weibull distribution with $\lambda_0(t) = \alpha \eta t^{\alpha-1}$, the conditional survival function is given by

$$S(t|\mathbf{Z}_i, b_i) = \exp\{-\eta t^\alpha \exp(\boldsymbol{\beta}^{\mathsf{T}} \mathbf{Z}_i + b_i)\}. \tag{7.10}$$

Based on the efficacy data $D_{\text{eff}}$, the conditional likelihood given random effects $\mathbf{b} = (b_1, \ldots, b_n)$ is

$$L(D_{\text{eff}}|\alpha, \eta, \boldsymbol{\beta}, \mathbf{b})$$
$$\propto \prod_{i=1}^{n} \{\alpha \eta x_i^{\alpha-1} \exp(\boldsymbol{\beta}^{\mathsf{T}} \mathbf{Z}_i + b_i)\}^{\Delta_i} \exp\{-\eta x_i^\alpha \exp(\boldsymbol{\beta}^{\mathsf{T}} \mathbf{Z}_i + b_i)\}.$$

### 7.12.2  Probit Model for Toxicity

Since toxicity is often ascertainable shortly after treatment, it is taken as a binary endpoint; that is, $Y_i = 1$ if patient $i$ has experienced toxicity, and $Y_i = 0$ otherwise. By introducing a latent normal random variable (Albert and Chib, 1993), $U_i \sim \mathrm{N}(\boldsymbol{\gamma}^{\mathsf{T}} \mathbf{Z}_i + b_i, 1)$, the probit model is given by

$$Y_i = \begin{cases} 1, & \text{if } U_i \geq 0, \\ 0, & \text{if } U_i < 0, \end{cases}$$

which is equivalent to

$$\Pr(Y_i = 1|\mathbf{Z}_i, b_i) = \Phi(\boldsymbol{\gamma}^{\mathsf{T}} \mathbf{Z}_i + b_i). \tag{7.11}$$

Based on the toxicity data $D_{\text{tox}}$, the conditional likelihood given random effects $\mathbf{b}$ is

$$L(D_{\text{tox}}|\boldsymbol{\gamma}, \mathbf{b}) \propto \prod_{i=1}^{n} \Phi(\boldsymbol{\gamma}^{\mathsf{T}} \mathbf{Z}_i + b_i)^{y_i} \{1 - \Phi(\boldsymbol{\gamma}^{\mathsf{T}} \mathbf{Z}_i + b_i)\}^{1-y_i}.$$

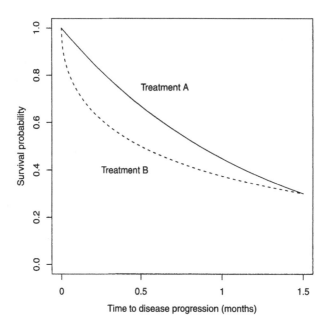

**Figure 7.6**   Times to disease progression with the same survival probability at $\tau = 1.5$ months, but different areas under the survival curves.

### 7.12.3   Efficacy and Toxicity Trade-offs

Under model (7.10), the survival probability at the end of the follow-up time $\tau$ can be used as a measure of treatment efficacy, which, however, ignores the entire path of the survival curve. Figure 7.6 shows that the survival curve under treatment B declines faster than that under treatment A, while both treatments yield the same survival probability at $\tau$. In this case, treatment A is preferred to treatment B because patients' qualities of life may be improved with delayed disease progression. The area under the survival curve captures the survival path toward $\tau$; the larger the area, the slower the survival curve declines. For subject $i$ assigned to treatment arm $k$, we define

$$p_{E,k} = \frac{1}{\tau} S(\tau | \mathbf{Z}_i, b_i) \int_0^\tau S(t | \mathbf{Z}_i, b_i) \, dt,$$

which simultaneously characterizes the survival probability at $\tau$ and the shape of the survival curve.

For each treatment arm $k$, we can construct a measure for efficacy and toxicity trade-offs,

$$\lambda_k = \frac{p_{E,k}}{p_{T,k}}, \quad k = 1, \dots, K,$$

where $p_{T,k}$ is the probability of toxicity given in (7.11). At each time of randomization, a patient will be assigned to arm $k$ with a probability of

$$\pi_k = \frac{\lambda_k}{\sum_{j=1}^{K} \lambda_j}, \quad k = 1, \ldots, K.$$

In contrast to the conventional AR that considers efficacy only, the efficacy-toxicity AR jointly models both endpoints. By modeling efficacy as time-to-event data, we allow for uninterrupted accrual and randomization and, more importantly, the trial duration is immensely shortened compared with that of using a full-length follow-up for efficacy evaluation.

## 7.13 FIXED OR ADAPTIVE RANDOMIZATION?

Although various AR procedures are available, the conventional fixed randomization (FR) remains its dominant role in clinical trials. In particular, ER (the FR with an allocation ratio of 1:1), which achieves nearly optimal power, appears to be the most sensible randomization scheme due to the state of equipoise. Notwithstanding the increasing trend of using AR to enhance trial ethics, the practical utility of AR has been challenged and debated. In general, AR and other adaptive designs in a much broader definition break the tradition and thus suffer from concerns as follows:

- Patients may not be balanced on certain covariates, especially those with possible time trends.

- Hypothesis tests during interim monitoring and at the trial completion are unconventional and difficult.

- Delayed outcomes may affect the practical implementation of AR.

In the comparison of AR and FR, Korn and Freidlin (2011) conduct simulations for typical two-arm trials, while assuming that patients' responses are dichotomous and immediately ascertainable. If FR with an allocation ratio of $K$:1 is used, patients will be randomized to the experimental arm with probability $K/(1 + K)$, and to the standard arm with probability $1/(1 + K)$. Through simulation studies, AR is compared with ER and FR with an allocation ratio of 2:1 (i.e., twice as many patients are randomly assigned to the experimental arm as those to the control arm). Based upon the required sample sizes and the numbers and proportions of nonresponders in the simulated trials, Korn and Freidlin (2011) conclude that AR may provide modest-to-no benefits over ER, and if the experimental treatment is believed to be more appealing to patients, FR with an allocation ratio of 2:1 is recommended. Albeit the numerical evidence, Berry (2011) argues that the light of AR shines brightest in complicated multi-arm settings, while the benefits of AR in a two-arm trial are limited but still real.

From a theoretical point of view, Yuan and Yin (2011c) further compare AR and FR in terms of reducing the number of nonresponders. Let $p_1$ and $p_2$ denote the response rates of the experimental and standard treatments, respectively. The optimal AR that minimizes the expected number of nonresponders should target the allocation ratio of $\sqrt{p_1}/\sqrt{p_2}$ between the experimental arm and the standard arm (Rosenberger et al., 2001). Denote $n_{\mathrm{AR}}$ as the expected number of nonresponders in the AR design, and $n_{\mathrm{FR}}$ as that in the FR design with the $K{:}1$ allocation ratio. We formulate the hypothesis testing as

$$H_0\colon p_1 = p_2 \quad \text{versus} \quad H_1\colon p_1 > p_2,$$

and construct a one-sided binomial test using normal approximation as discussed in Section 6.3.1. We control the type I error rate at $\alpha = 0.1$ and target a power of $1 - \beta = 90\%$. The minimum expected number of nonresponders for an AR design is

$$\min(n_{\mathrm{AR}}) = \frac{(z_\alpha + z_\beta)^2 \{\sqrt{p_1}(1 - p_1) + \sqrt{p_2}(1 - p_2)\}^2}{(p_1 - p_2)^2}, \quad p_1 \neq p_2,$$

where $z_\alpha$ is the $100(1 - \alpha)$th percentile of the standard normal distribution. It follows that when comparing AR and FR with an allocation ratio $K{:}1$, the maximum percentage of reduction in the number of nonresponders is given by

$$\max\left(\frac{n_{\mathrm{FR}} - n_{\mathrm{AR}}}{n_{\mathrm{FR}}}\right)$$
$$= 1 - \frac{K\{\sqrt{p_1}(1 - p_1) + \sqrt{p_2}(1 - p_2)\}^2}{\{p_1(1 - p_1) + Kp_2(1 - p_2)\}\{K(1 - p_1) + 1 - p_2\}}. \quad (7.12)$$

Figure 7.7 displays the maximum percentages of reduction of nonresponders for AR versus ER under various response rates. For practical relevance, we are only concerned with the cases that the improvement of the response rate by the experimental treatment over the standard treatment is less than 200%. Given a specific response rate of the standard treatment, the maximum possible gain (i.e., reduction in the number of nonresponders) using AR increases with respect to the response rate of the experimental treatment. In general, the reduction in the number of nonresponders is rather limited: When the response rate of the experimental treatment is higher than that of the standard treatment up to 50% (the solid segments of the curves), the maximum gain using AR is typically less than 1%; and even when the response rate of the experimental treatment doubles that of the standard treatment (the dashed segments of the curves), such gain is less than 3%.

Of course no design is perfect, while some designs could be more appropriate and informative under certain conditions. Whether to use ER or AR in a clinical trial depends on the real situation. If there is a long lag-time to observe response, AR may become impractical because it is difficult to learn about treatments

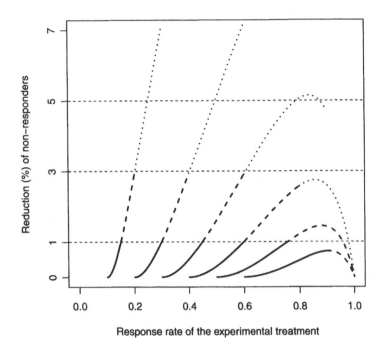

**Figure 7.7**    The maximum percentage of reduction in the number of nonresponders for response-adaptive randomization with respect to that for equal randomization. Curves from the left to the right correspond to the response rates of the standard treatment of $0.1, 0.2, \ldots, 0.6$. The solid, dashed, and dotted segments of each curve represent that the response rate of the experimental treatment is 0 to 50%, 50% to 100%, and 100% to 200% higher than that of the standard treatment, respectively.

effectively as patients enter the trial. Hence, long delay of response may negate the potential benefits of AR. On the other hand, early stopping for superiority or futility is another important feature of adaptive designs, which may diminish the advantages of using AR in a trial. When ER is equipped with early stopping, the design can separate out the treatment effects more efficiently.

The patient horizon includes the total number of patients in the trial and the future patients to be treated by the therapy with a greater proportion of favorable responses (Bather, 1981; 1985; Berry and Eick, 1995). Both patients in the trial and those outside the trial should be considered and weighed equally. The treatment effects should be sorted out as quickly as possible so that patients outside the trial will receive the better treatment sooner. If the disease is relatively common (i.e., the patient horizon is large), ER may be a preferred approach in order to draw a conclusion quickly. Nevertheless, if the condition is some type of rare cancer and the trial involves a substantial proportion of patients, AR designs may be more desirable such as to benefit more trial participants.

## EXERCISES

**7.1**   In a two-arm randomized trial, suppose that the outcome is a binary indicator of response or no response. The response rate for the new treatment is $p_1$ and that for the standard treatment is $p_2$. Derive Neyman's allocation ratio by minimizing the variance of the estimated difference between the two response rates. If the goal of the trial is to minimize the number of nonresponders while fixing the variance of the test statistic, derive the corresponding optimal allocation ratio.

**7.2**   For continuous outcomes, derive Neyman's allocation ratio and the optimal allocation ratio

$$r_{opt} = \frac{\sigma_1 \sqrt{\Phi\{(\mu_2 - c)/\sigma_2\}}}{\sigma_2 \sqrt{\Phi\{(\mu_1 - c)/\sigma_1\}}}.$$

**7.3**   For survival data, derive Neyman's allocation and the optimal allocation ratio under the exponential assumption,

$$r_{opt} = \frac{\lambda_1 \sqrt{\delta_2\{1 - \exp(-\lambda_2 c)\}}}{\lambda_2 \sqrt{\delta_1\{1 - \exp(-\lambda_1 c)\}}}.$$

**7.4**   In the comparison of fixed and adaptive randomization, derive the maximum percentage of reduction in the number of nonresponders in equation (7.12).

# CHAPTER 8

# LATE-ONSET TOXICITY

## 8.1 MISSING DATA WITH DELAYED OUTCOMES

In a typical phase I oncology trial, the primary objective is to identify the maximum tolerated dose (MTD) of an experimental drug. Most of the dose-finding methods require dose-limiting toxicities (DLTs) to be ascertainable shortly after treatment, so that the toxicity outcomes of all the previously treated patients are available by the time for the next dose assignment. However, DLTs may occur long after treatment or, relatively speaking, the occurrence of toxicity may not be as fast as the patient accrual. If the toxicity assessment cannot keep up with the accrual rate, the outcomes of those patients already under treatment might still be unobserved when a new cohort arrives. Such delayed toxicity outcomes often result in missing or censored data, which inevitably hinders dose assignment for incoming cohorts. For example, Muler et al. (2004) describe a phase I clinical trial in pancreatic cancer to determine the MTD of cisplatin in combination with gemcitabine and radiation therapy. In that trial, the accrual rate was one patient per week, while the follow-up time for each patient was nine weeks in order to fully assess toxicity.

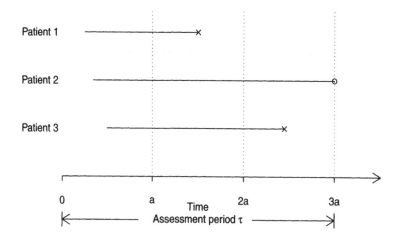

**Figure 8.1** Illustration of missing toxicity outcomes under fast patient accrual. For each patient, the horizontal line segment represents the length of the follow-up, at the end of which if toxicity occurs, it is indicated by a cross, otherwise censoring is noted by a circle.

Patients enter a trial sequentially and are followed for a fixed period of time $[0, \tau]$ to assess the drug's toxicity. The length of the evaluation period $\tau$ is chosen in a way that if a drug-related DLT occurs, it would occur within $[0, \tau]$; any toxicity event occurring after $\tau$ does not count. During this evaluation period, a binary toxicity outcome is taken for each subject $i$,

$$
Y_i = \begin{cases} 1, & \text{if a DLT is observed in } [0, \tau], \\ 0, & \text{if no DLT is observed in } [0, \tau]. \end{cases}
$$

Depending on the nature of the disease and treatment, $\tau$ may range from days to months.

Suppose that a new cohort arrives every time interval $a$, and $a$ is shorter than $\tau$, say $\tau = 3a$. Figure 8.1 shows that by the time for the next dose assignment, some of the patients who entered the trial earlier have only been followed partially and their toxicity outcomes have not yet been observed. For example, at time $2a$, the toxicity outcomes of patients 2 and 3 are unavailable (i.e., $Y_1 = 1$, but $Y_2$ and $Y_3$ are missing); and at time $3a$, the toxicity outcomes of all three patients are observed (i.e., $Y_1 = Y_3 = 1$ and $Y_2 = 0$). Intuitively, patients who will not experience toxicity in $[0, \tau]$ are more likely to produce missing data at the decision-making times. The amount of missing data due to late-onset toxicity depends on the ratio of the assessment period $\tau$ and the interarrival time $a$. The larger the value of $\tau/a$, the more missing data would be induced, because more patients would not have completed their toxicity assessment upon a new cohort's arrival.

The missing toxicity data pose immense difficulties in conducting a dose-finding trial. One possibility is simply to treat those subjects with missing toxicity outcomes as "no toxicity." However, this often underestimates the toxicity probabilities, because patients who have not experienced toxicity at the moment of dose assignment may yet experience toxicity later during the remaining follow-up. This naive strategy may lead to aggressive dose escalation, which in turn causes an undesirably large number of patients to be treated at excessively toxic doses. A "safer" approach would be to suspend the accrual and wait for each patient's outcome to be fully observed prior to the next dose assignment, which, however, may result in an unusually lengthy trial duration. Moreover, frequently suspending patient accrual is not practical, not only wasting resources but also causing tremendous administrative inconvenience.

To overcome the difficulties associated with late-onset toxicity, Yin and Zheng (2011) propose a fractional dose-finding scheme by modeling times to toxicity and redistributing censored data to the right. Each censored toxicity observation is split into two parts: One fraction stays at the censoring point and the other is somewhere larger than $\tau$. The fractional contributions can be naturally incorporated in the $3 + 3$ design and the continual reassessment method (CRM). An alternative approach is to use the weighted likelihood function of the CRM based on patients' exposure times (Cheung and Chappell, 2000; Braun, 2006). Furthermore, predictive risks may also be of help in monitoring trials with late-onset toxicity (Bekele et al., 2008). In a rigorous missing data framework, Yuan and Yin (2011d) develop an expectation-maximization (EM) approach to addressing the unobserved toxicity issues in dose finding. The rest of this chapter will provide deeper insights into the issues of late-onset toxicity and introduce each dose-finding method that is capable of accommodating delayed outcomes. The statistical methodologies discussed here can also be used to model other endpoints that are not immediately observable, such as the time-lagged efficacy event or delayed response.

## 8.2   FRACTIONAL 3 + 3 DESIGN

### 8.2.1   Redistributing Censored Data to the Right

Among various dose-finding methods, the $3 + 3$ design remains its popularity due to the ease of implementation. The $3 + 3$ design requires that toxicity be ascertainable shortly after treatment. Figure 8.2 displays that three patients are enrolled every time interval $a$, and they will be followed for a period of $\tau = 3a$ to assess toxicity. When a new cohort is ready for treatment, say at times $a$ and $2a$, the toxicity events of the patients under treatment may be censored but possibly will occur later during the rest of the follow-up.

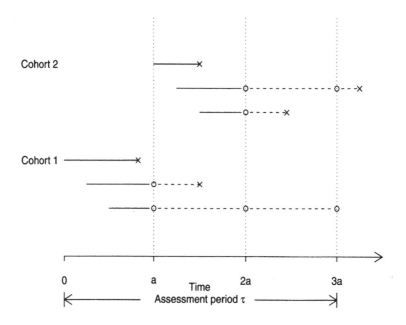

**Figure 8.2**   Illustration of censored toxicity outcomes with late-onset toxicity. Each cohort has three patients, with the horizontal line segment representing the follow-up time, along which toxicity is indicated by a cross and censoring by a circle.

To accommodate late-onset toxicity in the $3 + 3$ design, Yin and Zheng (2011) model the underlying times to toxicity through the Kaplan–Meier (1958) estimator by redistributing the mass of each censored observation to the right (Efron, 1967; Portnoy, 2003). Within the evaluation window $[0, \tau]$, if a patient experiences the DLT, we take the toxicity outcome $Y = 1$; if a patient has not experienced the DLT by the time of decision making, the toxicity event is censored and we split the point mass of 1 between the censoring point and somewhere that is larger than $\tau$. Only the weight assigned to the censoring time point within $[0, \tau]$ contributes to the estimation, and that assigned beyond $\tau$ does not.

For subject $i$, let $t_i$ denote the time to toxicity, and let $u_i$ $(u_i \leq \tau)$ denote the actual follow-up time that may censor $t_i$. We assume that $u_i$ is independent of $t_i$; that is, the time of dose assignment or the arrival time of a new cohort is independent of the time to toxicity due to patient staggered entry. The toxicity outcome is censored for patients who have not yet experienced toxicity $(u_i < t_i)$ and have not been fully followed up to $\tau$ $(u_i < \tau)$. If the toxicity event of subject

$i$ is censored, we can calculate his/her fractional contribution in the form of

$$\Pr(t_i < \tau | t_i > u_i) = \frac{\Pr(u_i < t_i < \tau)}{\Pr(t_i > u_i)}, \qquad (8.1)$$

which in fact is the conditional probability of the occurrence of toxicity in $(u_i, \tau)$ given that it has not occurred by $u_i$.

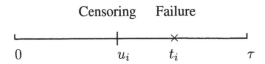

The fractional contribution for a censored toxicity outcome in (8.1) can be estimated by

$$\hat{y}_i = \frac{\hat{S}(u_i) - \hat{S}(\tau)}{\hat{S}(u_i)}, \qquad (8.2)$$

where $\hat{S}(\cdot)$ is the usual Kaplan–Meier estimator.

Suppose that $n_j$ patients have been treated at dose level $j$, at which we count the number of patients who have experienced toxicity ($y_i = 1$) and those who were censored with fractional contributions ($y_i = \hat{y}_i$). The estimate of the toxicity probability of dose $j$ is given by

$$\hat{p}_j = \frac{\sum_{i=1}^{n_j} y_i}{n_j}, \qquad (8.3)$$

where

$$y_i = \begin{cases} 0, & \text{if no toxicity has been observed by time } \tau, \\ 1, & \text{if toxicity is observed before } u_i, \\ \hat{y}_i, & \text{if } t_i \text{ is censored by } u_i. \end{cases}$$

### 8.2.2  Dose-Finding Algorithm with a Target

Let $\phi_T$ denote the target toxicity probability, and let $c_L$ and $c_U$ ($c_L < c_U$) denote the probability cutoffs for dose escalation and de-escalation, respectively. Patients are treated in a cohort size of three, and the first cohort is treated at the lowest dose. Before the fractional dose-finding scheme takes effect, there is a prephase of using the conventional $3 + 3$ design based on a full follow-up for each cohort. Once the first DLT is observed, we switch to the fractional $3 + 3$ dose-finding algorithm described as follows:

(1)  Suppose that the current dose level is $j$. Based on the accumulated data at dose level $j$, we can estimate the toxicity probability $\hat{p}_j$ as in (8.3), and

- if $\hat{p}_j > c_U$, de-escalate to dose level $j - 1$;
- if $\hat{p}_j < c_L$, escalate to dose level $j + 1$;
- otherwise, the dose stays at the same level $j$, for the next cohort of patients.

(2) Once the maximum sample size is reached, the dose with the toxicity probability closest to $\phi_T$ is selected as the MTD.

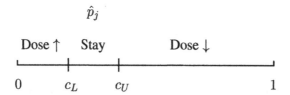

As shown by the above diagram, dose escalation, de-escalation, or staying at the same level depends on the comparisons of $\hat{p}_j$ with $c_L$ and $c_U$.

### 8.2.3   Simulation Study

We investigated the operating characteristics of the fractional 3+3 design through simulation studies. We considered six doses and took a maximum sample size of 36 patients. The cohort size was three, and the first cohort was treated at the lowest dose level. The toxicity assessment period was $\tau = 3$ months and the interarrival time between two consecutive cohorts was $a = 1$ month. We assumed that times to toxicity at dose level $j$ followed an exponential distribution with mean $1/\lambda_j$, $j = 1, \ldots, 6$. The hazards were monotonically increasing with respect to the doses, $\lambda_1 < \cdots < \lambda_J$; that is, a higher dose would induce toxicity sooner. In each scenario, we first specified all the $p_j$'s and then computed $\lambda_j$ from

$$p_j = 1 - \exp(-\lambda_j \tau), \quad j = 1, \ldots, 6,$$

so that a patient would experience the DLT with probability $p_j$ by the end of the evaluation period $\tau$. The target toxicity probability was $\phi_T = 30\%$, and we set $c_L = 0.2$ and $c_U = 0.4$. For comparison, we also implemented the standard 3+3 design (see Section 4.3), and the 3 + 3t design in which dose finding is based on the target, $c_L$, and $c_U$ as discussed in the last section, but without the fractional scheme. In both the 3 + 3 and 3 + 3t designs, we had to wait till observing all the toxicity outcomes of previously treated patients prior to assigning a dose to a new cohort. Under the fractional 3 + 3 design with a target (f3 + 3t), each cohort was treated immediately upon arrival without any delay. We simulated 10,000 trials for each case.

Table 8.1 presents the true toxicity probability, the selection percentage, and the number of patients treated at each dose, as well as the number of DLTs, the

**Table 8.1    Simulation Study Comparing the Fractional** $3 + 3$ **Design with a Target** **(f3 + 3t), the** $3 + 3$ **Design with a Target** $(3 + 3t)$**, and the Standard** $3 + 3$ **Design**

| Design | \multicolumn{6}{c}{Selection Percentage at Dose Level} | Total # Toxicity | Total # Patients | Trial Duration |
|---|---|---|---|---|---|---|---|---|---|
| | 1 | 2 | 3 | 4 | 5 | 6 | | | |
| Scenario 1 | 0.07 | 0.12 | 0.17 | 0.30 | 0.45 | 0.60 | | | |
| f3 + 3t | 4.4 | 11.4 | 23.3 | **41.1** | 15.2 | 1.8 | | | |
| # Patients | 3.8 | 5.6 | 7.7 | 10.0 | 5.8 | 2.1 | 9.1 | 35.0 | 20.4 |
| 3 + 3t | 4.3 | 12.2 | 23.4 | **42.8** | 14.2 | 1.3 | | | |
| # Patients | 3.9 | 5.2 | 8.3 | 10.9 | 5.9 | 1.2 | 9.0 | 35.4 | 35.4 |
| 3 + 3 | 8.2 | 16.4 | 29.6 | **31.4** | 11.5 | 1.2 | | | |
| # Patients | 3.7 | 3.9 | 3.8 | 3.2 | 1.5 | 0.3 | 3.1 | 16.4 | 16.4 |
| Scenario 2 | 0.04 | 0.08 | 0.12 | 0.15 | 0.30 | 0.50 | | | |
| f3 + 3t | 3.3 | 7.3 | 13.5 | 20.4 | **43.0** | 11.7 | | | |
| # Patients | 3.4 | 4.3 | 5.3 | 6.6 | 9.4 | 6.5 | 8.2 | 35.5 | 22.1 |
| 3 + 3t | 2.6 | 7.1 | 12.2 | 19.7 | **46.2** | 11.7 | | | |
| # Patients | 3.4 | 4.1 | 5.0 | 7.7 | 10.4 | 5.3 | 8.0 | 35.9 | 35.9 |
| 3 + 3 | 3.1 | 9.1 | 13.8 | 28.8 | **34.5** | 10.3 | | | |
| # Patients | 3.4 | 3.7 | 3.7 | 3.6 | 3.3 | 1.4 | 3.1 | 19.1 | 19.1 |
| Scenario 3 | 0.20 | 0.30 | 0.45 | 0.55 | 0.60 | 0.70 | | | |
| f3 + 3t | 16.4 | **43.7** | 14.3 | 2.5 | 0.5 | 0.1 | | | |
| # Patients | 7.1 | 12.5 | 6.1 | 1.7 | 0.4 | 0.1 | 9.5 | 27.9 | 15.8 |
| 3 + 3t | 11.1 | **43.5** | 14.5 | 2.1 | 0.2 | 0.0 | | | |
| # Patients | 8.4 | 11.5 | 7.1 | 1.7 | 0.2 | 0.0 | 9.4 | 28.9 | 28.9 |
| 3 + 3 | 36.7 | **34.8** | 12.7 | 1.7 | 0.1 | 0.0 | | | |
| # Patients | 4.6 | 3.5 | 1.7 | 0.4 | 0.0 | 0.0 | 2.9 | 10.2 | 10.2 |

total number of patients, and the average trial duration under the f3 + 3t, 3 + 3t, and 3 + 3 designs, respectively. In scenario 1, the MTD is at dose level 4; the f3 + 3t and 3 + 3t designs yielded similar selection percentages of the MTD, while the f3 + 3t design substantially shortened the trial duration. The 3 + 3 design took much fewer patients and thus had a much shorter trial duration, while the selection percentage of the MTD was about 10% less than the other two designs. Scenario 2 has the MTD at the fifth dose level; the f3 + 3t and 3 + 3t designs yielded much higher selection percentages of the MTD than the 3 + 3 design. In scenario 3, the second dose is the MTD; the f3 + 3t design performed similarly to the 3 + 3t design in terms of the MTD selection, but reduced the trial duration almost by half.

To meet the practical needs with late-onset toxicity, the fractional 3 + 3 design treats unobserved toxicity outcomes as censored data and estimates the conditional probability that toxicity occurs in the remaining follow-up given that it has not yet occurred. This approach is robust as it does not impose any parametric modeling structure. To incorporate the dose information, we may apply the proportional hazards model (Cox, 1972) or the local Kaplan–Meier estimator (Wang and Wang, 2009) to compute the fractional contribution for each censored observation. Generally speaking, the fractional design facilitates continual trial conduct and shortens the trial duration without sacrificing the trial performance much.

## 8.3  FRACTIONAL CONTINUAL REASSESSMENT METHOD

As discussed in Section 4.7, the CRM is a model-based approach to dose finding, which often outperforms the $3 + 3$ design by pooling all the information across different doses in search for the MTD. Under the monotone toxicity assumption, we need to prespecify the toxicity probability at each dose, denoted as $p_1 < \cdots < p_J$. Via a working dose–toxicity model, the true toxicity probability in the CRM is given by

$$\pi_j(\alpha) = p_j^{\exp(\alpha)}, \quad j = 1, \ldots, J, \tag{8.4}$$

where $\alpha$ is an unknown parameter. As more data are collected in the trial, the CRM continuously updates $\alpha$ and the toxicity probabilities of all the considered doses. When the maximum sample size is exhausted, the dose that has the estimated toxicity probability closest to the target $\phi_T$ will be recommended as the MTD.

However, the practical implementation of the CRM also requires fully observing the toxicity outcomes of all the patients who already entered the trial prior to the next dose assignment. Due to late-onset toxicity, patients' outcomes may not be immediately obtainable. As a result, missing data may be induced as the trial proceeds, which limits the general applicability of the CRM in dose finding.

To overcome the difficulty caused by missing data, we model toxicity as time-to-event data and redistribute censored observations to the right as discussed in the fractional $3 + 3$ design. For subject $i$, define

$$y_i = \begin{cases} 0, & \text{if no toxicity observed,} \\ 1, & \text{if toxicity observed,} \\ \Pr(t_i < \tau | t_i > u_i), & \text{if censored,} \end{cases} \tag{8.5}$$

where $\Pr(t_i < \tau | t_i > u_i)$ can be estimated by (8.2). For notational clarity, let $p_{j(i)} = p_j$ if subject $i$ is treated at dose level $j$, let $n$ be the number of patients treated in the trial thus far, and let $D$ denote the observed data. Based on the fractional scheme, the likelihood function is given by

$$L(D|\alpha) \propto \prod_{i=1}^{n} p_{j(i)}^{y_i \exp(\alpha)} \left\{ 1 - p_{j(i)}^{\exp(\alpha)} \right\}^{1-y_i},$$

where $y_i$ may take a value of 0, 1, or a fraction of 1 for a censored observation as defined in (8.5).

Once the censored data are fractionized, the rest of implementation of the fractional CRM is straightforward. We first specify a zero-mean normal prior distribution for $\alpha$. When a new cohort enters the trial, we update the posterior estimates of the toxicity probabilities of all the doses. The dose that has an estimated toxicity probability closest to the target $\phi_T$ is then recommended for the new cohort, under the restriction that the dose can only be escalated by one level at a time. The trial continues until the total sample size is exhausted, and finally the dose whose posterior estimate of the toxicity probability is closest to $\phi_T$ will be selected as the MTD. For safety, we terminate the trial early if the lowest dose under consideration is still overly toxic. The dose-finding algorithm of the fractional CRM basically follows that of the standard CRM; see Section 4.7 for details.

## 8.4    TIME-TO-EVENT CONTINUAL REASSESSMENT METHOD

### 8.4.1    Weighted Binomial Likelihood

Using patients' exposure times as weights, the time-to-event continual reassessment method (TITE-CRM) addresses the issues associated with late-onset toxicity based on a pseudo-binomial likelihood function (Cheung and Chappell, 2000). In a dose-finding trial, patients who have not experienced toxicity at the decision-making time are weighted by their follow-up times with respect to the specified evaluation period $\tau$. Intuitively, the longer the follow-up time, the more information a patient carries, and thus more weight should be given to this subject's currently observed outcome. In an extension, Braun (2006) accommodates both early- and late-onset toxicities by incorporating the dose information in phase I clinical trials. Mauguen, Le Deleya, and Zohar (2011) apply the same weighting scheme in the design of escalation with overdose control; see Section 4.9.

Let $u_i$ be the actual follow-up time for subject $i$, and let $y_i$ be the observed toxicity outcome at time $u_i$. As long as the toxicity event has not occurred, $y_i$ takes a value of 0, and otherwise 1. If a uniform weighting scheme is used to assign higher weights to subjects with longer exposure times, the weight takes the form of $w_i = u_i/\tau$. Patients who have experienced toxicity are given a full weight of 1. Under the CRM model (8.4), the pseudo-binomial likelihood function is given by

$$L(D|\alpha) \propto \prod_{i=1}^{n} \left\{ w_i p_{j(i)}^{\exp(\alpha)} \right\}^{y_i} \left\{ 1 - w_i p_{j(i)}^{\exp(\alpha)} \right\}^{1-y_i}$$

$$\propto \prod_{i=1}^{n} p_{j(i)}^{y_i \exp(\alpha)} \left\{ 1 - \left( \frac{u_i}{\tau} \right) p_{j(i)}^{\exp(\alpha)} \right\}^{1-y_i}.$$

Under this formulation, patients who have not experienced toxicity and have not been fully followed are treated as "no toxicity" with $y_i = 0$, although their data are in fact missing.

The TITE-CRM is built upon an exposure-time weighting scheme. The weight function can take a variety of forms, which may even depend on the unknown parameter $\alpha$. However, it is difficult to justify which weight function is more appropriate in practice. The uniform weight is simple, but using the same weight across all the doses may not be reasonable because it completely neglects the dose information. By contrast, the fractional CRM discussed in Section 8.3 takes a more rigorous approach to redistributing the probability mass for censored data to the right (Portnoy, 2003). This censoring redistribution scheme can be justified by the self-consistent property of the Kaplan–Meier estimator. As a result, the fractionized data can be treated as "complete" data and thus the CRM can proceed as usual.

### 8.4.2 Numerical Comparison

For comparison, we implemented both the fractional CRM (fCRM) and the TITE-CRM in the simulation study. In each trial, the maximum sample size was 36 patients, the cohort size was three, and the first cohort was treated at the lowest dose. Every month, a new cohort of patients would enter the trial, and the toxicity assessment period was $\tau = 3$ months. The target toxicity probability $\phi_T$ was 30%, and the prespecified toxicity probabilities of the six considered doses were $(p_1, \ldots, p_6) = (0.1, 0.2, 0.3, 0.4, 0.5, 0.6)$. We generated times to toxicity from Weibull distributions, and 10,000 simulations were carried out for each configuration.

In general, the selection percentages of the MTD, the numbers of patients, the numbers of toxicities, and the trial durations were all similar between the fCRM and TITE-CRM. Figure 8.3 displays the selection percentages of the MTD under the two designs in four scenarios. In scenario 1, the MTD is the last dose, while the TITE-CRM selected the fifth dose with the highest percentage. The MTD selection using the fCRM was 10% higher than that of using the TITE-CRM. The performance of the two designs in the other three scenarios was very close. In conclusion, both the fCRM and TITE-CRM are able to solve the issues of late-onset toxicity and thus facilitate continual trial conduct.

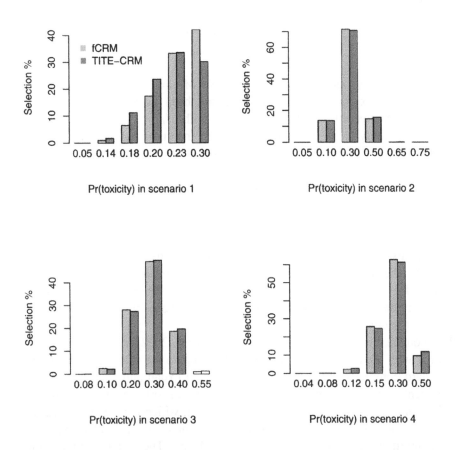

**Figure 8.3**   Dose selection percentages in the four scenarios with the target toxicity probability $\phi_T = 30\%$ using the fCRM and TITE-CRM, respectively.

## 8.5   EM CONTINUAL REASSESSMENT METHOD

### 8.5.1   EM Algorithm with Missing Data

As discussed before, late-onset toxicity often results in missing data during dose finding in phase I trials. Simply discarding such missing data may invalidate decision making on dose assignment, because not only does it cause bias and efficiency loss, but of greater consequence, it may also lead to overly aggressive dose escalation. To gain deeper insights into these issues, we denote $t_i$ as the time to toxicity for subject $i$, and set $t_i = \infty$ if subject $i$ will not experience toxicity in the evaluation window $[0, \tau]$. At the decision-making time for dose assignment, let $u_i$ $(0 \leq u_i \leq \tau)$ be the actual follow-up time, and let $M_i$ be the missing data indicator,

$$M_i = \begin{cases} 1, & \text{if } t_i > u_i \text{ and } u_i < \tau, \\ 0, & \text{if } t_i \leq u_i \text{ or } u_i = \tau. \end{cases} \qquad (8.6)$$

That is, the toxicity outcome is missing with $M_i = 1$ if patient $i$ has not yet experienced toxicity $(t_i > u_i)$ and has not been fully followed up to $\tau$ $(u_i < \tau)$; and the toxicity outcome is observed with $M_i = 0$ if he/she either has experienced toxicity $(t_i < u_i)$ or has completed the entire follow-up $(u_i = \tau)$ without experiencing toxicity. Correspondingly, the toxicity outcome of subject $i$ is

$$Y_i = \begin{cases} \text{missing}, & \text{if } t_i > u_i \text{ and } u_i < \tau, \\ 1, & \text{if } t_i \leq u_i \leq \tau, \\ 0, & \text{if } t_i > u_i = \tau. \end{cases}$$

Under the missing data mechanism (8.6), the probability of missingness of $Y_i$ depends on the underlying time to toxicity, and thus implicitly depends on the value of $Y_i$ itself. For patients who will not experience toxicity in $[0, \tau]$, their toxicity data are more likely to be missing compared with those who will experience toxicity.

Based on the missing data theory (Little and Rubin, 2002), a natural approach to dealing with the unobserved outcomes is to impute the missing data so that the standard complete-data method can be applied (Yuan and Yin, 2011d). In the frequentist paradigm, missing data problems are often tackled using the EM algorithm (Dempster, Laird, and Rubin, 1977), which is a general iterative procedure for maximizing the likelihood with incomplete data. Each iteration of the EM algorithm consists of an E step and an M step. The E step computes the conditional expectation of the missing data given the observed data and current parameter estimates. After substituting these expectations for the missing data, the M step maximizes the likelihood of the filled-in data to obtain the maximum likelihood estimators (MLEs) of the parameters.

As in the mixture cure rate model (Berkson and Gage, 1952), the patient population can be viewed as a mixture of patients who will experience toxicity $(Y_i = 1)$ and those who will not $(Y_i = 0)$. Under the CRM model (8.4), for subject $i$ treated at dose level $j$ we have

$$Y_i = \begin{cases} 1, & \text{with probability } \pi_j(\alpha), \\ 0, & \text{with probability } 1 - \pi_j(\alpha), \end{cases}$$

where $\pi_j(\alpha) = p_j^{\exp(\alpha)}$, and here we denote $p_{j(i)} = p_j$ to avoid ambiguity. Suppose that $n$ patients have been enrolled in a trial thus far, and denote the toxicity data as $\mathbf{y} = (y_1, \ldots, y_n)$. If all the $y_i$'s are completely observed (i.e., no missing data), the likelihood function is given by

$$L(\alpha) \propto \prod_{i=1}^{n} p_{j(i)}^{y_i \exp(\alpha)} \left\{ 1 - p_{j(i)}^{\exp(\alpha)} \right\}^{1-y_i}. \tag{8.7}$$

However, some of the $y_i$'s may be missing due to late-onset toxicity. In particular, let $\mathbf{y} = (\mathbf{y}_{\mathrm{obs}}, \mathbf{y}_{\mathrm{mis}})$, where $\mathbf{y}_{\mathrm{obs}}$ and $\mathbf{y}_{\mathrm{mis}}$ denote the observed and missing toxicity data, respectively.

For patients who will experience toxicity in $[0, \tau]$, we model their time-to-toxicity data. Suppose that there are $K$ distinct event times, sorted as $\tau_1 < \cdots < \tau_K$. Define the unknown discrete hazard at $\tau_k$ as $\lambda_k = \Pr(t = \tau_k | t \geq \tau_k)$, and $\boldsymbol{\lambda} = (\lambda_1, \ldots, \lambda_K)$.

At the $r$th iteration of the EM algorithm, the parameter estimates for $\alpha$ and $\boldsymbol{\lambda}$ are $\alpha^{(r)}$ and $\boldsymbol{\lambda}^{(r)}$, and the next iteration proceeds as follows:

- *E step*

  We replace the missing value of $y_i \in \mathbf{y}_{\mathrm{mis}}$ with its expectation so as to obtain the filled-in data,

$$
\begin{aligned}
\hat{y}_i &= \mathrm{E}(y_i | t_i > u_i, \alpha^{(r)}, \boldsymbol{\lambda}^{(r)}) \\
&= \Pr(y_i = 1 | t_i > u_i, \alpha^{(r)}, \boldsymbol{\lambda}^{(r)}) \\
&= \frac{\Pr(t_i > u_i | y_i = 1, \boldsymbol{\lambda}^{(r)}) \Pr(y_i = 1 | \alpha^{(r)})}{\Pr(y_i = 0 | \alpha^{(r)}) + \Pr(t_i > u_i | y_i = 1, \boldsymbol{\lambda}^{(r)}) \Pr(y_i = 1 | \alpha^{(r)})} \\
&= \frac{p_{j(i)}^{\exp(\alpha^{(r)})} \prod_{k:\tau_k < u_i} (1 - \lambda_k^{(r)})}{1 - p_{j(i)}^{\exp(\alpha^{(r)})} + p_{j(i)}^{\exp(\alpha^{(r)})} \prod_{k:\tau_k < u_i} (1 - \lambda_k^{(r)})}.
\end{aligned}
$$

- *M step*

  We update the estimate $\alpha^{(r+1)}$ by maximizing the likelihood function in (8.7) based on the filled-in data. Following the derivation in the mixture cure rate model (Taylor, 1995), the $k$th component of $\boldsymbol{\lambda}^{(r+1)}$ can be updated as

$$\lambda_k^{(r+1)} = \frac{d_k}{\sum_{j=k}^{K} (d_j + \sum_{i \in \mathcal{C}_j} \hat{y}_i)},$$

where $d_k$ is the number of events occurred at time $\tau_k$ and $\mathcal{C}_k$ is the set of censored observations in the interval $[\tau_k, \tau_{k+1})$.

### 8.5.2 Robust EM-CRM

The CRM, as discussed in Section 4.8, is sensitive to the prespecified toxicity probabilities $(p_1, \ldots, p_J)$. Due to a lack of toxicity information on a new drug, the values of the $p_j$'s are arbitrary and may deviate far from the true dose–toxicity curve and, consequently, the trial may select a wrong dose as the MTD. To enhance the robustness of the design, $m$ ($m > 1$) sets of toxicity probabilities may be simultaneously used in conjunction with model selection or model averaging.

Model selection identifies the best-fitting model among the candidates and the toxicity probability of each dose is estimated under the chosen model only. Commonly used model selection criteria include the Akaike (1973) information criterion (AIC) and the Bayesian information criterion (BIC). Under the CRM model,

$$\text{AIC} = -2 \log L(\alpha) + 2\nu,$$
$$\text{BIC} = -2 \log L(\alpha) + \nu \log n,$$

where $\log L(\alpha)$ is the log-likelihood in (8.7) and $\nu$ is the number of model parameters. The smaller the value of the AIC or BIC, the better the model fit. By contrast, model averaging explicitly accounts for the uncertainty of different models and draws inference based on all the competing models rather than one single model (Hoeting et al., 1999; Hjort and Claeskens, 2003). The frequentist model averaging estimate of the toxicity probability takes the form of

$$\bar{\pi}_j = \sum_{k=1}^{m} w_k \hat{\pi}_{kj}, \quad j = 1, \ldots, J,$$

where $\hat{\pi}_{kj}$ is the MLE of the toxicity probability at dose level $j$ under the $k$th CRM model, and the weight $w_k$ measures the relative influence of model $k$, for $k = 1, \ldots, m$. If we use a smoothed AIC estimator (Buckland et al., 1997), then

$$w_k = \frac{\exp(-\text{AIC}_k/2)}{\sum_{l=1}^{m} \exp(-\text{AIC}_l/2)}.$$

### 8.5.3 Dose-Finding Algorithm

The trial starts by treating the first cohort of patients at the lowest dose, and continues to escalate the dose until the first DLT occurs. Afterwards, we switch to the following dose-finding algorithm:

(1) Suppose that the current dose level is $j^{\text{curr}}$. Based on the accumulated data, we estimate the toxicity probabilities of all the doses, $\bar{\pi}_1, \ldots, \bar{\pi}_J$, using the EM algorithm coupled with the model selection or model averaging procedure.

(2) We find the dose level $j^*$ that has a toxicity probability closest to the target toxicity probability $\phi_T$; that is,

$$j^* = \underset{j \in \{1, \ldots, J\}}{\arg \min} |\bar{\pi}_j - \phi_T|,$$

and

- if $j^{\text{curr}} > j^*$, de-escalate to dose level $j^{\text{curr}} - 1$;
- if $j^{\text{curr}} < j^*$, escalate to dose level $j^{\text{curr}} + 1$;
- otherwise, the dose stays at the same level for the next cohort of patients.

(3) Once the maximum sample size is reached, the dose with the toxicity probability closest to $\phi_T$ is selected as the MTD.

For safety, we impose an early stopping rule based on the 90% confidence interval for the toxicity probability of the lowest dose. If the lower bound of the confidence interval is greater than $\phi_T$, the trial will be terminated.

### 8.5.4 Simulation Study

We investigated the performance of the EM-CRM designs in conjunction with model selection or model averaging by simulating four scenarios as listed in Table 8.2. The maximum number of patients was 36, and patients were treated sequentially in a cohort size of 3. We took the target toxicity probability $\phi_T = 30\%$, the toxicity assessment period $\tau = 3$ months, and the interarrival time $a = 1$ month. For patients who would experience toxicity in $[0, \tau]$, their times to toxicity were generated from Weibull distributions.

Figure 8.4 presents the three sets of prespecified toxicity probabilities:

$$(p_1, \ldots, p_6) = \begin{cases} (0.05, 0.14, 0.18, 0.22, 0.26, 0.30), & \text{skeleton 1}, \\ (0.08, 0.12, 0.20, 0.30, 0.40, 0.50), & \text{skeleton 2}, \\ (0.20, 0.30, 0.40, 0.50, 0.60, 0.70), & \text{skeleton 3}, \end{cases}$$

which were used for model selection (EM-CRM$_{\text{Sel}}$) and model averaging (EM-CRM$_{\text{Avg}}$). Under the EM-CRMs, each cohort was treated immediately upon arrival. For comparison, we also implemented the standard CRM, in which every

**Table 8.2    Four Simulation Scenarios with True Toxicity Probabilities at Six Increasing Dose Levels**

| Scenario | Dose Level | | | | | |
|---|---|---|---|---|---|---|
|  | 1 | 2 | 3 | 4 | 5 | 6 |
| 1 | 0.05 | 0.14 | 0.18 | 0.22 | 0.26 | **0.30** |
| 2 | 0.08 | 0.10 | 0.12 | **0.30** | 0.50 | 0.60 |
| 3 | 0.06 | 0.08 | 0.10 | 0.15 | **0.30** | 0.45 |
| 4 | 0.05 | 0.10 | **0.30** | 0.50 | 0.60 | 0.70 |

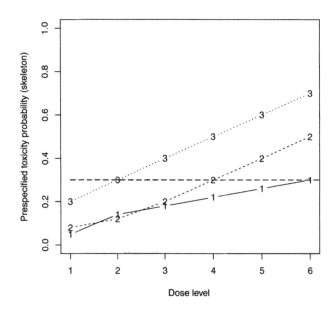

**Figure 8.4**   Three different skeletons in the EM-CRM coupled with model selection or model averaging with the target toxicity probability $\phi_T = 30\%$.

patient was fully followed until all the toxicity data were completely observed prior to the next dose assignment. We refer to the individual CRM using each of the three skeletons as CRM 1, 2, and 3, and denote EM-CRM 1, 2, and 3 for the CRMs coupled with the EM algorithm, respectively. We carried out 10,000 simulated trials for each configuration.

Figure 8.5 displays the selection percentages of the MTD under the designs of (CRM 1, EM-CRM 1), ..., (CRM 3, EM-CRM 3), and (EM-CRM$_{\text{Sel}}$, EM-CRM$_{\text{Avg}}$), respectively. In scenario 1, the MTD is the last dose; the three standard CRMs and corresponding EM-CRMs using skeletons 1, 2, and 3 yielded very different selection percentages of the MTD. The designs using skeleton 1 performed substantially better than those based on the other two skeletons, indicating that both the CRM and EM-CRM are sensitive to the prespecified skeleton. The MTD selection percentages using the EM-CRMs were slightly lower but very close to those of the CRMs, while the trial duration was dramatically reduced from 37 to 21 months. Using multiple skeletons coupled with model selection or model averaging, both the EM-CRM$_{\text{Sel}}$ and EM-CRM$_{\text{Avg}}$ satisfactorily strengthened the robustness of the designs. Scenario 2 has the MTD at the fourth dose level; CRM 1 behaved much worse than the other two CRMs, and the EM-CRMs performed similarly to the CRMs in terms of the MTD

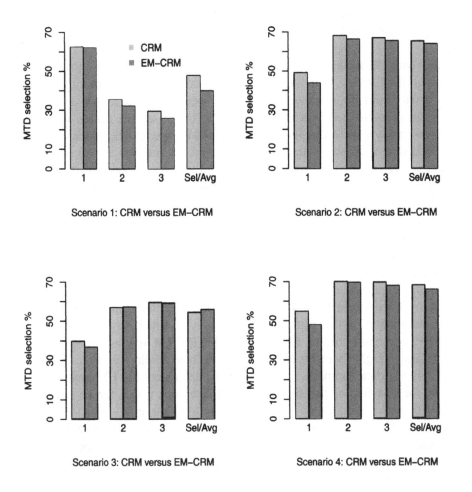

**Figure 8.5**    Selection percentages of the MTD in the order of using the CRM and EM-CRM under skeletons 1, 2, and 3, respectively. The last two bars correspond to the EM-CRM in conjunction with model selection (EM-CRM$_{Sel}$) and model averaging (EM-CRM$_{Avg}$).

selection, but yielded much shorter trial durations. Scenario 3 has the MTD at the fifth dose level; CRM 1 and EM-CRM 1 had the lowest MTD selection, whereas both the EM-CRM$_{Sel}$ and EM-CRM$_{Avg}$ recommended the MTD with much higher percentages. Had the first skeleton been used to conduct the trial in scenarios 2 and 3, the performance of the design could have been compromised. Similar conclusions can be drawn from scenario 4: The EM-CRMs immensely shortened the trial duration without sacrificing the trial performance much, and when coupled with model selection or model averaging the designs became more robust.

By employing the model selection and model averaging procedures, the EM-CRM$_{Sel}$ and EM-CRM$_{Avg}$ automatically lean toward the best-performing skeleton, and greatly limit the influence of those poor-performing skeletons. Hence, as long as there is one good-performing skeleton in the set, the design would perform reasonably well. As an alternative to the EM approach, the missing data may be treated as unknown "parameters" in the model, and the Bayesian data argumentation can be used to draw the unobserved toxicity outcomes from their full conditional distributions together with other model parameters (Tanner and Wong, 1987). After filling in the missing data with their posterior samples, the posterior samples of the model parameters can be easily obtained through the standard MCMC procedure.

In this chapter, we have introduced several statistical designs to meet the practical needs when toxicity outcomes cannot be observed quickly in a dose-finding study. In particular, by redistributing the censored data to the right, the fractional $3+3$ design and the fCRM naturally fractionize the point mass of each censored observation, so that patients whose toxicity events have not happened yet may still contribute to dose finding. The TITE-CRM applies a weighting scheme to assign higher weights to patients with longer follow-up times. In a rigorous missing data approach, the EM-CRM implements the EM algorithm coherently for dose finding based on the incomplete data, which can be further coupled with model selection or model averaging to enhance the robustness of the design. Unlike the standard $3 + 3$ design and the CRM which require the toxicity outcome to be ascertainable shortly after treatment, these methods allow for delayed response and fast and continuous accrual and, most importantly, they substantially shorten the trial duration.

## EXERCISES

**8.1**  In the fractional $3 + 3$ design, derive the local Kaplan–Meier estimator to incorporate the dose information, and compute the fractional contribution for each censored observation.

**8.2**  Following the notation of the EM-CRM in Section 8.5, show that the $k$th component of the hazard estimate $\boldsymbol{\lambda}^{(r+1)}$ in the $(r + 1)$th EM iteration is

$$\lambda_k^{(r+1)} = \frac{d_k}{\sum_{j=k}^{K}\left(d_j + \sum_{i \in \mathcal{C}_j} \hat{y}_i\right)}.$$

# CHAPTER 9

# DRUG-COMBINATION TRIALS

## 9.1 WHY ARE DRUGS COMBINED?

Human diseases are very complicated and often involve various biological mechanisms. In particular, cancer cells are the most difficult to tackle due to many intricate disease pathways. To optimize the treatment strategy, a combination of drugs or treatment interventions may be simultaneously used to target multiple and related disease pathways. Traditionally, a phase I clinical trial only evaluates one single treatment at a time. Given the tremendous advances in medicine, many new drugs are available for testing in different combinations. Compared with single-agent treatments, combination therapies may

- lead to synergistic treatment effects,

- target tumor cells with differing drug susceptibilities, and

- achieve higher dose intensities with nonoverlapping toxicities.

In the development of combination therapies, it is essential to study the joint actions of multiple drugs and pin down their interactive effects. For simplicity, we consider a two-drug combination study. Let $D_A$ denote the dose of drug A

*Clinical Trial Design.* By Guosheng Yin

and let $D_B$ denote the dose of drug B that would produce the same toxicity (or efficacy) effect, when each drug is administered alone. When drug A and drug B are combined, let $d_A$ denote the dose of drug A and let $d_B$ denote that of drug B, such that the dose combination would achieve the same toxicity/efficacy effect as that of $D_A$ or $D_B$ when each drug is administered alone. Many statistical models can be used to characterize the drug–drug interactive effects; for example, the Bliss (1939) independence model implies that in a two-drug combination study each drug behaves independently of each other.

The Loewe (1953) additivity model defines the interaction index as

$$\tau = \frac{d_A}{D_A} + \frac{d_B}{D_B}. \tag{9.1}$$

To understand the meaning of $\tau$, we rewrite (9.1) as

$$d_A + \rho d_B = \tau D_A,$$

where $\rho = D_A/D_B$ is the relative potency of drug B versus drug A (Morgan, 1992). When $\tau = 1$, then $d_A + \rho d_B = D_A$, that is, the combined doses of $d_A$ and $d_B$ induce the same effect as that when drug A is used alone, indicating additivity of the combined doses. When $\tau < 1$, then $d_A + \rho d_B < D_A$, that is, the total amount of dosage is less than that when drug A is administered alone, indicating synergy of the combination doses $d_A$ and $d_B$. When $\tau > 1$, then $d_A + \rho d_B > D_A$, that is, the total amount of dosage is more than that when drug A is given alone, indicating antagonism of the combination doses $d_A$ and $d_B$.

In an alternative formulation, Plackett and Hewlett (1967) study the model of

$$\left(\frac{d_A}{D_A}\right)^\alpha + \left(\frac{d_B}{D_B}\right)^\alpha = 1.$$

When $0 < \alpha < 1$, the effects of drug A and drug B are synergistic; when $\alpha = 1$, the effects of the two drugs are additive; and when $\alpha > 1$, the effects of the two drugs are antagonistic. Tan et al. (2003) propose modeling the synergy of combined drugs based on uniform designs to reduce the variability, and Lee et al. (2007) review and expand on the estimation of the interaction index.

Treating patients with a combination of agents is becoming commonplace. To embrace this growing trend, this chapter mainly focuses on dose finding in phase I drug-combination trials, in which the goal is to find the maximum tolerated dose (MTD) combination. For example, Lokich (2001) combines four doses of topotecan with two doses of irinotecan in a clinical trial to treat advanced malignancy. Single-agent trials often assume that toxicity monotonically increases with the dose, and the order of toxicity is known along the one-dimensional dose searching line. By contrast, for a two-drug combination study as shown in Figure 9.1, there are up to eight adjacent doses in the two-dimensional searching plane, and the toxicity order is *not* known along the off-diagonal directions. That

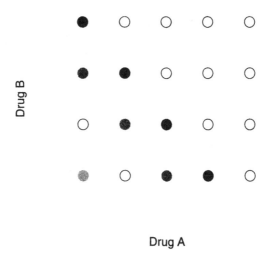

**Figure 9.1** Dose pairs in a two-drug combination study where the toxicity order is unknown alone the off-diagonal direction.

is, the monotonic toxicity assumption may still hold when fixing one drug at a certain dose level, but it is not clear whether the joint toxicity would increase when lowering the dose of one drug and increasing that of the other. Of greater importance is the need to prevent patients from experiencing excessive toxicities when they are treated with multiple agents.

**EXAMPLE 9.1**

A phase I drug-combination trial was designed to study the safety of the combination of bortezomib and gemcitabine plus doxorubicin in the treatment of metastatic urothelial cancer. Bortezomib works by entering cancer cells and interfering with cell division. Gemcitabine and doxorubicin, given together and thus considered as one drug for dose-finding purposes, are chemotherapeutic agents that disrupt the growth and cause the death of cancer cells. Combining bortezomib with chemotherapies is expected to induce drugs' synergistic effects and to enhance treatment efficacy. In this drug-combination trial, each drug had eight prespecified dose levels, leading to an $8 \times 8$ matrix of dose pairs. The primary objective was to determine the MTD combination of bortezomib and chemotherapies with a target toxicity rate of 30%.

Trial designs for drug combinations can be extended to broader applications, for example, to simultaneously determine the optimal dose level and dose schedule for a single agent (Braun et al., 2007; Li et al., 2008). When a drug is given at the same dose but on a more intense or frequent administration schedule, the patient response to treatment may improve (Braun, Yuan, and Thall, 2005). Hence, optimizing the dose schedule at different dose levels may also be viewed as a two-dimensional dose-finding problem, in which one dimension is the dose level and the other is the administration schedule (e.g., frequency and duration of treatment). As the third kind of two-dimensional dose finding, patients may be classified into ordered groups such as good or poor prognosis, and the group-specific MTDs may be identified (O'Quigley and Paoletti, 2003).

## 9.2   NEW CHALLENGES

Consider a two-drug combination trial in which drug A has $J$ dose levels, denoted as $A_1 < \cdots < A_J$, and drug B has $K$ dose levels, denoted as $B_1 < \cdots < B_K$. Let $(A_j, B_k)$ denote the combination of drug A at dose level $j$ and drug B at dose level $k$, for $j = 1, \ldots, J$ and $k = 1, \ldots, K$. When two or more drugs are given in combination, drug–drug interactive effects may be very complex and often lead to unknown toxicity patterns. As a result, dose finding with combined agents poses many new challenges that are beyond the scope of single-agent trial designs:

(1) In a drug-combination trial, the toxicity order of dose combinations is only partially known. For example, the dose combination of $(A_2, B_3)$ is more toxic than $(A_2, B_2)$, while along the off-diagonal direction, the toxicity order of $(A_2, B_3)$ and $(A_3, B_2)$ is unknown. Therefore, if the current dose combination can be well tolerated, it is not clear which dose pair should be assigned to the next cohort of patients.

(2) The dimension of the dose searching space expands multiplicatively with respect to the number of drugs in the combination. For instance, in a two-drug combination study with eight dose levels for each drug, the search space involves 64 dose pairs. This rapid increment of dose combinations inevitably calls for an increase of sample size in order to cover the whole search space, notwithstanding limited resources in a phase I trial.

(3) Due to MTD equivalence contours, multiple MTD combinations may exist in the two-dimensional dose space. Dose finding may lack the opportunity to explore the entire space if trapped in a local region.

These difficulties severely limit direct applications of single-agent dose-finding methods to drug-combination trials.

As more drug-combination studies emerge, many statistical methods are developed for combined therapies. Early work on modeling the combination of agents can be found in Ashford (1981) and Abdelbasit and Plackett (1982). By

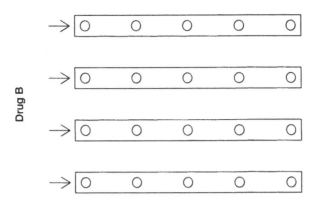

Drug A

**Figure 9.2**    Independent parallel dose finding for drug combinations by searching through the doses of drug A while fixing the dose of drug B.

introducing a graphical tolerable dose diagram, Korn and Simon (1993) provide guidance to target specific MTD combinations. Conaway, Dunbar, and Peddada (2004) study both the simple and partial orders for drug combinations based on the pool-adjacent-violators algorithm (Barlow et al., 1972). Figure 9.2 shows that single-agent trial designs may be applied to a two-dimensional dose-finding study, if we fix drug B at each given dose and search through the doses of drug A for the MTD. In each of the $K$ one-dimensional subtrials, the monotonic toxicity order is preserved (Kuzuya et al., 2001). However, such an independent parallel trial design only utilizes the simple toxicity order within each subtrial and completely ignores the partial orders across these subtrials. Not only this strategy causes efficiency loss, but it also requires a large sample size because almost every dose combination needs to be visited. Of more severe consequence is that many patients may be treated at doses that are either excessively toxic or can be well tolerated and thus are presumably ineffective. If we are interested in finding only *one* MTD combination, we can simply choose the one whose toxicity probability is closest to the target from the $K$ identified MTD combinations. On the other hand, we may choose a subset of dose combinations by including only the dose pairs with a known toxicity order. Figure 9.3 exhibits that the two-dimensional dose-finding space is reduced into a one-dimensional searching line (Kramar, Lebecq, and Candalh, 1999).

In contrast to dimension reduction of the dose searching space, we may directly model the joint toxicity probability at each dose pair to guide dose escalation

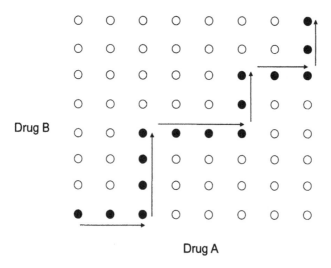

**Figure 9.3** Selection of a subset of dose combinations that maintains the monotonic toxicity order.

or de-escalation throughout the trial. Let $Z_{A_j}$ and $Z_{B_k}$ denote the standardized doses for the dose combination $(A_j, B_k)$. Under the usual logistic regression, the joint toxicity probability at $(A_j, B_k)$ can be modeled as

$$\pi_{jk} = \frac{\exp(\beta_0 + \beta_1 Z_{A_j} + \beta_2 Z_{B_k} + \beta_3 Z_{A_j} Z_{B_k})}{1 + \exp(\beta_0 + \beta_1 Z_{A_j} + \beta_2 Z_{B_k} + \beta_3 Z_{A_j} Z_{B_k})},$$

where the interaction term $\beta_3 Z_{A_j} Z_{B_k}$ captures the drug–drug interactive effects. Through a different modeling structure, Thall et al. (2003) propose a six-parameter regression model in the form of

$$\pi_{jk} = \frac{\alpha_1 Z_{A_j}^{\beta_1} + \alpha_2 Z_{B_k}^{\beta_2} + \alpha_3 (Z_{A_j}^{\beta_1} Z_{B_k}^{\beta_2})^{\beta_3}}{1 + \alpha_1 Z_{A_j}^{\beta_1} + \alpha_2 Z_{B_k}^{\beta_2} + \alpha_3 (Z_{A_j}^{\beta_1} Z_{B_k}^{\beta_2})^{\beta_3}},$$

to characterize the joint toxicity probability $\pi_{jk}$ at the dose combination $(A_j, B_k)$. Their model, however, appears to be nonparsimonious and thus sheds doubt on the stability of parameter estimates, especially with a small sample size. If the actual doses of drug A and drug B are replaced by the prespecified toxicity probabilities, $p_1 < \cdots < p_J$ and $q_1 < \cdots < q_K$, the joint toxicity probability may be modeled as

$$\pi_{jk} = 1 - (1 - p_j)^{\alpha}(1 - q_k)^{\beta + \gamma \log(1 - p_j)}, \qquad (9.2)$$

where $\alpha$, $\beta$, and $\gamma$ are unknown parameters (Wang and Ivanova, 2005). For clarity, we can rewrite (9.2) as

$$\log(1 - \pi_{jk}) = \alpha \log(1 - p_j) + \beta \log(1 - q_k) + \gamma \log(1 - p_j) \log(1 - q_k),$$

where $\gamma$ captures drugs' interaction. If the two drugs act independently on patients, then $\gamma = 0$, and $\pi_{jk} = 1 - (1 - p_j)^{\alpha}(1 - q_k)^{\beta}$.

Since combination therapies become increasingly important, more efficient statistical designs are developed to model the unforeseen toxicity order of dose combinations. In the next few sections, we will provide in-depth discussions on the most updated dose-finding methods for drug-combination trials. In particular, Yuan and Yin (2008) propose a simple sequential dose-finding scheme based upon both the simple and partial orders of dose combinations. By making use of the copula regression structure, Yin and Yuan (2009b) explicitly incorporate the single-agent toxicity information to model the joint toxicity probability. In a different route, Yin and Yuan (2009c) introduce a latent $2 \times 2$ contingency table for each dose combination and construct a binomial likelihood for combination doses of two drugs. Braun and Wang (2010) propose Bayesian hierarchical modeling for the joint toxicity probability of two therapeutic agents. In a phase I/II drug-combination trial, Yuan and Yin (2011b) investigate seamless transition between these two consecutive phases coupled with adaptive randomization.

## 9.3  SEQUENTIAL DOSE-FINDING SCHEME

The simplest approach to two-dimensional dose finding is based on a sequential scheme, which utilizes both simple and partial toxicity orders (Yuan and Yin, 2008). Denote $A_{(s \to t)}B_k$ as the $k$th subtrial, in which the dose level of drug A increases from $s$ to $t$ $(s < t)$ and drug B is fixed at dose level $k$. We divide the entire two-dimensional trial into several groups of one-dimensional subtrials: The first group consists of $\{A_{(1 \to J)}B_1, A_{(1 \to J)}B_2, A_{(1 \to J)}B_3\}$, the second includes $\{A_{(1 \to J)}B_4, A_{(1 \to J)}B_5, A_{(1 \to J)}B_6\}$, and so on. Each group is composed of three subtrials, while the last group may contain one or two subtrials. Within each group, we refer to the subtrial at the lower dose level of drug B as the low-dose subtrial; that at the higher dose level of drug B as the high-dose subtrial; and that at the intermediate dose level of drug B as the intermediate-dose subtrial. These subtrials are conducted in a specific order, such that the MTD that has been determined in the completed subtrial can be used as the truncation boundary to shrink the searching space of other subtrials that have not been carried out yet.

Consider an example of combining drug A with six dose levels and drug B with three dose levels, as illustrated in Figure 9.4. Under the sequential design, the intermediate-dose subtrial $A_{(1 \to 6)}B_2$ is conducted first, and suppose that the dose combination $(A_3, B_2)$ is identified as the MTD. Based on the monotonic

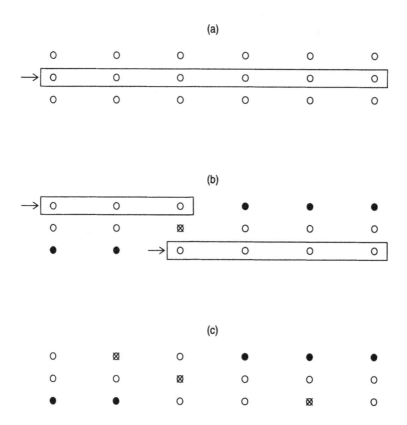

**Figure 9.4**    For the first group of subtrials $\{A_{(1 \to 6)}B_1, A_{(1 \to 6)}B_2, A_{(1 \to 6)}B_3\}$, the sequential design proceeds in the order of (a) running the intermediate-dose subtrial, (b) conducting the low-dose and high-dose subtrials simultaneously in the reduced searching spaces based on the MTD previously found, and (c) identifying a total of three MTDs. Crosses denote the MTDs, open circles in the box represent the dose combinations under consideration, and solid circles are those removed from the subsequent subtrials.

order of toxicity, we immediately know that if we fix drug B at dose level 1, the MTD level of drug A cannot be lower than dose level 3; and if we fix drug B at dose level 3 or higher, the MTD level of drug A cannot exceed dose level 3. In other words, after $(A_3, B_2)$ is determined as the MTD in the subtrial of $A_{(1 \to 6)}B_2$, we can shrink the full-length subtrials $A_{(1 \to 6)}B_1$ and $A_{(1 \to 6)}B_3$ to $A_{(3 \to 6)}B_1$ and $A_{(1 \to 3)}B_3$, respectively. As a result, the dose searching spaces of the subsequent subtrials are substantially reduced.

In a more general setup, the first group of subtrials under the sequential scheme is conducted as follows:

(1) Run the intermediate-dose subtrial $A_{(1 \to J)} B_2$ to find the MTD, which is denoted by $A_{j_2^*} B_2$.

(2) Run the low-dose and high-dose subtrials in the reduced dose-finding spaces simultaneously; that is, $A_{(j_2^* \to J)} B_1$ and $A_{(1 \to j_2^*)} B_3$.

(3) If the MTD in $A_{(1 \to J)} B_2$ does not exist because all the doses are overly toxic, run the low-dose subtrial $A_{(1 \to J)} B_1$ only.

Suppose that the MTD of the high-dose subtrial in the first group is determined as $A_{j_3^*} B_3$, then run the second group of subtrials in a similar way, but with appropriately truncated dose levels of drug A.

The most appealing feature of the sequential scheme is that it can be coupled with any single-agent dose-find method for a drug-combination trial without extra effort. In a sequential order, single-agent dose-find methods, such as the $3 + 3$ design or the CRM, can be easily applied to each of the subtrials. The identified MTDs in the completed subtrials will be used to shrink the dose searching space of those subtrials yet to conduct. The low-dose subtrial tends to have more futile doses, whereas the high-dose subtrial tends to include more excessively toxic doses. Based on the location of the MTD in the intermediate-dose subtrial, we are able to efficiently remove futile and over-toxic doses from subsequent subtrials. Consequently, fewer patients would be allocated to suboptimal dose combinations compared with the independent parallel dose-finding method as shown in Figure 9.2.

By adaptively shortening the dose searching length of each subtrial based on the MTDs determined in the previous subtrials, the sequential design leads to substantial savings in sample size. This, in turn, shortens the overall trial time, since patient accrual is often the bottleneck of trial conduct. For each subtrial, the sample size may be determined by allocating one cohort of patients at each dose—for example, with a cohort size of three. The sequential design identifies all the $K$ MTD combinations by fixing drug $B$ at each dose level $k$, $k = 1, \ldots, K$. If the goal is to find only one MTD combination, we can simply choose the dose combination that has an estimated toxicity probability closest to the target.

## 9.4    DOSE FINDING WITH COPULA-TYPE REGRESSION

### 9.4.1    Clayton-Type Model

Before any drug-combination trial is carried out, each drug must have been thoroughly studied when administered alone. These single-agent trials naturally provide rich prior information to design a drug-combination study. For ease of exposition, we consider combining two drugs, say drug A with $J$ doses and drug B with $K$ doses. Let $p_j$ be the prespecified toxicity probability for $A_j$, the $j$th dose of drug A, satisfying $p_1 < \cdots < p_J$; and let $q_k$ be that of $B_k$, the $k$th dose of drug B, satisfying $q_1 < \cdots < q_K$. Typically, the maximum dose for each drug in the combination should not exceed the individual MTD that has already be determined in the previous single-agent trials. That is, the highest doses $A_J$ and $B_K$ are the MTDs or the doses below the MTDs for drug A and drug B, respectively. The toxicity probabilities of the MTDs of drugs A and B are known, and thereby naturally set the corresponding upper bounds for $p_J$ and $q_K$. As a result, instead of arbitrarily choosing a sequence of values in $(0, 1)$, the prespecified toxicity probabilities for drug A and drug B can be more precisely chosen from $(0, p_J)$ and $(0, q_K)$, respectively.

When two or more drugs are combined as a treatment, it is unrealistic to assume that each drug acts independently on the patient, because the drug–drug interactive effects may have a strong influence on the joint toxicity probability. Although each drug has its own toxicity profile, the individual drug information cannot be delineated in a combination trial. To enhance the flexibility and accommodate the uncertainty of the prespecified $p_j$ and $q_k$, we incorporate a power parameter to each toxicity probability in the form of $(p_j^\alpha, q_k^\beta)$ with $\alpha > 0$ and $\beta > 0$. By borrowing the structure of the Clayton (1978) copula, the joint toxicity probability at $(A_j, B_k)$ is modeled as

$$\pi_{jk} = 1 - \{(1 - p_j^\alpha)^{-\gamma} + (1 - q_k^\beta)^{-\gamma} - 1\}^{-1/\gamma}, \qquad (9.3)$$

where $\gamma > 0$ characterizes the drug–drug interactions. Nevertheless, it worths emphasizing that model (9.3) is in fact *not* a copula because it does not characterize any bivariate distribution with marginal distributions (Yin and Yuan, 2010b). In a drug-combination trial, we only observe one single dose-limiting toxicity (DLT) outcome for combined agents, in contrast to the bivariate outcomes in the usual copula sense. More specifically, for a patient treated at the dose combination $(A_j, B_k)$, there is only a single toxicity outcome $Y$ that takes a value of 1 with probability $\pi_{jk}$, and 0 with probability $1 - \pi_{jk}$.

Model (9.3) satisfies three intuitive conditions:

(1) If $p_j^\alpha = 0$ and $q_k^\beta = 0$, then $\pi_{jk} = 0$. That is, if the toxicity probabilities of both drugs are zero (essentially no drugs), the joint toxicity probability is zero.

(2) If $p_j^\alpha = 0$, then $\pi_{jk} = q_k^\beta$; and if $q_k^\beta = 0$, then $\pi_{jk} = p_j^\alpha$. When the toxicity probability of one drug is zero, the joint toxicity probability reduces to a single-agent case.

(3) If either $p_j^\alpha \to 1$ or $q_k^\beta \to 1$, then $\pi_{jk} \to 1$. In other words, if either drug causes the DLT with probability one, the joint toxicity probability is one.

As characterized by the three model parameters $(\alpha, \beta, \gamma)$ in (9.3), the toxicity probability surface may have various shapes. In particular, for $\alpha = \beta = 2$

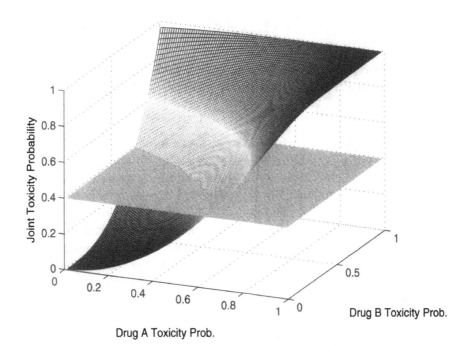

**Figure 9.5**    Toxicity probability surface and MTD equivalence contour under the Clayton copula-type model.

and $\gamma = 1.5$, Figure 9.5 displays the joint toxicity probability surface in the two-dimensional probability space. If the target toxicity probability is 40%, as indicated by the horizontal plane, there exists an intersection curve that represents the MTD equivalence contour for the two drugs. Therefore, multiple MTD combinations may exist in a drug-combination trial.

Depending on the dosage, cancer drugs often induce multiple toxicities of different levels of severity, for example, fatigue, nausea, vomiting, diarrhea of different grades, and so on. If one of these toxicities exceeds its threshold such as to be qualified as the DLT, then the toxicity outcome $Y$ takes a value of 1; only if none of these toxicities exceeds the DLT threshold, then $Y = 0$. Although it may happen that certain types of toxicities diminishes or neutralize each other when two drugs are administered together, it is rare in reality that all types of toxicity effects induced by the two drugs are antagonistic.

Suppose that among $n_{jk}$ patients treated at the dose combination $(A_j, B_k)$, $y_{jk}$ of them have experienced toxicity, for $j = 1, \ldots, J$ and $k = 1, \ldots, K$.

Based on the binomial distribution, the likelihood function is given by

$$L(D|\alpha, \beta, \gamma) \propto \prod_{j=1}^{J} \prod_{k=1}^{K} \pi_{jk}^{y_{jk}} (1 - \pi_{jk})^{n_{jk} - y_{jk}},$$

where $D$ denotes the observed data. Given the prior distribution $f(\alpha, \beta, \gamma)$ for all the model parameters, the joint posterior distribution is

$$f(\alpha, \beta, \gamma|D) \propto L(D|\alpha, \beta, \gamma) f(\alpha, \beta, \gamma).$$

Since the toxicity information when each drug is administered alone is available, the specification of $p_j$ and $q_k$ is relatively accurate. In contrast, much less information can be elicited for the drug interaction effect. Therefore, relatively informative prior distributions may be assigned to $\alpha$ and $\beta$ compared with $\gamma$; for example, $\alpha, \beta \sim \text{Ga}(2, 2)$ and $\gamma \sim \text{Ga}(0.1, 0.1)$ if we take independent prior distributions for $\alpha$, $\beta$, and $\gamma$. The full conditional distributions of the model parameters can be easily derived, from which posterior samples can be drawn using the Gibbs sampler in a straightforward way. Upon each new cohort's arrival, we update the posterior estimates of $\pi_{jk}$ in light of the cumulative toxicity data, and determine dose assignment accordingly.

### 9.4.2   Multiple Drugs in Combination

In practice, a drug-combination trial typically involves a pair of agents, while it may be more beneficial to treat patients with three or more drugs combined. As the dimensionality of the dose-finding space grows, it becomes much more challenging to search for the MTD across multiple drugs. Nevertheless, the copula-type design can be easily extended to accommodate higher dimensional dose-finding problems.

If three drugs are combined, in addition to $p_j$ of drug A and $q_k$ of drug B as defined before, we further specify $v_l$ as the toxicity probability of the $l$th dose of drug C for $l = 1, \ldots, L$. Apparently, the dose searching space grows multiplicatively to a three-dimensional cube of size $J \times K \times L$. The triplet $(p_j, q_k, v_l)$ represents the prespecified toxicity probabilities associated with the combined doses $(A_j, B_k, C_l)$, and thus the joint toxicity probability is given by

$$\pi_{jkl} = 1 - \{(1 - p_j^{\alpha})^{-\gamma} + (1 - q_k^{\beta})^{-\gamma} + (1 - v_l^{\eta})^{-\gamma} - 2\}^{-1/\gamma},$$

where all the parameters $\alpha$, $\beta$, $\eta$, and $\gamma$ are positive, and $\gamma$ characterizes the synergism among the three drugs.

### 9.4.3   Dose-Finding Algorithm

At the early stage of a trial, very limited information is available, and thus the posterior estimates of the toxicity probabilities for dose combinations may not

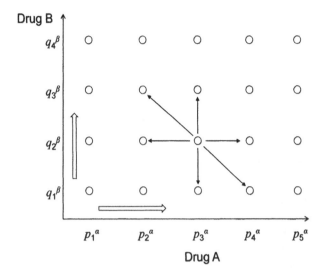

**Figure 9.6**    Dose escalation or de-escalation in a matrix of $5 \times 4$ dose combinations.

be reliable. To alleviate the difficulty associated with sparse data, we initiate a prephase: First along the vertical direction, escalate the dose of drug B while fixing drug A at dose level 1 until the first DLT occurs; then along the horizontal direction, escalate the dose of drug A while fixing drug B at dose level 1 until another DLT is observed. Based on the data collected in this prephase, we can estimate the toxicity probabilities of all the dose combinations. The starting point for the copula-type dose-finding procedure is the dose combination whose toxicity probability is closest to the target $\phi_T$.

Suppose that the current cohort is treated at the dose combination $(A_j, B_k)$ with the toxicity probability of $\pi_{jk}$. For safety, we restrict the next dose assignment within the neighborhood of $(A_j, B_k)$ as shown in Figure 9.6, while simultaneous escalation or de-escalation of both agents along the diagonal direction is prohibited. Let $c_e$ and $c_d$ $(c_e + c_d > 1)$ denote the fixed probability cutoffs for dose escalation and de-escalation, respectively. The Bayesian copula-type dose-finding algorithm is described as follows:

(1) If at the current dose combination,

$$\Pr(\pi_{jk} < \phi_T | D) > c_e,$$

escalate to the adjacent dose combination whose toxicity probability is higher than $\pi_{jk}$ and closest to $\phi_T$. If the current dose combination is $(A_J, B_K)$, the doses stay the same.

(2) If at the current dose combination,

$$\Pr(\pi_{jk} > \phi_T | D) > c_d,$$

de-escalate to the adjacent dose combination whose toxicity probability is lower than $\pi_{jk}$ and closest to $\phi_T$. If the current dose combination is $(A_1, B_1)$, the trial is terminated.

(3) Otherwise, treat the next cohort of patients at the same dose combination.

(4) Once the maximum sample size is exhausted, the dose combination with a toxicity probability closest to $\phi_T$ is selected as the MTD combination.

### 9.4.4  Simulation Study

We examined the performance of the Bayesian copula-type design by simulating four scenarios listed in Table 9.1. Drug A had five dose levels, drug B had four, and the numbers and locations of the MTD combinations varied from one scenario to another. The target toxicity probability was $\phi_T = 40\%$, the maximum sample size was 60, and patients were treated in a cohort size of three. When each drug was administered alone, the toxicity probability of the MTD of drug A was 0.4 and that of drug B was 0.3. Bounded by these two values, we specified $(p_1, \ldots, p_5) = (0.08, 0.16, 0.24, 0.32, 0.4)$ and $(q_1, \ldots, q_4) = (0.075, 0.15, 0.225, 0.3)$. We set $c_e = 0.8$ for dose escalation and $c_d = 0.45$ for dose de-escalation. In the Markov chain Monte Carlo (MCMC) procedure, we recorded 2,000 posterior samples of the model parameters after 100 burn-in iterations. We simulated 2,000 trials under each scenario.

Table 9.1 presents the selection percentage of each dose combination and the sum of those of the MTD combinations under the Bayesian copula-type design. In the four scenarios, we explored the cases with two, three, or four MTD combinations, and clearly the overall performance of the Bayesian copula-type design was satisfactory. The selection percentages of the MTD combinations were the highest among all the dose combinations. Approximately, there was a 50% of chance to identify a true MTD combination in each scenario, and most of the patients were treated at the MTD or the nearby dose combinations. The simulation study demonstrates the advantages of directly modeling the joint toxicity probabilities and freely assigning doses across the entire drug-combination space.

Not only does the copula-type model fully evaluate the joint toxicity profile of the combined drugs, but it also preserves the single-agent property and reduces to the usual CRM if only one drug is tested. Based on the accumulated data, the toxicity probabilities of the dose combinations can be continuously estimated and efficiently ordered, so that each new cohort of patients will be treated at the most appropriate dose combination.

**Table 9.1    Simulation Study Using the Bayesian Copula-Type Dose-Finding Method under Four Scenarios for Two-Drug Combination Trials with a Target Toxicity Probability of 40%**

| Sc. | Pr{toxicity at $(A_j, B_k)$} | | | | | Selection Percentage | | | | | Sum (%) |
|-----|------|------|------|------|------|------|------|------|------|------|------|
| 1 | 0.54 | 0.67 | 0.75 | 0.81 | 0.86 | 0.9 | 0.1 | 0.0 | 0.0 | 0.0 | 44.0 |
|   | 0.48 | 0.59 | 0.68 | 0.75 | 0.81 | 10.2 | 1.7 | 0.1 | 0.0 | 0.0 | |
|   | **0.40** | 0.45 | 0.59 | 0.67 | 0.74 | **24.9** | 11.6 | 1.7 | 0.1 | 0.0 | |
|   | 0.24 | **0.40** | 0.47 | 0.56 | 0.64 | 3.1 | **19.1** | 6.2 | 0.3 | 0.0 | |
| 2 | 0.49 | 0.58 | 0.68 | 0.75 | 0.81 | 5.0 | 1.5 | 0.0 | 0.0 | 0.0 | 48.0 |
|   | **0.40** | 0.49 | 0.59 | 0.68 | 0.75 | **17.6** | 11.6 | 1.4 | 0.1 | 0.0 | |
|   | 0.27 | **0.40** | 0.45 | 0.59 | 0.67 | 7.3 | **19.2** | 9.3 | 1.7 | 0.1 | |
|   | 0.18 | 0.29 | **0.40** | 0.47 | 0.56 | 0.1 | 5.1 | **11.2** | 5.0 | 0.3 | |
| 3 | 0.31 | **0.40** | 0.50 | 0.61 | 0.75 | 3.8 | **11.7** | 8.5 | 1.3 | 0.1 | 52.2 |
|   | 0.23 | 0.34 | **0.40** | 0.53 | 0.67 | 0.7 | 5.9 | **12.7** | 8.0 | 1.2 | |
|   | 0.16 | 0.25 | 0.34 | **0.40** | 0.52 | 0.0 | 0.7 | 3.5 | **12.0** | 10.3 | |
|   | 0.09 | 0.16 | 0.18 | 0.22 | **0.40** | 0.0 | 0.0 | 0.3 | 3.5 | **15.8** | |
| 4 | **0.40** | 0.52 | 0.72 | 0.75 | 0.84 | **10.2** | 8.7 | 0.9 | 0.0 | 0.0 | 52.5 |
|   | 0.29 | **0.40** | 0.51 | 0.60 | 0.68 | 5.3 | **16.7** | 5.9 | 0.5 | 0.0 | |
|   | 0.20 | 0.31 | **0.40** | 0.50 | 0.59 | 0.4 | 4.7 | **14.1** | 8.3 | 1.0 | |
|   | 0.12 | 0.21 | 0.30 | **0.40** | 0.47 | 0.1 | 0.2 | 5.8 | **11.5** | 5.3 | |

Note: Sc. stands for Scenario, and Sum (%) is the sum of the selection percentages of all the MTD combinations.

## 9.5  LATENT CONTINGENCY TABLE APPROACH

### 9.5.1  Bivariate Binary Outcomes

Combining multiple drugs may help to achieve a higher dose intensity by exploiting nonoverlapping toxicities of different agents. Ideally, the toxicities of the two drugs in combination can be explicitly distinguished, such that we can formulate a $2 \times 2$ contingency table to accommodate the bivariate binary toxicity data.

As defined before, let $p_j$ be the prespecified toxicity probability for $A_j$, and let $q_k$ be the prespecified toxicity probability for $B_k$. By incorporating two unknown power parameters $\alpha > 0$ and $\beta > 0$, the marginal toxicity probabilities for $A_j$ and $B_k$ are given by $p_j^\alpha$ and $q_k^\beta$, respectively. For patients treated at the dose combination $(A_j, B_k)$, if we observe the DLT from drug A, then $X_{jk} = 1$, otherwise $X_{jk} = 0$; if we observe the DLT from drug B, then $Y_{jk} = 1$, otherwise $Y_{jk} = 0$. As shown in Figure 9.7, we can formulate a $2 \times 2$ contingency table at

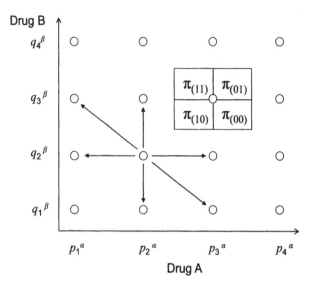

**Figure 9.7**    In a two-drug combination trial, given the marginal toxicity probabilities $p_j^\alpha$ and $q_k^\beta$, we construct a latent $2 \times 2$ probability table at each dose pair.

each dose combination $(A_j, B_k)$ for $j = 1, \ldots, J$ and $k = 1, \ldots, K$,

$$
\begin{array}{c c}
 & \begin{array}{cc} p_j^\alpha & \quad 1 - p_j^\alpha \end{array} \\
\begin{array}{c} q_k^\beta \\[1em] 1 - q_k^\beta \end{array} &
\begin{array}{|c|c|}
\hline
\pi_{jk(11)} & \pi_{jk(01)} \\
\hline
\pi_{jk(10)} & \pi_{jk(00)} \\
\hline
\end{array}
\end{array}
\tag{9.4}
$$

where each cell $\pi_{jk(xy)}$ represents the joint toxicity probability associated with the bivariate binary outcomes $(X_{jk} = x, Y_{jk} = y)$ for $x = 0, 1; y = 0, 1$.

Based on the Gumbel model (Murtaugh and Fisher, 1990), the joint toxicity probability for the bivariate outcomes $(x, y)$ is given by

$$
\begin{aligned}
\pi_{jk(xy)} = {}& p_j^{\alpha x}(1 - p_j^\alpha)^{1-x} q_k^{\beta y}(1 - q_k^\beta)^{1-y} \\
& + (-1)^{x+y} p_j^\alpha (1 - p_j^\alpha) q_k^\beta (1 - q_k^\beta) \frac{e^\gamma - 1}{e^\gamma + 1},
\end{aligned}
\tag{9.5}
$$

where the association parameter $\gamma$ characterizes drugs' synergistic effect. If $\gamma = 0$, model (9.5) reduces to the independent case.

Suppose that among $n_{jk}$ patients treated at the dose combination $(A_j, B_k)$, $n_{jk(11)}$ patients have experienced DLTs from both drugs, $n_{jk(10)}$ patients have experienced DLTs from drug A only, $n_{jk(01)}$ patients have experienced DLTs from drug B only, and $n_{jk(00)}$ patients have not experienced any DLTs. Following a multinomial distribution, the likelihood function is given by

$$L(D|\alpha,\beta,\gamma) \propto \prod_{j=1}^{J} \prod_{k=1}^{K} \prod_{x=0}^{1} \prod_{y=0}^{1} \{\pi_{jk(xy)}\}^{n_{jk(xy)}},$$

which, however, is based on an imaginary situation that the DLTs from the two agents can always be distinguished.

### 9.5.2  Latent Contingency Table

In reality, the toxicities from the two drugs in combination are often partially overlapping as shown in Figure 9.8. For example, a side effect of hypertension can only be induced by drug A, and an elevated lipid level is only caused by drug B, while nausea, fatigue, and vomiting are the common toxicities from both drugs.

When an overlapping DLT is observed, it is usually impossible to determine whether the toxicity was caused by drug A ($X_{jk} = 1$), drug B ($Y_{jk} = 1$), or both drugs ($X_{jk} = Y_{jk} = 1$), and also what proportion of toxicity is from each drug. Nevertheless, we can introduce a *latent* $2 \times 2$ toxicity probability table as in (9.4) for the combined doses ($A_j, B_k$). The strategy is to collapse the three indistinguishable cells with probabilities of $\pi_{jk(11)}$, $\pi_{jk(10)}$, and $\pi_{jk(01)}$ into a single cell, representing the probability of *any* toxicity (Yin and Yuan, 2009c). The observed data can be modeled using a binomial distribution instead of a multinomial distribution due to a lack of information on the toxicities

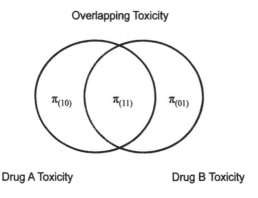

**Figure 9.8**    When two drugs are combined, some toxicities may be unique to each drug and others may be common to them; $\pi_{(10)}$ is for drug A, $\pi_{(01)}$ is for drug B, and $\pi_{(11)}$ corresponds to both drugs.

attributed to each drug. Let $n_{jk(00)}$ denote the number of patients who have not experienced any toxicity among those $n_{jk}$ patients treated at $(A_j, B_k)$. The binomial likelihood function is then given by

$$L(D|\alpha, \beta, \gamma) \propto \prod_{j=1}^{J} \prod_{k=1}^{K} \{1 - \pi_{jk(00)}\}^{n_{jk} - n_{jk(00)}} \{\pi_{jk(00)}\}^{n_{jk(00)}}.$$

The underlying rationale is that once a patient has experienced toxicity, regardless of whether the toxicity was caused by drug A, drug B, or their combination, the outcome would fall into the collapsed cell associated with probability $1 - \pi_{jk(00)}$; only the cell with probability $\pi_{jk(00)}$ corresponds to the patients with no toxicity.

In the Bayesian paradigm, let $f(\alpha, \beta, \gamma)$ denote the prior distribution for all the model parameters, and then the joint posterior distribution is given by

$$f(\alpha, \beta, \gamma|D) \propto L(D|\alpha, \beta, \gamma) f(\alpha, \beta, \gamma).$$

Based on the accumulated data, we sample from the full conditional distributions using the Gibbs sampler, and estimate the toxicity probabilities $1 - \pi_{jk(00)}$ under model (9.5). The dose-finding algorithm is the same as that of the Bayesian copula-type design described in Section 9.4.3, except that dose escalation or de-escalation in the $2 \times 2$ table design is guided by $1 - \pi_{jk(00)}$ .

### 9.5.3   Simulation Study

We examined the latent $2 \times 2$ table dose-finding procedure by simulating four scenarios listed in Table 9.2. Each drug had four dose levels, and the target toxicity probability $\phi_T$ was 30%. The total sample size was 60, and patients were treated in a cohort size of three. We specified the same toxicity probabilities for drug A and drug B; that is, $(p_1, \ldots, p_4) = (q_1, \ldots, q_4) = (0.075, 0.15, 0.225, 0.3)$. Under each scenario, 2,000 trials were simulated.

Table 9.2 presents the selection percentage of each dose combination and the sum of those for the true MTD combinations. Scenario 1 has four MTD combinations, which were all selected with much higher percentages than other dose combinations. There are three MTD combinations at different locations in scenarios 2 and 3, respectively; and their selection percentages were substantially higher than other dose combinations. There are two MTD combinations in scenario 4, and the $2 \times 2$ table design also performed well.

In conclusion, the toxicities of combined drugs are usually overlapping, but we cannot recover the information on which drug has produced what proportion of the common toxicities. Through latent $2 \times 2$ contingency tables, the correlation between the bivariate binary outcomes can be easily incorporated. We collapse the three indistinguishable probability cells so as to derive a binomial likelihood function. The $2 \times 2$ table design integrates all the data for decision making, and also provides the freedom for dose assignment across the entire dose-combination space, which would help to pin down the MTD combination faster.

**Table 9.2    Simulation Study Using the Latent $2 \times 2$ Table Design with a Target Toxicity Probability of 30%**

| Scenario | Pr{toxicity at $(A_j, B_k)$} | | | | Selection Percentage | | | | Sum (%) |
|---|---|---|---|---|---|---|---|---|---|
| 1 | **0.30** | 0.50 | 0.60 | 0.70 | **19.9** | 8.8 | 0.1 | 0.0 | 65.0 |
| | 0.15 | **0.30** | 0.52 | 0.60 | 5.6 | **21.5** | 4.6 | 0.2 | |
| | 0.10 | 0.20 | **0.30** | 0.55 | 0.3 | 5.3 | **13.3** | 3.7 | |
| | 0.08 | 0.14 | 0.19 | **0.30** | 0.0 | 0.3 | 5.7 | **10.3** | |
| | | | | | | | | | |
| 2 | **0.30** | 0.50 | 0.55 | 0.60 | **20.0** | 9.4 | 0.8 | 0.1 | 53.0 |
| | 0.12 | **0.30** | 0.50 | 0.55 | 3.9 | **19.9** | 6.2 | 1.2 | |
| | 0.10 | 0.15 | **0.30** | 0.45 | 0.1 | 3.8 | **13.1** | 9.9 | |
| | 0.08 | 0.12 | 0.16 | 0.18 | 0.0 | 0.0 | 2.6 | 8.6 | |
| | | | | | | | | | |
| 3 | 0.50 | 0.55 | 0.60 | 0.70 | 2.5 | 0.3 | 0.0 | 0.0 | 67.7 |
| | **0.30** | 0.50 | 0.55 | 0.60 | **27.3** | 7.3 | 0.2 | 0.0 | |
| | 0.12 | **0.30** | 0.50 | 0.55 | 5.5 | **22.9** | 6.8 | 0.2 | |
| | 0.10 | 0.15 | **0.30** | 0.45 | 0.0 | 5.6 | **17.5** | 2.6 | |
| | | | | | | | | | |
| 4 | 0.48 | 0.52 | 0.55 | 0.58 | 0.5 | 0.1 | 0.0 | 0.0 | 49.8 |
| | 0.42 | 0.45 | 0.50 | 0.52 | 7.9 | 1.0 | 0.2 | 0.0 | |
| | **0.30** | 0.40 | 0.48 | 0.50 | **27.1** | 8.1 | 1.2 | 0.1 | |
| | 0.15 | **0.30** | 0.40 | 0.45 | 4.7 | **22.7** | 7.3 | 0.6 | |

Note: Sum (%) is the sum of the selection percentages of all the MTD combinations.

## 9.6    PHASE I/II DRUG-COMBINATION TRIAL

### 9.6.1    Motivation

To expedite drug development and reduce the associated cost, the trend of integrating phase I and phase II trials has grown. The majority of phase I/II seamless designs focus on single-agent clinical trials, while treating patients with combination therapies is common. In a two-drug combination trial, multiple MTD combinations with similar toxicity may exist due to the toxicity equivalence contour in the two-dimensional dose searching space. As a consequence, we need to determine which MTD combination among those identified in phase I should be carried forward to a subsequent phase II trial for efficacy evaluation. Huang et al. (2007) propose modifying the $3 + 3$ design in phase I and applying adaptive randomization in phase II for the combination of low-dose decitabine with Ara-C in the treatment of leukemia patients. Yuan and Yin (2011b) first employ the copula-type dose-finding method to identify all the admissible dose combinations in phase I, and then seamlessly move to the adaptively randomized phase II trial for efficacy evaluation.

**EXAMPLE 9.2**

A phase I/II trial was designed to find the most effective and safe doses for decitabine and peginterferon Alfa-2b when used in combination to treat melanoma patients. Decitabine is a DNA methyltransferase inhibitor, which has shown clinical activities in leukemia and myelodysplastic syndrome (MDS) patients. MDS are bone marrow stem cell disorders characterized by dysfunctional production of myeloid blood cells and risk of transformation to myelogenous leukemia. Peginterferon Alfa-2b is a derivative of recombinant interferon, which has been used to treat patients with advanced solid tumors. *In vitro* and *in vivo* data suggest that decitabine and interferon synergize and cause apoptosis of melanoma cancer cells by direct cytotoxic mechanisms. This joint action motivated the combination of decitabine and peginterferon Alfa-2b to enhance patient response in clinical settings. Patients were treated for three cycles in a total of 12 weeks to assess their clinical responses, which included stable disease, partial response, and complete response. The MTDs of decitabine and peginterferon Alfa-2b when each is administered alone were already determined in previous single-agent trials. This trial combined two doses of decitabine and three doses of peginterferon Alfa-2b below their respective MTDs.

### 9.6.2  Phase I/II Seamless Design

In a phase I/II drug-combination trial, phase I may follow the Bayesian copula-type design as discussed in Section 9.4 to identify the admissible doses, and phase II subsequently evaluates efficacy of these admissible treatments using adaptive randomization. Suppose that $m$ admissible doses have been found in phase I, and they will be moved in parallel to phase II for further investigation. Let $\theta_i$ denote the response rate of the $i$th admissible dose for $i = 1, \ldots, m$. If we observe $y_i$ responses among $n_i$ patients treated in arm $i$, the Bayesian hierarchical model can be naturally applied to borrow information across multiple arms,

$$y_i | \theta_i \sim \text{Bin}(n_i, \theta_i),$$
$$\theta_i | (\alpha, \beta) \sim \text{Beta}(\alpha, \beta),$$
$$\alpha \sim \text{Ga}(\xi, \xi),$$
$$\beta \sim \text{Ga}(\xi, \xi),$$

where the hyperparameter $\xi$ may take a small value, say $\xi = 0.01$, such as to induce noninformative prior distributions. In the phase II component of the trial, we continuously update the posterior estimates of $\theta_i$ and apply the moving-reference adaptive randomization described in Section 7.11.3.

Let $\phi_T$ be the toxicity upper limit and $\phi_E$ be the efficacy lower limit, which together set the drug's therapeutic window. Let $n_1$ and $n_2$ be the maximum sample sizes for phase I and phase II of the trial, respectively. In addition, we denote $c_e$, $c_d$ ($c_d < c_e$), $c_a$, and $c_f$ as the probability cutoffs corresponding to dose escalation, de-escalation, admissibility, and futility. The seamless phase I/II design is displayed in Figure 9.9 and described as follows:

### Phase I

(1) Treat the first cohort of patients at the lowest dose combination $(A_1, B_1)$.

(2) Suppose that the current dose combination is $(A_j, B_k)$, and let $D$ denote the accumulated data thus far.

   (i) If $\Pr(\pi_{jk} < \phi_T | D) > c_e$, escalate to the adjacent dose combination whose toxicity probability is higher than $\pi_{jk}$ and closest to $\phi_T$. If the current dose combination is $(A_J, B_K)$, the next cohort will be treated at the same doses.

   (ii) If $\Pr(\pi_{jk} < \phi_T | D) < c_d$, de-escalate to the adjacent dose combination whose toxicity probability is lower than $\pi_{jk}$ and closest to $\phi_T$. If the current dose combination is $(A_1, B_1)$, the trial will be terminated.

   (iii) Otherwise, the next cohort of patients will be treated at the same dose combination $(A_j, B_k)$.

(3) Once the sample size in the phase I component, $n_1$, is reached, all the dose combinations that satisfy $\Pr(\pi_{jk} < \phi_T | D) > c_a$ are considered admissible and will be carried forward in parallel to phase II.

### Phase II

(1) The moving-reference adaptive randomization is invoked immediately in phase II to randomize patients among the $m$ admissible treatment arms. For $i = 1, \ldots, m$, let $\pi_i$ denote the toxicity probability of treatment $i$ (i.e., the $i$th admissible dose combination). If either of the following two criteria is met:

$$\text{Safety stopping: } \Pr(\pi_i < \phi_T | D) < c_a,$$
$$\text{Futility stopping: } \Pr(\theta_i > \phi_E | D) < c_f,$$

then arm $i$ will be terminated.

(2) Once the sample size in the phase II component, $n_2$, is reached, the dose combination that has the highest efficacy rate will be recommended as the best dose.

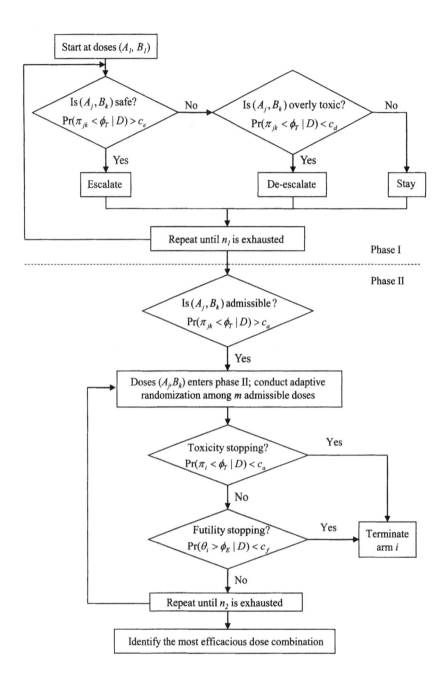

**Figure 9.9** Diagram of the seamless phase I/II drug-combination trial design.

**Table 9.3    Four Simulation Scenarios for Two-Drug Combinations with Three Doses of Drug A and Two Doses of Drug B**

| Sc. | Pr(toxicity) | | | Pr(efficacy) | | | Selection % | | | # Patients | | |
|-----|------|------|------|------|------|------|------|------|------|------|------|------|
| 1 | 0.10 | **0.20** | 0.50 | 0.20 | **0.40** | 0.55 | 4.0 | **44.5** | 2.8 | 11.3 | **21.2** | 8.1 |
|   | 0.05 | 0.15 | 0.40 | 0.10 | 0.30 | 0.50 | 0.3 | 24.0 | 19.2 | 9.7 | 15.8 | 11.4 |
| 2 | 0.10 | 0.15 | **0.20** | 0.20 | 0.30 | **0.50** | 1.7 | 7.0 | **67.1** | 8.3 | 10.9 | **31.3** |
|   | 0.05 | 0.10 | 0.15 | 0.10 | 0.20 | 0.40 | 0.0 | 1.9 | 19.8 | 8.2 | 7.9 | 11.9 |
| 3 | 0.10 | 0.40 | 0.60 | 0.30 | 0.50 | 0.60 | 16.3 | 25.4 | 0.2 | 16.1 | 15.1 | 3.7 |
|   | 0.05 | **0.20** | 0.50 | 0.20 | **0.40** | 0.55 | 3.9 | **46.2** | 3.1 | 14.2 | **22.3** | 5.7 |
| 4 | 0.10 | **0.20** | 0.50 | 0.20 | **0.40** | 0.50 | 4.2 | **41.8** | 9.3 | 10.6 | **20.3** | 10.7 |
|   | 0.05 | 0.15 | **0.20** | 0.10 | 0.30 | **0.40** | 0.5 | 10.7 | **29.8** | 9.5 | 12.1 | **15.0** |

Note: Sc. stands for Scenario. The target toxicity and efficacy probabilities are $\phi_T = 33\%$ and $\phi_E = 20\%$, respectively. The target dose combinations are in boldface.

### 9.6.3  Simulation Study

We conducted simulation studies to examine the operating characteristics of the seamless phase I/II drug-combination design. The maximum sample size was 80 patients, with $n_1 = 20$ for phase I and $n_2 = 60$ for phase II. We specified the toxicity upper limit $\phi_T = 0.33$ and the efficacy lower limit $\phi_E = 0.2$. We set $c_e = 0.8$ and $c_d = 0.45$ to direct dose escalation and de-escalation, respectively; $c_a = 0.45$ to define admissibility; and $c_f = 0.1$ for futility stopping. The decisions on dose assignment and adaptive randomization were made upon observing the outcomes of every patient. In phase I, we adopted the copula-type model in (9.3), and assigned noninformative prior distributions to all the model parameters. We simulated 1,000 trials, and for each trial we took 2,000 posterior samples after 100 burn-in iterations in the MCMC procedure.

Under each scenario in Table 9.3, the target dose combination is the one that is admissible and has the highest efficacy rate. In scenario 1, the target dose combination was selected with the highest percentage, at which most of the patients were treated. The target dose combination in scenario 2 is the highest doses of both drugs; its selection percentage was close to 70%, and almost half of the patients were treated at that dose combination. Scenario 4 is an interesting case with two target dose combinations: Both of them were selected with higher percentages than other dose combinations, and they were also used to treat more patients.

To gain more insights into the design, Table 9.4 displays (i) the percentage that each dose combination is selected into the admissible set and (ii) the average number of admissible doses, $\bar{m}$, at the completion of the phase I portion. In most

**Table 9.4  Selection Percentages of Admissible Doses and Average Numbers of Selected Admissible Doses, $\bar{m}$**

| Admissible Dose (%) | | | $\bar{m}$ | Admissible Dose (%) | | | $\bar{m}$ |
|---|---|---|---|---|---|---|---|
| Scenario 1 | | | | Scenario 2 | | | |
| 97.9 | 92.2 | 38.2 | 4.9 | 99.6 | 99.0 | 91.8 | 5.9 |
| 98.8 | 98.2 | 72.6 | | 99.7 | 99.7 | 98.3 | |
| Scenario 3 | | | | Scenario 4 | | | |
| 93.3 | 75.9 | 14.6 | 4.2 | 97.9 | 94.6 | 55.6 | 5.3 |
| 96.5 | 94.9 | 52.1 | | 98.8 | 98.5 | 86.1 | |

Note: The true admissible doses are in shaded areas.

of the cases, the selection percentages of the admissible doses were higher than 90%, and the average number of admissible doses was close to the true value.

Due to the existence of toxicity equivalence contours in a dose-combination space, multiple MTD combinations with similar toxicity may be identified in a phase I trial. With no preference to any of these MTD combinations, they are all moved forward to phase II testing. Adaptive randomization in a phase II trial tends to assign more patients to more effective doses. As opposed to conducting these two phases of trials separately, it appears more natural to seamlessly bridge phase I and phase II trials in order to identify the most appropriate dose combination. The phase I/II drug-combination design adopts the copula-type model to select admissible doses and the moving-reference adaptive randomization to evaluate efficacy, which provides a smooth transition from phase I to phase II.

## 9.7  SUMMARY

This chapter has covered a broad range of statistical methods for dose finding in drug-combination trials. The sequential scheme is the most straightforward approach to designing a two-drug combination trial, which can be coupled with any single-agent dose-finding method. The sequential scheme can efficiently shrink the dose searching space by utilizing the partial order across different subtrials. The copula-type design has an elegant structure, which reduces to the single-agent CRM if only one drug is tested. The latent $2 \times 2$ table approach can easily incorporate correlations or interactions between the two drugs in combination, but the likelihood degenerates to a binomial distribution due to a lack of information on toxicities attributable to each drug. In a phase I/II drug-combination trial, we model both toxicity and efficacy, which in fact is more natural because we need to determine the most effective one among multiple identified MTD combinations due to toxicity equivalence contours. Although we have focused on combinations of two drugs, the two-dimensional dose-finding methods can also be applied to two other situations: One is to jointly search for the optimal dose level and dose schedule, and the other is dose finding with ordered groups. If more than two drugs are combined, dose finding becomes much more difficult, while the copula-type design may still be applicable as discussed in Section 9.4.2.

## EXERCISES

**9.1**    Design a two-drug combination trial using the $3 + 3$ design coupled with the sequential dose-finding scheme in Section 9.3.

**9.2**    The Gumbel–Hougaard copula (Hougaard, 1986) takes the form of

$$C_\gamma(u, v) = \exp\left[-\{(-\log u)^{1/\gamma} + (-\log v)^{1/\gamma}\}^\gamma\right],$$

where $C_\gamma(\cdot\,,\,\cdot)$ is a distribution function on $[0, 1]^2$ with an association parameter $\gamma$. Based on the Gumbel–Hougaard copula, construct a copula-type regression model to link the joint toxicity probability $\pi_{jk}$ with the toxicity probabilities $(p_j^\alpha, q_k^\beta)$, such that all the three model conditions in Section 9.4 are satisfied.

**9.3**    For a three-drug combination trial as discussed in Section 9.4.2, derive the likelihood function. Specify appropriate prior distributions for model parameters, and then derive the joint posterior distribution.

# CHAPTER 10

# TARGETED THERAPY DESIGN

## 10.1 CYTOSTATIC AGENTS

Despite various classifications based on tumor diagnosis and histology, patients in the same prognostic group may still be heterogeneous in many aspects. This in turn causes patients to respond differentially to the same treatment. To treat patients in a more effective way, there is a new trend of developing molecularly targeted therapy in the modern era of personalized medicine. Targeted therapies are typically developed along with important biomarkers that regulate cell signaling, malignant transformation, and proliferation.

Traditional cancer treatments, such as chemotherapy, are cytotoxic, which may not be able to distinguish rapidly dividing normal cells and cancer cells and thus will eradicate both blindly. As a result, cytotoxic agents often induce various adverse effects due to their harm to normal tissues as well. Because both toxicity and efficacy are assumed to increase with respect to the dose, cytotoxic agents are often administered at the maximum tolerated dose (MTD), which would help to achieve the maximum therapeutic effect of the drug. Cytotoxic agents may be given in a pulsed way with multiple cycles of on-and-off treatment periods. Such intermittent drug administration allows normal tissues to recover

*Clinical Trial Design.* By Guosheng Yin
Copyright © 2012 John Wiley & Sons, Inc.

after acute cellular damage. By contrast, targeted agents follow the drug-receptor cytostatic scheme. Because these molecular-based drugs target specific proteins that upregulate in malignant transformation, they are more selective and less toxic to normal cells. To achieve optimal therapeutic effects, targeted agents may be administered continuously as opposed to periodically. In addition, a low dose of a cytostatic agent may be as effective as a high dose.

In accordance, clinical trial designs for cytostatic agents are very different from those for cytotoxic agents. In a phase I trial with a cytostatic agent, the primary objective is to find the optimum biological dose (OBD) characterized by an efficacy endpoint as opposed to the MTD based on a toxicity endpoint. The OBD achieves the maximum therapeutic effect of the drug, which, however, may be far below the MTD. For cytotoxic agents, the toxicity and therapeutic effects are assumed to be parallel to each other, so searching for the MTD is equivalent to finding the maximum effective dose that is still tolerable. However, this is not true for cytostatic agents—using toxicity alone cannot underpin the searching for the OBD. Hunsberger et al. (2005) propose the $3 + 3$ type of designs for molecularly targeted agents that have little or no toxicity in the therapeutic dose range.

In a phase II trial with a cytostatic agent, the goal is still to evaluate the drug's short-term efficacy effect. However, the meaning of efficacy could be very different from that of a cytotoxic agent. Targeted agents may prevent tumor growth by blocking certain disease pathways without directly shrinking the tumor. Hence, the usual clinical response characterized by a certain percentage of decrease in the measurable lesions may not be applicable. It is more sensible to use some feasible endpoints, such as the time to disease progression, the inhibition of the target, or the measurement on the tumor biomarker. Moreover, phase II trials for cytostatic agents are often randomized to compare multiple treatments instead of using a single-arm study design (Korn et al., 2001). In a phase III trial with a cytostatic drug, we aim for a definitive evaluation of the drug's therapeutic effect, and the randomized controlled phase III design remains as the gold standard.

## 10.2 PROGNOSTIC AND PREDICTIVE BIOMARKERS

A biomarker is a single trait or a signature of multiple traits, which is often assessed by immunohistochemistry, fluorescent in situ hybridization, microarrays, and proteomics technologies (Mandrekar and Sargent, 2009). In the development of targeted agents, it is essential to identify and validate important biomarkers for therapeutic use—for example, to select molecular targets, screen patients, and evaluate clinical endpoints (Simon, 2009). A biomarker is called a prognostic marker if it reflects patients' prognosis such as their health conditions, tumor stages, or disease status. Prognostic markers are associated with the disease outcome regardless of the presence of the treatment. A biomarker is called a predictive marker if it can be used to predict differential treatment effects for patients belonging to different marker groups. For example, if only marker-positive patients will benefit from a particular treatment while marker-negative patients will not, this biomarker is predictive for the treatment effect.

**EXAMPLE 10.1**

In breast cancer, estrogen receptor (ER) overexpression may be used as a prognostic marker because ER-positive patients have longer survival in the absence of systematic therapy. In addition, the ER status may also be used as a predictive marker because ER-positive patients would benefit from anti-estrogens such as tamoxifen, while ER-negative patients may benefit more from some cytotoxic chemotherapies. Another important predictive marker in breast cancer is the human epidermal growth factor receptor 2 (HER2) amplification, as only HER2-positive patients may benefit from trastuzumab. In colorectal cancer, patients with KRAS mutations appear to be poor candidates for treatment with epidermal growth factor receptor (EGFR) antibodies. As a result, cetuximab and panitumumab only benefit colorectal cancer patients with the wild-type KRAS gene status, but not those with mutant KRAS.

To better understand the differences between prognostic and predictive biomarkers, we consider a study with two treatments—standard therapy and targeted therapy. Based on a single biomarker expression, patients can be classified as marker positive or marker negative. Suppose that the primary endpoint is dichotomous indicating whether a patient has responded to the treatment, and a response rate of 10% or less is considered of no clinical interest, and that of 30% or more is considered clinically relevant. To discriminate prognostic and predictive biomarkers, we create four $2 \times 2$ contingency tables, in which each cell represents the response rate of that specific group.

- The biomarker is neither prognostic nor predictive, if

|  | Marker − | Marker + |
|---|---|---|
| Standard therapy | 0.1 | 0.1 |
| Targeted therapy | 0.1 | 0.1 |

- The biomarker is prognostic but not predictive, if

|  | Marker − | Marker + |
|---|---|---|
| Standard therapy | 0.1 | 0.3 |
| Targeted therapy | 0.1 | 0.3 |

- The biomarker is predictive but not prognostic, if

|                   | Marker − | Marker + |
| ----------------- | -------- | -------- |
| Standard therapy  | 0.1      | 0.1      |
| Targeted therapy  | 0.1      | 0.3      |

- The biomarker is both prognostic and predictive, if

|                   | Marker − | Marker + |
| ----------------- | -------- | -------- |
| Standard therapy  | 0.1      | 0.3      |
| Targeted therapy  | 0.2      | 0.6      |

## 10.3 PREDICTIVE BIOMARKER VALIDATION

### 10.3.1 Marker-by-Treatment Interaction Design

With rapid technological advance in genomics and proteomics, a large amount of biomarker information can be collected in a fast and cost-effective way. Identifying and validating important biomarkers for therapeutic use have become the key issues in clinical trials for targeted agents. A biomarker has predictive value for a treatment if patients with a higher (or lower) value of that marker benefit more from the treatment. Sargent et al. (2005) describe a marker-by-treatment interaction design and a marker-based strategy design for clinical trials involving biomarker development. These designs are known as all-comers or unselected approaches, because all of the eligible patients are enrolled regardless of their marker status.

The marker-by-treatment interaction design uses the marker status for stratification, and within each stratum (marker positive or negative) patients are randomized to the targeted or the standard therapy as shown in Figure 10.1. At the end of the trial, the final analysis may test

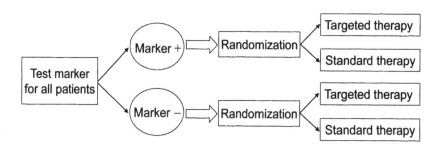

**Figure 10.1**   Marker-by-treatment interaction design.

- whether there is a treatment difference between the targeted and the standard therapy, separately within each biomarker group, and

- whether there is a significant interaction between the biomarker and treatment.

### 10.3.2   Targeted Therapy Design with Marker-Based Strategy

To utilize the biomarker information during treatment assignment, the marker-based or marker-assisted strategy can be implemented. As shown in Figure 10.2, patients are first randomized to a group with marker-assisted treatment strategy or that without such assistance. In the marker-assisted group, patients with positive marker values are given the targeted agent, and those with negative marker values are treated by the standard therapy. In the other group with no marker assistance, all of the patients are given the standard of care. Hence, randomization only takes place at the first enrollment, while treatment assignment is fully determined once patients are recruited into marker-based or non-marker-based groups. At the end of the study, we can make a comparison between marker-based and non-marker-based groups. The biomarker is said to has predictive value if the response rate in the marker-based group is higher than that in the non-marker-based group.

The marker-based strategy in Figure 10.2 does not allow marker negative patients to be treated by the targeted therapy, and thus it cannot evaluate whether the treatment is superior in all the patients regardless of their marker status. As shown in Figure 10.3, this design can be slightly modified by further randomizing patients in the non-marker-based strategy group to either the targeted or the

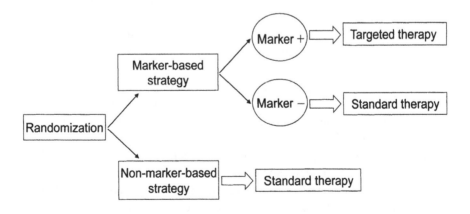

**Figure 10.2**   Targeted therapy design with the marker-based strategy.

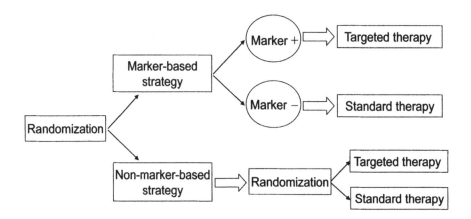

**Figure 10.3**  Modified targeted therapy design with the marker-based strategy.

standard therapy. Nevertheless, when comparing the marker-based and non-marker-based groups, the overall detectable difference could be diluted because a substantial number of patients are also treated by the targeted agent in the non-marker-based group.

## 10.4  RANDOMIZED DISCONTINUATION DESIGN

Among a large number of potential targeted agents, only those showing the most promise may pass through the phase II screening for further evaluation, while nonactive agents should be filtered out. During the early development of targeted agents, it is difficult to select patients in a reliable way for a certain target, while inclusion of nonresponding patients might significantly dilute the detectable treatment effect.

It is possible to identify and enrich certain patient subgroups that are more likely to benefit from the treatment, such as treating more patients of HER2-positive status with trastuzumab in breast cancer, or enriching patients with rapidly increasing PSA levels in prostate cancer. The randomized discontinuation design (RDD) belongs to the family of enrichment designs, in which only a selected more homogeneous subset of patients are randomized. In particular, patients who have adhered to the treatment with stable disease and have not experienced excessive toxicity will be randomized to continue or discontinue the treatment, while other patients will be taken off the study (Kopec, Abrahamowicz, and Esdaile, 1993; Rosner, Stadler, and Ratain, 2002; Freidlin and Simon, 2004). As shown in Figure 10.4, the RDD consists of two stages:

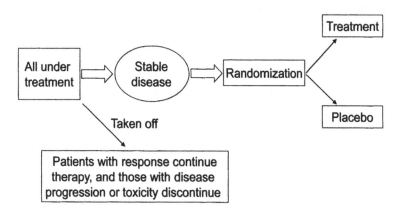

**Figure 10.4**  Randomized discontinuation design.

- *Stage 1*
  All the enrolled patients are treated by the cytostatic agent; that is, everyone is exposed to the new treatment initially, which makes the RDD more attractive to trial participants.

- *Stage 2*
  After a fixed period of follow-up, patients who have responded will continue the treatment; those who had disease progression or experienced excessive toxicity will be taken off the study; and those with stable disease will be randomized to a group that continues the treatment or that off the treatment for observation only (the placebo group).

Therefore, in the RDD only the patients with stable disease are randomized in the second stage, and after randomization, this subset of patients will be followed for another fixed period of time. At the completion of stage 2, we compare the proportions of patients maintaining stable disease between the continual and discontinued treatment groups during the randomization period.

Based on numerical comparisons of the RDD with the upfront randomization design, Freidlin and Simon (2004) conclude that proper enrichment may improve trial efficiency and power when there is no reliable assay to select sensitive patients. Nevertheless, there are limitations associated with the RDD; for example, there might be some carryover effects or drug resistance following the treatment in the first stage.

## 10.5  ADAPTIVE SIGNATURE DESIGN

### 10.5.1  Split-Sample Approach

By monitoring a large number of gene expressions simultaneously, our knowledge and understanding of tumors are immensely expanded at genomic scales. Not only can the genomic information help to identify important genes, but it may also provide the potential of classifying different tumor types and disease status. Molecularly targeted therapies may only benefit a subset of patients who are characterized by certain gene expressions. This subgroup of patients, however, might be overlooked if traditional trial designs and hypothesis tests are used.

Freidlin and Simon (2005) propose an adaptive signature design to identify sensitive patients through an assay or a signature (known as the gene-expression classifier). The adaptive signature trial follows two sequential stages. Suppose that there are $G$ genes that can be used to identify sensitive patients who are responsive to the treatment and their gene expression levels are denoted by $(X_{i1}, \ldots, X_{iG})$ for subject $i$. Let $p_i$ be the probability of response, and let $Z_i$ be the treatment indicator with $Z_i = 1$ for the experimental treatment and $Z_i = 0$ for the control. Based on the data collected in stage 1, a gene signature classifier is developed to predict which patient is more likely to benefit from the new treatment.

- *Stage 1*
  For each gene $g$, the single-gene logistic model is applied to the data in stage 1,

  $$\log\left(\frac{p_i}{1 - p_i}\right) = \beta_0 + \beta_1 Z_i + \gamma_g Z_i X_{ig}, \quad g = 1, \ldots, G,$$

  where $\beta_1$ represents the treatment main effect and $\gamma_g$ characterizes the interaction between the treatment and gene profiling. At a specified significance level $\eta$, all the genes that have significant treatment-gene interactions can be identified. The maximum likelihood estimators of $\beta_1$ and $\gamma_g$ are denoted as $\hat{\beta}_1$ and $\hat{\gamma}_g$, respectively.

- *Stage 2*
  For patients enrolled in stage 2, if patient $i$ has a predicted experimental versus control odds ratio

  $$\exp(\hat{\beta}_1 + \hat{\gamma}_g X_{ig}) > c,$$

  where $c$ is a prespecified cutoff, for at least $S$ genes $(S \leq G)$, then this subject is considered a "sensitive" patient.

The gene-expression classifier developed using patients in stage 1 is prospectively applied to the patients in stage 2 to identify a subset of sensitive patients.

The tuning parameters $(\eta, c, S)$ can be empirically chosen using the leave-one-out cross-validation method.

The adaptive signature design can achieve three goals:

(1) to identify the subset of patients who are most likely to benefit from the new agent;

(2) to maintain a properly powered test of an overall treatment effect at the end of the trial using all randomized patients; and

(3) to test the treatment effect for the subset of sensitive patients selected from the patients enrolled in stage 2.

At the conclusion of the trial, two tests will be performed in a sequential order. To maintain an overall significance level at $\alpha = 0.05$, we split $\alpha = \alpha_1 + \alpha_2$; for example, $\alpha_1 = 0.04$ and $\alpha_2 = 0.01$. The first test compares the experimental treatment and the control for all the subjects at the significance level of $\alpha_1$. If the null hypothesis (no treatment difference) is rejected, we stop and claim that the experimental treatment works for all patients. Otherwise, we compare treatment effects for the subset of sensitive patients from those enrolled in stage 2 at the significance level of $\alpha_2$. By choosing the subset of sensitive patients, we try to eliminate the nonresponders who would dilute the treatment effect. Hence in this more homogeneous subgroup of patients, the treatment effect is expected to be much stronger than that in the overall study population. Therefore, even using a more stringent significance level, such as $\alpha_2 = 0.01$, the test may still possess adequate power to detect the treatment difference. The gene-signature development and verification are carried out on two nonoverlapping subsamples, which thus preserves the overall significance level of the test at the nominal level of $\alpha$.

The adaptive signature design incorporates prospective development of the sensitive patient classifier in a properly powered test procedure for the overall treatment effect. If the experimental treatment is broadly effective to all patients, the adaptive signature design has a similar power to detect the overall treatment effect as the traditional design. If the proportion of sensitive patients is low and thus the effectiveness of the experimental treatment is much weakened in the general patient population, the signature design reduces the chance of overlooking a truly effective treatment.

### 10.5.2  Cross-Validation Approach

In the adaptive signature design of Freidlin and Simon (2005), approximately one-half of the data is used to develop the gene signature in stage 1, and the other half is used for validation in stage 2. However, such a half–half split of the sample may incur power loss and lead to low trial efficiency, especially when the proportion of sensitive patients in the study population is small and there is a large number of genes to evaluate.

To enhance efficiency of the adaptive signature design, Freidlin, Jiang, and Simon (2010) propose a cross-validation approach to prospectively developing the sensitive patient classifier as well as testing for the overall treatment effect. In a $K$-fold cross-validation procedure, the total data $D$ are divided into $K$ nonoverlapping verification subsets, $D = \{V_1, \ldots, V_K\}$. Let $D_k$ denote the developmental subset containing the rest of the data excluding $V_k$ from $D$; that is, $D = D_k \cup V_k$ for $k = 1, \ldots, K$. We develop the predictive gene signature based on $D_k$, which is then used to identify the sensitive patients in $V_k$. This procedure is repeated for each $k$ to identify all of the sensitive patients in the entire sample. Because each patient exactly appears once in the validation cohorts, all of the patients will be classified as sensitive or nonsensitive at the end of the cross-validation procedure.

Among the selected sensitive patients, the experimental treatment is compared with the control. Due to the use of cross validation, the standard asymptotic theory may not work for hypothesis testing. For valid statistical inference, we may apply the permutation to simulate the null distribution of the test statistic by randomly switching treatment labels. After performing a large number of permutations, say $J$ times, the original test statistic $T_n$ is compared with the permuted test statistics $T_1^*, \ldots, T_J^*$, which yields

$$p\text{-value} = \frac{1 + \sum_{j=1}^{J} I(T_j^* \geq T_n)}{1 + J}.$$

The cross-validation approach maximizes the number of patients contributing to the gene signature development, and thus sensitive patients can be selected in a more reliable way. As a result, the power of the adaptive signature design is considerably improved.

## 10.6 ADAPTIVE THRESHOLD DESIGN

Targeted agents for cancer are often putative or tumor growth-inhibitory. Suppose that we compare an experimental agent with a control, and the primary endpoint is the time to disease progression. The experimental treatment only benefits patients with a high expression of a certain biomarker, which is measured by a continuous biomarker variable. However, there is no binary classifier to categorize patients into marker positive (biomarker expression is above a cutoff value) or marker negative (biomarker expression is below a cutoff value) groups. In this situation, Jiang, Freidlin, and Simon (2007) propose two different procedures for hypothesis testing, which are described as follows.

For $i = 1, \ldots, n$, let $Z_i$ be the treatment indicator taking a value of 1 if subject $i$ is treated by the experimental drug, and 0 for the control. If we denote the biomarker expression value as $X_i$, those subjects with $X_i > c$ are considered sensitive patients who would respond to the experimental treatment, where $c$ is an unknown threshold for classification of marker positive or marker negative. The Cox proportional hazards model is used to compare patients' survival times in different groups,

$$\lambda(t|Z_i, X_i) = \lambda_0(t) \exp\{\beta Z_i + \gamma I(X_i > c) + \theta Z_i I(X_i > c)\}, \qquad (10.1)$$

where $\lambda_0(t)$ is the baseline hazard function, $\beta$ represents the treatment main effect, $\gamma$ stands for the main effect for the dichotomous biomarker status, and $\theta$ corresponds to the interaction between the treatment and biomarker status. Based on hypothesis testing, if $\gamma$ is significantly different from zero, the biomarker is a prognostic marker; and if $\theta$ is significantly different from zero, the biomarker is a predictive marker. For simplicity, we are only interested in testing whether the marker has any predictive value; that is, $\gamma = 0$, and model (10.1) reduces to

$$\lambda(t|Z_i, X_i) = \lambda_0(t) \exp\{\beta Z_i + \theta Z_i I(X_i > c)\}. \qquad (10.2)$$

If $\beta = 0$ in (10.2), then the experimental treatment does not work for all patients; furthermore, if $\beta = 0$ but $\theta \neq 0$, then the treatment only works for a subset of sensitive patients whose biomarker expression levels are above $c$. If $\beta = 0$, the logarithm of the hazard ratio between the experimental and the control arms is

$$\log\left\{\frac{\lambda(t|Z_i = 1, X_i)}{\lambda(t|Z_i = 1, X_i)}\right\} = \begin{cases} 0, & \text{if biomarker expression } X_i \text{ is below } c, \\ \theta, & \text{if biomarker expression } X_i \text{ is above } c. \end{cases}$$

The first strategy takes two sequential tests by splitting the overall type I error rate $\alpha = \alpha_1 + \alpha_2$ to maintain the overall significance level at $\alpha = 0.05$. It is recommended using $\alpha_1 = 0.04$ and $\alpha_2 = 0.01$ to perform the two tests, respectively.

- *Stage 1*
  We first compare the outcomes of all patients between the experimental and the control arms at the significance level of $\alpha_1$. If the test is significant, we stop and claim that the new treatment is effective for all patients.

- *Stage 2*
  Otherwise, we determine a cutoff value $c$ for the biomarker expression in a way that the treatment difference between the experimental and control groups is maximized, if the analysis is restricted only to those patients whose biomarker levels are higher than $c$.

Suppose that the biomarker expression lies in $(0, 1)$. We consider the hypothesis testing of

$$H_0: \theta = 0 \quad \text{versus} \quad H_1: \theta \neq 0,$$

for the selected subset of patients with $X_i > c$ only. For each chosen value of $c$, we calculate the log-likelihood ratio statistic $R_n(c)$ and take the test statistic $T_n = \max_{0.5 < c < 1} R_n(c)$; that is, the test statistic maximizes the difference between the experimental treatment and the control.

The second strategy combines the test for the overall treatment effect and that for the subset treatment effect by accounting for the correlation between the two test statistics. For each value of $c$, we fit model (10.1) to the data and compute the log-likelihood ratio statistic, $R_n(c)$. We test whether there is a treatment difference for the subset of patients whose biomarker values are higher than $c$. If $c = 0$, $R_n(c)$ reduces to testing for the overall treatment effect. The final test statistic is the maximum of all the test statistics over the chosen values of $c$,

$$T_n = \max\{R_n(0) + 2.2, \ \max_{0 < c < 1} R_n(c)\},$$

where the constant 2.2 is recommended to balance between the overall and subset tests.

To determine the statistical significance of the test, the null distribution of $T_n$ is simulated by randomly permuting the treatment labels. The permutation procedure avoids inflating the type I error rate and thus leads to a valid statistical test. We repeat the permutation for a large number of times, say $J$, and then construct the permuted versions of the test statistics, $T_1^*, \ldots, T_J^*$. As a result, the $p$-value is given by

$$p\text{-value} = \frac{1 + \sum_{j=1}^{J} I(T_j^* \geq T_n)}{1 + J}.$$

By profiling the likelihood function $L(\beta, \gamma, \theta, c)$ based on (10.1), $c$ can be estimated by

$$\hat{c} = \arg\max_c \log L_p(c),$$

where the profile log-likelihood is

$$\log L_p(c) = \max_{\beta, \gamma, \theta} \log L(\beta, \gamma, \theta, c).$$

The confidence interval for the optimal cutoff value $c$ can be constructed by the bootstrap method.

With the rapid development of targeted therapy in oncology, the drug discovery is marching toward personalized medicine. From a large number of biomarkers, we aim to identify the prognostic or predictive markers that are therapeutically useful. Through appropriate subgroup analysis, we can examine whether the treatment effects are the same or greater in patients with certain features or disease characteristics, so that more marker-specific treatment decisions can be made.

## EXERCISES

**10.1**    What are the main differences between cytotoxic agents and cytostatic agents? How do these differences affect clinical trial designs?

**10.2**    Describe how to obtain a $p$-value through permutation. How is the permutation procedure related to bootstrap?

**10.3**    Describe the cross-validation procedure.

# REFERENCES

Abdelbasit, K. M. and Plackett, R. L. (1982). Experimental design for joint action. *Biometrics* **38**, 171–179.

Akaike, H. (1973). Information theory and an extension of the maximum likelihood principle. In: *Second International Symposium on Information Theory*, B. N. Petrov and F. Csaki (eds.), pp. 267–281. Budapest: Akademiai Kiado.

Albert, J. H. and Chib, S. (1993). Bayesian analysis of binary and polychotomous response data. *Journal of the American Statistical Association* **88**, 669–679.

Andersen, P. K. and Gill, R. D. (1982). Cox's regression model for counting processes: A large-sample study. *The Annals of Statistics* **10**, 1100–1120.

Angrist, J. D., Imbens, G. W., and Rubin, D. B. (1996). Identification of causal effects using instrumental variables (with discussion). *Journal of the American Statistical Association* **91**, 444–472.

Antognini, A. B. and Giovagnoli, A. (2004). A new biased coin design for the sequential allocation of two treatments. *Journal of the Royal Statistical Society, Series C* **53**, 651–664.

Ashford, J. R. (1981). General models for the joint action of mixtures of drugs. *Biometrics* **37**, 457–474.

Babb, J., Rogatko, A., and Zacks, S. (1998). Cancer phase I clinical trials: Efficient dose escalation with overdose control. *Statistics in Medicine* **17**, 1103–1120.

Bang, H. and Davis, C. E. (2007). On estimating treatment effects under noncompliance in randomized clinical trials: Are intent-to-treat or instrumental variables analyses perfect solutions? *Statistics in Medicine* **26**, 954–964.

Barker, A. D., Sigman, C. C., Kelloff, G. J., Hylton, N. M., Berry, D. A., and Esserman, L. J. (2009). I-SPY 2: An adaptive breast cancer trial design in the setting of neoadjuvant chemotherapy. *Clinical Pharmacology & Therapeutics* **86**, 97–100.

Barlow, R. E., Bartholomew, D. J., Bremner, J. M., and Brunk, H. D. (1972). *Statistical Inference under Order Restrictions: The Theory and Application of Isotonic Regression*. New York: Wiley.

Bather, J. A. (1981). Randomized allocation of treatments in sequential medical trials (with discussion). *Journal of the Royal Statistical Society, Series B* **43**, 265–292.

Bather, J. A. (1985). On the allocation of treatments in sequential medical trials (with discussion). *International Statistical Review* **53**, 1–13.

Bauer, P. and Köhne, K. (1994). Evaluation of experiments with adaptive interim analyses. *Biometrics* **50**, 1029–1041.

Bekele, B. N., Ji, Y., Shen, Y., and Thall, P. F. (2008). Monitoring late-onset toxicities in phase I trials using predicted risks. *Biostatistics* **9**, 442–457.

Bekele, B. N. and Shen, Y. (2005). A Bayesian approach to jointly modeling toxicity and biomarker expression in a phase I/II dose-finding trial. *Biometrics* **61**, 343–354.

Berger, J. O. (1985). *Statistical Decision Theory and Bayesian Analysis*. New York: Springer-Verlag.

Berkson, J. and Gage, R. P. (1952). Survival curve for cancer patients following treatment. *Journal of the American Statistical Association* **47**, 501–515.

Berry, D. A. (2006). Bayesian clinical trials. *Nature Reviews Drug Discovery* **5**, 27–36.

Berry, D. A. (2011). Adaptive clinical trials: The promise and the caution. *Journal of Clinical Oncology* **29**, 606–609.

Berry, D. A. and Eick, S. G. (1995). Adaptive assignment versus balanced randomization in clinical trials: A decision analysis. *Statistics in Medicine* **14**, 231–246.

Berry, S. M., Carlin, B. P., Lee, J. J., and Müller, P. (2010). *Bayesian Adaptive Methods for Clinical Trials*. Chapman & Hall/CRC, Boca Raton.

Biswas, S., Liu, D. D., Lee, J. J., and Berry, D. A. (2009). Bayesian clinical trials at the University of Texas M. D. Anderson Cancer Center. *Clinical Trials* **6**, 205–216.

Biswas, A. and Mandal, S. (2004). Optimal adaptive designs in phase III clinical trials for continuous responses with covariates. In: *Advances in Model-Oriented Design and Analysis - mODa 7*, A. D. Bucchianico, H. Läuter, and H. P. Wynn (eds.), pp. 51–59. Heidelberg: Physica-Verlag.

Blackwell, D. H. and Hodges, J. L. (1957). Design for the control of selection bias. *Annals of Mathematical Statistics* **28**, 449–460.

Bliss, C. I. (1939). The toxicity of poisons applied jointly. *Annals of Applied Biology* **26**, 585–615.

Braun, T. M. (2002). The bivariate continual reassessment method: extending the CRM to phase I trials of two competing outcomes. *Controlled Clinical Trials* **23**, 240–256.

Braun, T. M. (2006). Generalizing the TITE-CRM to adapt for early- and late-onset toxicities. *Statistics in Medicine* **25**, 2071–2083.

Braun, T. M., Thall, P. F., Nguyen, H., and de Lima, M. (2007). Simultaneously optimizing dose and schedule of a new cytotoxic agent. *Clinical Trials* **4**, 113–124.

Braun, T. M. and Wang, S. (2010). A hierarchical Bayesian design for phase I trials of novel combinations of cancer therapeutic agents. *Biometrics* **66**, 805–812.

Braun, T. M., Yuan, Z., and Thall, P. F. (2005). Determining a maximum tolerated schedule of a cytotoxic agent. *Biometrics* **61**, 335–343.

Breslow, N. E. (1974). Contribution to the discussion of the paper by D. R. Cox. *Journal of the Royal Statistical Society, Series B* **34**, 187–220.

Buckland, S. T., Burnham, K. P., and Augustin, N. H. (1997). Model selection: An integral part of inference. *Biometrics* **53**, 603–618.

Carlin, B. P. and Louis, T. (2008). *Bayesian Methods for Data Analysis.* 3rd ed. Boca Raton, FL: Chapman & Hall/CRC.

Casella, G. and Berger, R. L. (2001). *Statistical Inference.* 2nd ed. Pacific Grove, CA: Duxbury Press.

Chang, M. (2008). *Adaptive Design Theory and Implementation Using SAS and R.* Boca Raton, FL: Chapman & Hall/CRC.

Chang, M. N., Therneau, T. M., Wieand, H. S., and Cha, S. S. (1987). Designs for group sequential phase II clinical trials. *Biometrics* **43**, 865–874.

Chen, M., Shao, Q., and Ibrahim, J. G. (2000). *Monte Carlo Methods in Bayesian Computation.* New York: Springer.

Chernozhukov, V. and Hong, H. (2003). An MCMC approach to classical estimation. *Journal of Econometrics* **115**, 293–346.

Cheung, Y. K. (2011). *Dose Finding by the Continual Reassessment Method.* Boca Raton, FL: Chapman & Hall/CRC.

Cheung, Y. K. and Chappell, R. (2000). Sequential designs for phase I clinical trials with late-onset toxicities. *Biometrics* **56**, 1177–1182.

Chevret, S. (2006). *Statistical Methods for Dose-Finding Experiments.* Chichester, England: John Wiley & Sons.

Chow, S.-C. and Chang, M. (2006). *Adaptive Design Methods in Clinical Trials.* Boca Raton, FL: Chapman & Hall/CRC.

Chow, S.-C., Shao, J., and Chang, M. (2007). *Sample Size Calculations in Clinical Research,* 2nd ed. New York: Marcel Dekker.

Clayton, D. G. (1978). A model for association in bivariate life tables and its application in epidemiological studies of familial tendency in chronic disease incidence. *Biometrika* **65**, 141–152.

Collett, D. (1994). *Modelling Survival Data in Medical Research.* Boca Raton, FL: Chapman & Hall/CRC.

Colton, T. and McPherson, K. (1976). Two-stage plans compared with fixed-sample-size and Wald SPRT plans. *Journal of the American Statistical Association* **71**, 80–86.

Conaway, M. R., Dunbar, S., and Peddada, S. D. (2004). Designs for single- or multiple-agent phase I trials. *Biometrics* **60**, 661–669.

Conaway, M. R. and Petroni, G. R. (1996). Designs for phase II trials allowing for a trade-off between response and toxicity. *Biometrics* **52**, 1375–1386.

Connor, E. M., Sperling, R. S., Gelber, R., et al. (1994). Reduction of maternal-infant transmission of human immunodeficiency virus type 1 with zidovudine treatment. *The New England Journal of Medicine* **331** 1173–1180.

Cowles, M. K. and Carlin, B. P. (1996). Markov chain Monte Carlo convergence diagnostics: A comparative review. *Journal of the American Statistical Association* **91**, 883–904.

Cox, D. R. (1972). Regression models and life-tables (with discussion). *Journal of the Royal Statistical Society, Series B* **34**, 187–220.

Cox, D. R. (1975). Partial likelihood. *Biometrika* **62**, 269–276.

Cui, L. Hung, H. M. J., and Wang, S. J. (1999). Modification of sample size in group sequential clinical trials. *Biometrics* **55**, 853–857.

Daimon, T., Zohar, S., and O'Quigley, J. (2011). Posterior maximization and averaging for Bayesian working model choice in the continual reassessment method. *Statistics in Medicine* **30**, 1563–1573.

Dale, J. R. (1986). Global cross-ratio models for bivariate, discrete, ordered responses. *Biometrics* **42**, 909–917.

DeMets, D. L. and Ware, J. H. (1980). Group sequential methods for clinical trials with a one-sided hypothesis. *Biometrika* **67**, 651–660.

DeMets, D. L. and Ware, J. H. (1982). Asymmetric group sequential boundaries for monitoring clinical trials. *Biometrika* **69**, 661–663.

Dempster, A. P., Laird, N. M., and Rubin, D. B. (1977). Maximum likelihood from incomplete data via the EM algorithm (with discussion). *Journal of the Royal Statistical Society, Series B* **39**, 1–38.

Desai, S. P., Ben-Josef, E., Normolle, D. P., et al. (2007). Phase I study of oxaliplatin, full-dose gemcitabine, and concurrent radiation therapy in pancreatic cancer. *Journal of Clinical Oncology* **25**, 4587–4592.

Diggle, J. P., Heagerty, P., Liang, K. Y., and Zeger, S. L. (2002). *Analysis of Longitudinal Data,* 2nd ed. New York: Oxford University Press.

Durham, S. D., Flournoy, N., and Rosenberger, W. F. (1997). A random walk rule for phase I clinical trials. *Biometrics* **53**, 745–760.

Efron, B. (1967). The two-sample problem with censored data. In: *Proceedings, Fifth Berkeley Symposium in Mathematical Statistics, IV,* L. Le Cam and J. Neyman, eds., pp. 831–853. New York: Prentice-Hall.

Efron, B. (1971). Forcing sequential experiments to be balanced. *Biometrika* **58**, 403–417.

Eick, S. G. (1988). The two-armed bandit with delayed responses. *The Annals of Statistics* **16**, 254–264.

Eisele, J. R. (1994). The doubly adaptive biased coin design for sequential clinical trials. *Journal of Statistical Planning and Inference* **38**, 249–262.

Eisele, J. R. and Woodroofe, M. (1995). Central limit theorems for doubly adaptive biased coin designs. *The Annals of Statistics* **23**, 234–254.

Elashoff, J. D. and Reedy, T. J. (1984). Two-stage clinical trial stopping rules. *Biometrics* **40**, 791–795.

Estey, E. H., Shen, Y., and Thall, P. F. (2000). Effect of time to complete remission on subsequent survival and disease-free survival time in AML, RAEB-t, and RAEB. *Blood* **95**, 72–77.

Faries, D. (1994). Practical modification of the continual reassessment methods for phase I cancer clinical trials. *Journal of Biopharmaceutical Statistics* **4**, 147–164.

Fisher, R. A. (1926). The arrangement of field experiments. *Journal of the Ministry of Agriculture* **33**, 503–513.

Fisher, L. D. (1998). Self-designing clinical trials. *Statistics in Medicine* **17**, 1551–1562.

Fisher, L. D., Dixon, D. O., Herson, J., Frankowski, R. K., Hearon, M. S., and Pearce, K. E. (1990). Intention to treat in clinical trials. In: *Statistical Issues in Drug Research and Development*, K. E. Pearce, ed., pp. 331–350. New York: Marcel Dekker.

Fleming, T. R. (1982). One-sample multiple testing procedure for phase II clinical trials. *Biometrics* **38**, 143–151.

Fleming, T. R. and Harrington, D. (1991). *Counting Processes and Survival Analysis*. New York: John Wiley & Sons.

Freidlin, B., Jiang, W., and Simon, R. (2010). The cross-validated adaptive signature design. *Clinical Cancer Research* **16**, 691–698.

Freidlin, B. and Simon, R. (2004). Evaluation of randomized discontinuation design. *Journal of Clinical Oncology* **23**, 5094–5098.

Freidlin, B. and Simon, R. (2005). Adaptive signature design: An adaptive clinical trial design for generating and prospectively testing a gene expression signature for sensitive patients. *Clinical Cancer Research* **11**, 7872–7878.

Friedman, L. M., Furberg, C. D., and DeMets, D. L. (1998). *Fundamentals of Clinical Trials*, 3rd ed. New York: Springer.

Gasparini, M. and Eisele, J. (2000). A curve-free method for phase I clinical trials. *Biometrics* **56**, 609–615.

Gehan, E. A. (1961). The determination of the number of patients required in a follow-up trial of a new chemotherapeutic agent. *Journal of Chronic Diseases* **13**, 346–353.

Gelfand, A. E. and Smith, A. F. M. (1990). Sampling-based approaches to calculating marginal densities. *Journal of the American Statistical Association* **85**, 398-409.

Gelman, A., Carlin, J. B., Stern, H. S. and Rubin, D. B. (2003). *Bayesian Data Analysis*, 2nd ed. Boca Raton, FL: Chapman & Hall/CRC.

Gelman, A. and Rubin, D. B. (1992). Inference from iterative simulation using multiple sequences. *Statistical Science* **7**, 457–511.

Geman, S. and Geman, D. (1984). Stochastic relaxation, Gibbs distributions and the Bayesian restoration of images. *IEEE Transactions on Pattern Analysis and Machine Intelligence* **6**, 721–741.

Geweke, J. (1992). Evaluating the accuracy of sampling-based approaches to the calculation of posterior moments. In: *Bayesian Statistics 4*, J. M. Bernardo, J. Berger, A. P. Dawid, and A. F. M. Smith (eds.), pp. 169–193. Oxford: Oxford University Press.

Gezmu, M. and Flournoy, N. (2006). Group up-and-down designs for dose-finding. *Journal of Statistical Planning and Inference* **136**, 1749–1764.

Gilks, W. R., Best, N. G., and Tan, K. K. C. (1995). Adaptive rejection Metropolis sampling within Gibbs sampling. *Journal of the Royal Statistical Society, Series C* **44**, 455–472.

Glasser, S. P., Salas, M., and Delzell, E. (2007). Importance and challenges of studying marketed drugs: What is a phase IV study? Common clinical research designs, registries, and self-reporting systems. *The Journal of Clinical Pharmacology* **47**, 1074–1086.

Goodman, S. N., Zahurak, M. L., and Piantadosi, S. (1995). Some practical improvements in the continual reassessment method for phase I studies. *Statistics in Medicine* **14**, 1149–1161.

Gooley, T. A., Martin, P. J., Fisher, L. D., and Pettinger, M. (1994). Simulation as a design tool for phase I/II clinical trial: An example from bone marrow transplantation. *Controlled Clinical Trial* **15**, 450–462.

Gould, A. L. (1992). Interim analyses for monitoring clinical trials that do not materially affect the type I error rate. *Statistics in Medicine* **11**, 55–66.

Gould, A. L. (2001). Sample size re-estimation: recent developments and practical considerations. *Statistics in Medicine* **20**, 2625–2643.

Gould, A. L. and Pecore, V. J. (1982). Group sequential methods for clinical trials allowing early acceptance of $H_0$ and incorporating costs. *Biometrika* **69**, 75–80.

Greenwood, M. (1926). The natural duration of cancer. Reports on Public Health and Medical Subjects, No. 33, His Majesty's Stationery Office.

Hall, A. R. (2005). *Generalized Method of Moments*. New York: Oxford University Press.

Hansen, L. P. (1982). Large sample properties of generalized method of moments estimators. *Econometrica* **50**, 1029–1054.

Hansen, L. P., Heaton, J., and Yaron, A. (1996). Finite-sample properties of some alternative GMM estimators. *Journal of Business & Economic Statistics* **14**, 262–280.

Harville, D. A. (1977). Maximum likelihood approaches to variance component estimation and to related problems. *Journal of the American Statistical Association* **72**, 320–338.

Hastings, W. K. (1970). Monte Carlo sampling methods using Markov chains and their applications. *Biometrika* **57**, 97–109.

Hedaya, M. A. (2007). *Basic Pharmacokinetics*. Boca Raton, FL: CRC Press.

Heyd, J. M. and Carlin, B. P. (1999). Adaptive design improvements in the continual reassessment method for phase I studies. *Statistics in Medicine* **18**, 1307–1321.

Hill, A. V. (1910). The possible effects of the aggregation of the molecules of haemoglobin on its dissociation curves. *The Journal of Physiology* **40**, iv–vii.

Hjort, N. L. and Claeskens, G. (2003). Frequentist model average estimators (with discussion). *Journal of the American Statistical Association* **98**, 879–899.

Hochberg, Y. (1988). A sharper Bonferroni procedure for multiple tests of significance. *Biometrika* **75**, 800–802.

Hoeting, J. A., Madigan, D., Raftery, A. E., and Volinsky, C. T. (1999). Bayesian model averaging: A tutorial. *Statistical Science* **14**, 382–401.

Hogg, R. V., McKean, J. W., and Craig, A. T. (2005). *Introduction to Mathematical Statistics*. Upper Saddle River, NJ: Pearson Prentice Hall.

Holm, S. (1979). A simple sequentially rejective multiple test procedure. *Scandinavian Journal of Statistics* **6**, 65–70.

Hougaard, P. (1986). A class of multivariate failure time distributions. *Biometrika* **73**, 671–678.

Hu, F. and Rosenberger, W. F. (2003). Optimality, variability, power: Evaluating response-adaptive randomization procedures for treatment comparisons. *Journal of the American Statistical Association* **98**, 671–678.

Hu, F. and Rosenberger, W. F. (2006). *The Theory of Response-Adaptive Randomization in Clinical Trials*. New York: Wiley.

Hu, F. and Zhang, L. X. (2004). Asymptotic properties of doubly adaptive biased coin designs for multitreatment clinical trials. *The Annals of Statistics* **32**, 268–301.

Huang, X., Biswas, S., Oki, Y., Issa, J. P., and Berry, D. A. (2007). A parallel phase I/II clinical trial design for combination therapies. *Biometrics* **63**, 429–436.

Huang, Y. and Hsu, J. C. (2007). Hochberg's step-up method: Cutting corners off Holm's step-down method. *Biometrika* **94**, 965–975.

Hunsberger, S., Rubinstein, V. L., Dancey, J., and Korn, E. L.(2005). Dose escalation trial designs based on a molecularly targeted endpoint. *Statistics in Medicine* **24**, 2171–2181.

Ibrahim, J. G., Chen, M., and Sinha, D. (2001). *Bayesian Survival Analysis*. New York: Springer.

Inoue, L. Y. T., Thall, P. F., and Berry, D. A. (2002). Seamlessly expanding a randomized phase II trial to phase III. *Biometrics* **58**, 823–831.

Ishizuka, N. and Ohashi, Y. (2001). The continual reassessment method and its applications: A Bayesian methodology for phase I cancer clinical trials. *Statistics in Medicine* **20**, 2661–2681.

Ivanova, A. (2003). A play-the-winner type urn model with reduced variability. *Metrika* **58**, 1–13.

Jeffreys, H. (1961), *Theory of Probability*, 3rd ed. London: Oxford University Press.

Jennison, C. and Turnbull, B. W. (1989). Interim analyses: The repeated confidence interval approach (with discussion). *Journal of the Royal Statistical Society, Series B* **51**, 305–361.

Jennison, C. and Turnbull, B. W. (1997). Group-sequential analysis incorporating covariate information. *Journal of the American Statistical Association* **92**, 1330–1341.

Jennison, C. and Turnbull, B. W. (2000). *Group Sequential Methods with Applications to Clinical Trials*. Boca Raton, FL: Chapman & Hall/CRC.

Ji, Y. and Bekele, B. N. (2009). Adaptive randomization for multi-arm comparative clinical trials based on joint efficacy/toxicity outcomes. *Biometrics* **65**, 876–884.

Ji, Y., Li, Y., and Bekele, B. N. (2007). Dose-finding in phase I clinical trials based on toxicity probability intervals. *Clinical Trials* **4**, 235–244.

Ji, Y., Li, Y., and Yin, G. (2007). Bayesian dose finding in phase I clinical trials based on a new statistical framework. *Statistica Sinica* **17**, 531–547.

Jiang, W., Freidlin, B., and Simon, R. (2007). Biomarker-adaptive threshold design: A procedure for evaluating treatment with possible biomarker-defined subset effect. *Journal of National Cancer Institute* **99**, 1036–1043.

Julious, S. A. (2010). *Sample Sizes for Clinical Trials*. Boca Raton, FL: Chapman & Hall/CRC.

Kalbfleisch, J. D. and Prentice, R. L. (2002). *The Statistical Analysis of Failure Time Data*, 2nd ed. New York: John Wiley.

Kaplan, E. L. and Meier, P. (1958). Non-parametric estimation from incomplete observations. *Journal of the American Statistical Association* **53**, 457–481.

Kass, R. E. and Raftery, A. E. (1995). Bayes factors. *Journal of the American Statistical Association* **90**, 773–795.

Kelly, J. A., Spielberg, F., and McAuliffe, T. L. (2008). Defining, designing, implementing, and evaluating phase 4 HIV prevention effectiveness trials for vulnerable populations. *Journal of Acquired Immune Deficiency Syndromes* **47**, 28–33.

Kim, J.-Y. (2002). Limited information likelihood and Bayesian analysis. *Journal of Econometrics* **107**, 175–193.

Kopec, J. A., Abrahamowicz, M., and Esdaile, J. M. (1993). Randomized discontinuation trials: Utility and efficiency. *Journal of Clinical Epidemiology* **46**, 959–971.

Korn, E. L. (2004). Nontoxicity endpoints in phase I trial designs for targeted, non-cytotoxic agents. *Journal of the National Cancer Institute* **96**, 977–978.

Korn, E. L. and Freidlin, B. (2011) Outcome–adaptive randomization: Is it useful? *Journal of Clinical Oncology* **29**, 771–776.

Korn, E. L. and Simon, R. (1993). Using the tolerable-dose diagram in the design of Phase I combination chemotherapy trials. *Journal of Clinical Oncology* **11**, 794–801.

Korn, E. L., Arbuck, S. G., Pluda, J. M., Simon, R., Kaplan, R. S., and Christian, M. C. (2001). Clinical trial designs for cytostatic agents: Are new approaches needed? *Journal of Clinical Oncology* **19**, 265–272.

Kramar, A., Lebecq, A., and Candalh, E. (1999). Continual reassessment methods in phase I trials of the combination of two drugs in oncology. *Statistics in Medicine* **18**, 1849–1864.

Kuk, A. Y. C. and Chen, C. H. (1992). A mixture model combining logistic regression with proportional hazards regression. *Biometrika* **79**, 531–541.

Kuzuya, K., Ishikawa, H., Nakanishi, T., et al. (2001). Optimal doses of paclitaxel and carboplatin combination chemotherapy for ovarian cancer: A phase I modified continual reassessment method study. *International Journal of Clinical Oncology* **6**, 271–278.

Lachin, J. M. and Foulkes, M. A. (1986). Evaluation of sample size and power for analyses of survival with allowance for nonuniform patient entry, losses to follow-up, noncompliance, and stratification. *Biometrics* **42**, 507–519.

Lakatos, E. (1988). Sample sizes based on the log-rank statistic in complex clinical trials. *Biometrics* **44**, 229–241.

Lan, K. K. G. and DeMets, D. L. (1983). Discrete sequential boundaries for clinical trials. *Biometrika* **70**, 659–663.

Lee, J. J., Gu, X., and Liu, S. (2010). Bayesian adaptive randomization designs for targeted agent development. **7**, 584–596.

Lee, J. J., Kong, M., Ayers, G. D., and Lotan, R. (2007). Interaction index and different methods for determining drug interaction in combination therapy. *Journal of Biopharmaceutical Statistics* **17**, 461–480.

Lee, J. J. and Liu, D. D. (2008). A predictive probability design for phase II cancer clinical trials *Clinical Trials* **5**, 93–106.

Lehmacher, W. and Wassmer, G. (1999). Adaptive sample size calculations in group sequential trials. *Biometrics* **55**, 1286–1290.

Lei, X., Yuan, Y., and Yin, G. (2011). Bayesian phase II clinical trial design with time-to-event adaptive randomization. *Lifetime Data Analysis* **17**, 156–174.

Leung, D. H.-Y. and Wang, Y.-G. (2002). An extension of the continual reassessment method using decision theory. *Statistics in Medicine* **21**, 51–63.

Li, Y., Bekele, B. N., Ji, Y., and Cook, J. D. (2008). Dose-schedule finding in phase I/II clinical trials using a Bayesian isotonic transformation. *Statistics in Medicine* **27**, 4895–4913.

Liang, K. Y. and Zeger, S. L. (1986). Longitudinal data analysis using generalized linear models. *Biometrika* **73**, 13–22.

Lin, Y. and Shih, W. J. (2001). Statistical properties of the traditional algorithm-based designs for phase I cancer clinical trials. *Biostatistics* **2**, 203–215.

Lind, J. (1753). *A Treatise of the Scurvy*. Edinburgh: Sands, Murray, Cochran. Reprinted in *Lind's Treatise on Scurvy*, C. P. Stewart and D. Guthrie, eds. Edinburgh: Edinburgh University Press.

Lindley, D. V. and Phillips, L. D. (1976). Inference for a Bernoulli process (a Bayesian view). *American Statistician* **30**, 112–119.

Little, R. J. A. and Rubin, D. B. (2002). *Statistical Analysis with Missing Data*, 2nd ed. New York: Wiley.

Liu, A., Shih, W. J., and Gehan, E. A. (2002). Sample size and power determination for clustered repeated measurements. *Statistics in Medicine* **21**, 1787–1801.

Liu, G. and Liang, K. Y. (1997). Sample size calculations for studies with correlated observations. *Biometrics* **53**, 937–947.

Liu, Q. and Chi, G. Y. H. (2001). On sample size and inference for two-stage adaptive designs. *Biometrics* **57**, 172–177.

Liu, Q. and Pledger, G. W. (2005). Phase 2 and 3 combination designs to accelerate drug development. *Journal of the American Statistical Association* **100**, 493–502.

Loewe, S. (1953). The problem of synergism and antagonism of combined drugs. *Arzeim Forsch* **3**, 285–290.

Lokich, J. (2001). Phase I clinical trial of weekly combined topotecan and irinotecan. *American Journal Clinical Oncology* **24**, 336–340.

Louis, T. A. (1977). Sequential allocation in clinical trials comparing two exponential survival curves. *Biometrics* **33**, 627–634.

Madigan, D. and Raftery, A. E. (1994). Model selection and accounting for model uncertainty in graphical models using Occam's window. *Journal of the American Statistical Association* **89**, 1535–1546.

Maller, R. A. and Zhou, X. (1996). *Survival Analysis with Long-Term Survivors*. New York: Wiley.

Mandrekar, S. J. and Sargent, D. J. (2009). Clinical trial designs for predictive biomarker validation: Theoretical considerations and practical challenges. *Journal of Clinical Oncology* **27**, 4027–4034.

Marcus, R., Peritz, E., and Gabriel, K. R. (1976). On closed testing procedures with special reference to ordered analysis of variance. *Biometrika* **63**, 655–660.

Mauguen, A., Le Deleya, M. C., and Zohar, S. (2011). Dose-finding approach for dose escalation with overdose control considering incomplete observations. *Statistics in Medicine* **30**, 1584–1594.

McCullagh, P. (1983). Quasi-likelihood function. *The Annals of Statistics* **11**, 59-67.

McCullagh, P. and Nelder, J. A. (1989). *Generalized Linear Models*, 2nd ed. London: Chapman & Hall.

Medical Research Council (1948). Streptomycin treatment of pulmonary tuberculosis. *British Medical Journal* **2**, 769–782.

Melfi, V., Page, C., and Geraldes, M. (2001). An adaptive randomized design with application to estimation. *Canadian Journal of Statistics* **29**, 107–116.

Metropolis, N., Rosenbluth, A. W., Rosenbluth, M. N., Teller, A. H., and Teller, E. (1953). Equations of state calculations by fast computing machines. *Journal of Chemical Physics* **21**, 1087–1092.

Mok, T. S., Wu, Y.-L., Thongprasert, S., et al. (2009). Gefitinib or carboplatin–paclitaxel in pulmonary adenocarcinoma. *The New England Journal of Medicine* **361**, 947–957.

Møller, S. (1995). An extension of the continual reassessment methods using a preliminary up-and-down design in a dose finding study in cancer patients, in order to investigate a greater range of doses. *Statistics in Medicine* **14**, 911–922.

Morgan, B. J. T. (1992). *Analysis of Quantal Response Data*. London: Chapman & Hall.

Moyé, L. A. (2003) *Multiple Analyses in Clinical Trials: Fundamentals for Investigators*. New York: Springer-Verlag.

Muler, J. H., McGinn, C. J., Normolle, D. Lawrence, T., Brown, D., Hejna, G., and Zalupski, M. M. (2004). Phase I trial using a time-to-event continual reassessment strategy for dose escalation of cisplatin combined with gemcitabine and radiation therapy in pancreatic cancer. *Journal of Clinical Oncology* **22**, 238–243.

Müller, H.-H. and Schäfer, H. (2001). Adaptive group sequential designs for clinical trials: Combining the advantages of adaptive and of classical group sequential approaches. *Biometrics* **57**, 886–891.

Murtaugh, P. A. and Fisher, L. D. (1990). Bivariate binary models of efficacy and toxicity in dose-ranging trials. *Communications in Statistics, Theory and Methods* **19**, 2003–2020.

Nelsen, R. B. (1999). *An Introduction to Copulas*. New York: Springer-Verlag.

Ning, J. and Huang, X. (2010). Response-adaptive randomization for clinical trials with adjustment for covariate imbalance. *Statistics in Medicine* **29**, 1761–1768.

O'Brien, P. C. and Fleming, T. R. (1979). A multiple testing procedure for clinical trials. *Biometrics* **35**, 549–556.

O'Quigley, J. and Chevret, S. (1991). Methods for dose finding studies in cancer clinical trials: A review and results of a Monte Carlo study. *Statistics in Medicine* **10**, 1647–1664.

O'Quigley, J., Hughes, M. D., and Fenton, T. (2001). Dose-finding designs for HIV studies. *Biometrics* **57**, 1018–1029.

O'Quigley, J. and Paoletti, X. (2003). Continual reassessment method for ordered groups. *Biometrics* **59**, 430-440.

O'Quigley, J., Pepe, M., and Fisher, L. D. (1990). Continual reassessment method: A practical design for Phase I clinical trials in cancer. *Biometrics* **46**, 33–48.

O'Quigley, J. and Shen, L. Z. (1996). Continual reassessment method: A likelihood approach. *Biometrics* **52**, 673–684.

Piantadosi, S. (2005). *Clinical Trials: A Methodologic Perspective.* 2nd ed. New York: John Wiley & Sons.

Piantadosi, S., Fisher, J., and Grossman, S. (1998). Practical implementation of a modified continual reassessment method for dose finding trials. *Cancer Chemotherapy and Pharmacology* **41**, 429–436.

Plackett, R. L. and Hewlett, P. S. (1967). A comparison of two approaches to the construction of models for quantal responses to mixtures of drugs. *Biometrics* **23**, 27–44.

Pocock, S. J. (1977). Group sequential methods in the design and analysis of clinical trials. *Biometrika* **64**, 191–199.

Pocock, S. J. and Simon, R. (1975). Sequential treatment assignment with balancing for prognostic factors in the controlled clinical trials. *Biometrics* **31**, 103–115.

Portnoy, S. (2003). Censored regression quantiles. *Journal of the American Statistical Association* **98**, 1001–1012.

Posch, M. and Bauer, P. (2000). Interim analysis and sample size reassessment. *Biometrics* **56**, 1170–1176.

Proschan, M. A. and Hunsberger, S. A. (1995). Designed extension of studies based on conditional power. *Biometrics* **51**, 1315–1324.

Raftery, A. E., Madigan, D., and Hoeting, J. A. (1997). Bayesian model averaging for linear regression models. *Journal of the American Statistical Association* **92**, 179–191.

Ratain, M. J. and Sargent, D. J. (2009). Optimising the design of phase II oncology trials: the importance of randomisation. *European Journal of Cancer* **45**, 275–280.

Robbins, H. (1952). Some aspects of the sequential design of experiments. *Bulletin of the American Mathematical Society* **58**, 527–535.

Rochon, J. (1991). Sample size calculations for two-group repeated-measures experiments. *Biometrics* **47**, 1383–1398.

Rosenberger, W. F. (1996). New directions in adaptive designs. *Statistical Science* **11**, 137–149.

Rosenberger, W. F. and Lachin, J. M. (2002). *Randomization in Clinical Trials: Theory and Practice.* New York: John Wiley & Sons.

Rosenberger, W. F., Stallard, N., Ivanova, A., Harper, C., and Ricks, M. (2001). Optimal adaptive designs for binary response trials. *Biometrics* **57**, 909–913.

Rosner, G. L., Stadler, W., and Ratain, M. J. (2002). Randomized discontinuation design: Application to cytostatic antineoplastic agents. *Journal of Clinical Oncology* **20**, 4478–4484.

Saijo, N., Takeuchi, M., and Kunitoh, H. (2009). Reasons for response differences seen in the V15-32, INTEREST and IPASS trials. *Nature Reviews Clinical Oncology* **6**, 287–294.

Sargent, D. J., Conley, B. A., Allegra, C., and Collette, L. (2005). Clinical trial designs for predictive marker validation in cancer treatment trials. *Journal of Clinical Oncology* **23**, 2020–2027.

Sarkar, S. (1998). Some probability inequalities for ordered MTP2 random variables: A proof of the Simes conjecture. *The Annals of Statistics* **26**, 494–504.

Scharfstein, D. O., Tsiatis, A. A., and Robins, J. M. (1997). Semiparametric efficiency and its implication on the design and analysis of group sequential studies. *Journal of the American Statistical Association* **92**, 1342–1350.

Schoenfeld, D. (1981). The asymptotic properties of nonparametric tests for comparing survival distributions. *Biometrika* **68**, 316–319.

Self, S. G. and Mauritsen, R. H. (1988). Power/sample size calculations for generalized linear models. *Biometrics* **44**, 79–86.

Sen, P. K. and Singer, J. M. (1993). *Large Sample Methods in Statistics*. New York: Chapman & Hall.

Sessa, C. Capri, G., Gianni, L., Peccatori, F., Grasselli, G., Bauer, J., Zucchetti, M., Vigano, L., Gatti, A., Minoia, C., Liati, P., Van den Bosch, S., Bernareggi, A. and Camboni, G., and Marsoni, S. (2000). Clinical and pharmacological phase I study with accelerated titration design of a daily times five schedule of BBR3464, a novel cationic triplatinum complex. *Annals of Oncology* **11**, 977–983.

Shao, J., Yu, X., and Zhong, B. (2010). A theory for testing hypotheses under covariate-adaptive randomization. *Biometrika* **97**, 347–360.

Shen, L. Z. and O'Quigley, J. (1996). Consistency of continual reassessment method under model misspecification. *Biometrika* **83**, 395–405.

Shen, Y. and Fisher, L. (1999). Statistical inference for self-designing clinical trials with a one-sided hypothesis. *Biometrics* **55**, 190–197.

Shih, W. J. (1992). Sample size reestimation in clinical trials. In: *Biopharmaceutical Sequential Statistical Applications*, pp. 285–301. New York: Marcel Dekker.

Shih, W. J. (2001). Sample size re-estimation—journey for a decade. *Statistics in Medicine* **20**, 515–518.

Shun, Z., Yuan, W., Brady, W., and Hsu, H. (2001). Type I error in sample size re-estimations based on observed treatment difference. *Statistics in Medicine* **20**, 497–513.

Simon, R. (1979). Restricted randomization in clinical trials. *Biometrics* **35**, 503–512.

Simon, R. (1989). Optimal two-stage designs for phase II clinical trials. *Controlled Clinical Trials* **10**, 1–10.

Simon, R. (2009). Advances in clinical trial designs for predictive biomarker discovery and validation. *Current Breast Cancer Reports* **1**, 216–221.

Simon, R., Freidlin, B., Rubinstein, L. V., Arbuck, S., Collins, J., and Christian, M. (1997). Accelerated titration designs for phase I clinical trials in oncology. *Journal of the National Cancer Institute* **89**, 1138–1147.

Storer, B. E. (1989). Design and analysis of Phase I clinical trials. *Biometrics* **45**, 925–937.

Spiegelhalter, D. J., Abrams, K. R., and Myles, J. P. (2004). *Bayesian Approaches to Clinical Trials and Health-Care Evaluation*. England: John Wiley & Sons.

Spiegelhalter, D. J., Best, N. G., Carlin, B. P., and van der Linde, A. (2002). Bayesian measures of model complexity and fit. *Journal of the Royal Statistical Society, Series B* **64**, 583–616.

Strom, B. L. (2006). How the US drug safety system should be changed. *Journal of American Medical Association* **295**, 2072–2074.

Stylianou, M. and Flournoy, N. (2002). Dose finding using the biased coin up-and-down design and isotonic regression. *Biometrics* **58**, 171–177.

Sun, J. (2006). *The Statistical Analysis of Interval-Censored Failure Time Data*. New York: Springer.

Tan, M., Fang, H., Tian, G., and Houghton, P. J. (2003). Experimental design and sample size determination for testing synergism in drug combination studies based on uniform measures. *Statistics in Medicine* **22**, 2091–2100.

Tanner, M. A. and Wong, W. H. (1987). The calculation of posterior distributions by data augmentation (with discussion). *Journal of the American Statistical Association* **82**, 528–550.

Taves, D. R. (1974). Minimization: A new method of assigning patients to treatment and control groups. *Clinical Pharmacology and Therapeutics* **15**, 443-453.

Taylor, J. M. G. (1995). Semi-parametric estimation in failure time mixture models. *Biometrics* **51**, 899–907.

Thall, P. F. and Cook, J. (2004). Dose-finding based on toxicity-efficacy trade-offs. *Biometrics* **60**, 684–693.

Thall, P. F., Millikan, R. E., Müller, P., and Lee, S.-J. (2003). Dose-finding with two agents in phase I oncology trials. *Biometrics* **59**, 487–496.

Thall, P. F. and Russell, K. E. (1998). A strategy for dose-finding and safety monitoring based on efficacy and adverse outcomes in phase I/II clinical trials. *Biometrics* **54**, 251–264.

Thall, P. F. and Simon, R. (1994). Practical Bayesian guidelines for phase IIB clinical trials. *Biometrics* **50**, 337–349.

Thall, P. F., Simon, R., and Estey, E. H. (1995). Bayesian sequential monitoring designs for single-arm clinical trials with multiple outcomes. *Statistics in Medicine* **14**, 357–379.

Thall, P. F. and Wathen, K. J. (2007). Practical Bayesian adaptive randomisation in clinical trials. *European Journal of Cancer* **43**, 859–866.

Thompson, W. R. (1933). On the likelihood that one unknown probability exceeds another in the revises of the evidence of the two samples. *Biometrika* **25**, 275–294.

Therneau, T. M. (1993) How many stratification factors are "too many" to use in a randomization plan? *Controlled Clinical Trials* **14**, 98–108.

Ting, N. (2006). *Dose Finding in Drug Development*. New York: Springer.

Tsiatis, A. A. and Mehta, C. (2003). On the inefficiency of the adaptive design for monitoring clinical trials. *Biometrika* **90**, 367–378.

Tsodikov, A. (1998). A proportional hazards model taking account of long-term survivors. *Biometrics* **54**, 1508–1516.

Vieta, E., Martinez-Aran, A., Goikolea, J. M., Torrent, C., Colom, F., Benabarre, A., and Reinares, M. (2002). A randomized trial comparing paroxetine and venlafaxine in the treatment of bipolar depressed patients taking mood stabilizers. *Journal of Clinical Psychiatry* **63**, 508–512.

Vonesh, E. F. and Schork, M. A. (1986). Sample sizes in the multivariate analysis of repeated measurements. *Biometrics* **42**, 601–610.

Wang, H. and Wang, L. (2009). Locally weighted censored quantile regression. *Journal of the American Statistical Association* **104**, 1117–1128.

Ware, J. H. and Hamel, M. B. (2011). Pragmatic trials—guides to better patient care? *The New England Journal of Medicine* **364**, 1685–1687.

Wassmer, G. (1998). A comparison of two methods for adaptive interim analyses in clinical trials. *Biometrics* **54**, 696–705.

Wang, K. and Ivanova, A. (2005). Two-dimensional dose finding in discrete dose space. *Biometrics* **61**, 217–222.

Wang, S. K. and Tsiatis, A. A. (1987). Approximately optimal one-parameter boundaries for group sequential trials. *Biometrics* **43**, 193–199.

Wedderburn, R. W. M. (1974). Quasi-likelihood functions, generalized linear models, and the Gauss-Newton method. *Biometrika* **61**, 439–447.

Wei, L. J. (1978). The adaptive biased coin design for sequential experiments. *The Annals of Statistics* **6**, 92-100.

Wei, L. J. and Durham, S. (1978). The randomized play-the-winner rule in medical trials. *Journal of the American Statistical Association* **73**, 840–843.

Whitehead, J. and Brunier, H. (1995). Bayesian decision procedures for dose determining experiments. *Statistics in Medicine* **14**, 885–893.

Whitehead, J. and Stratton, I. (1983). Group sequential clinical trials with triangular continuation regions. *Biometrics* **39**, 227–236.

Wilson, T. W., Lacourcière, Y., and Barnes, C. C. (1998). The antihypertensive efficacy of losartan and amlodipine assessed with office and ambulatory blood pressure monitoring. *Canadian Medical Association Journal* **159**, 469–476.

Yakovlev, A. Y., Asselain, B., Bardou, V. J., Fourquet, A., Hoang, T., Rochefediere, A., and Tsodikov, A. D. (1993). A simple stochastic model of tumour recurrence and its applications to data on premenopausal breast cancer. In: *Biometrie et Analyse de Dormees Spatio-Temporelles*, **12**, B. Asselain, M. Boniface, C. Duby, C. Lopez, J. P. Masson, and J. Tranchefort, (eds.), pp. 66–82. Société Francaise de Biométrie, ENSA Renned, France.

Yin, G. (2009). Bayesian generalized method of moments (with discussion). *Bayesian Analysis* **4**, 191–208; and Rejoinder, 217–222.

Yin, G., Chen, N., and Lee, J. J. (2012). Phase II trial design using Bayesian adaptive randomization and predictive probability. *Journal of the Royal Statistical Society, Series C*, in press.

Yin, G. and Ibrahim, J. (2005). Cure rate models: A unified approach. *Canadian Journal of Statistics* **33**, 559–570.

Yin, G., Li, Y., and Ji, Y. (2006). Bayesian dose-finding in phase I/II trials using toxicity and efficacy odds ratio. *Biometrics* **62**, 777–784.

Yin, G., Ma, Y., Liang, F., and Yuan, Y. (2011). Stochastic generalized method of moments. *Journal of Computational and Graphical Statistics* **20**, 714–727.

Yin, G. and Shen, Y. (2005a). Adaptive design and estimation in randomized clinical trials with correlated observations. *Biometrics* **61**, 362–369.

Yin, G. and Shen, Y. (2005b). Self-designing trial combining with classical group sequential monitoring. *Journal of Biopharmaceutical Statistics* **15**, 667–675.

Yin, G. and Yuan, Y. (2009a). Bayesian model averaging continual reassessment method in phase I clinical trials. *Journal of the American Statistical Association* **104**, 954–968.

Yin, G. and Yuan, Y. (2009b). Bayesian dose-finding in oncology for drug combinations by copula regression. *Journal of the Royal Statistical Society, Series C* **58**, 211–224.

Yin, G. and Yuan, Y. (2009c). A latent contingency table approach to dose-finding for combinations of two agents. *Biometrics* **65**, 866–875.

Yin, G. and Yuan, Y. (2010a). Bayesian approach for adaptive design. In: *Handbook of Adaptive Designs in Pharmaceutical and Clinical Development*, A. Pong, and S.-C. Chow, (eds.), Chapter 3. pp. (3-1)–(3-19). Boca Raton, FL: Chapman & Hall/CRC.

Yin, G. and Yuan, Y. (2010b). Correspondence "Bayesian dose-finding in oncology for drug combinations by copula regression" by M. Gasparini, Bailey, S. and Neuenschwander, B. *Journal of Royal Statistical Society, Series C* **59**, 544–546.

Yin, G. and Zheng, S. (2011). Fractional dose-finding methods with incomplete outcomes in phase I clinical trials. *Technical report*, Department of Statistics and Actuarial Science at The University of Hong Kong.

Yuan, Y., Huang, X., and Liu, S. (2011). A Bayesian response-adaptive covariate-balanced randomization design with application to a leukemia clinical trial. *Statistics in Medicine* **30**, 1218–1229.

Yuan, Y. and Yin, G. (2008). Sequential continual reassessment method for two-dimensional dose finding. *Statistics in Medicine* **27**, 5664–5678.

Yuan, Y. and Yin, G. (2009). Bayesian dose finding by jointly modeling toxicity and efficacy as time-to-event outcomes. *Journal of Royal Statistical Society, Series C* **58**, 719–736.

Yuan, Y. and Yin, G. (2011a). Bayesian hybrid dose-finding design in phase I oncology clinical trials. *Statistics in Medicine* **30**, 2098–2108.

Yuan, Y. and Yin, G. (2011b). Phase I/II adaptively randomized oncology trials with combined drugs. *Annals of Applied Statistics* **5**, 924–942.

Yuan, Y. and Yin, G. (2011c). On the usefulness of outcome-adaptive randomization. *Journal of Clinical Oncology* **29**, e390–e392.

Yuan, Y. and Yin, G. (2011d). Robust EM continual reassessment method in oncology dose finding. *Journal of the American Statistical Association* **106**, 818–831.

Yuan, Z., Chappell, R., and Bailey, H. (2007). The continual reassessment method for multiple toxicity grades: A Bayesian quasi-likelihood approach. *Biometrics* **63**, 173–179.

Zelen, M. (1969). Play the winner rule and the controlled clinical trial. *Journal of the American Statistical Association* **64**, 131–146.

Zelen, M. and Wei, L. J. (1995). Foreword. In: *Adaptive Designs*. N. Flournoy and W. F. Rosenberger, (eds.), Hayward, CA: Institute of Mathematical Statistics.

Zellner, A. (1997). The Bayesian method of moments (BMOM): Theory and applications. *Advances in Econometrics* **12**, 85–105.

Zellner, A., Tobias, J., and Ryu, H. (1997). Bayesian method of moments (BMOM) analysis of parametric and semiparametric regression models. In *Proceedings of the Section on Bayesian Statistical Science*, pp. 211–216. Alexandria, VA: American Statistical Association.

Zhang, L. and Rosenberger, W. F. (2006). Response-adaptive randomization in clinical trials with continuous outcomes. *Biometrics* **62**, 562–569.

Zhang, L. and Rosenberger, W. F. (2007). Response–adaptive randomization for survival trials: the parametric approach. *Journal of Royal Statistical Society, Series C* **56**, 153–165.

Zhang, L. X., Chan, W. S., Cheung, S. H., and Hu, F. (2007). A generalized drop-the-loser urn for clinical trials with delayed responses. *Statistica Sinica* **17**, 387–409.

Zhou, X., Liu, S. Kim, E. S., Herbstc, R. S., and Lee J. J. (2008). Bayesian adaptive design for targeted therapy development in lung cancer—a step toward personalized medicine. *Clinical Trials* **5**, 181–193.

# AUTHOR INDEX

*Clinical Trial Design*. By Guosheng Yin
Copyright © 2012 John Wiley & Sons, Inc.

# SUBJECT INDEX

*Clinical Trial Design.* By Guosheng Yin
Copyright © 2012 John Wiley & Sons, Inc.

**333**

# WILEY SERIES IN PROBABILITY AND STATISTICS

ESTABLISHED BY WALTER A. SHEWHART AND SAMUEL S. WILKS

Editors: *David J. Balding, Noel A. C. Cressie, Garrett M. Fitzmaurice,*
*Harvey Goldstein, Iain M. Johnstone, Geert Molenberghs, David W. Scott,*
*Adrian F. M. Smith, Ruey S. Tsay, Sanford Weisberg*
Editors Emeriti: *Vic Barnett, J. Stuart Hunter, Joseph B. Kadane, Jozef L. Teugels*

The ***Wiley Series in Probability and Statistics*** is well established and authoritative. It covers many topics of current research interest in both pure and applied statistics and probability theory. Written by leading statisticians and institutions, the titles span both state-of-the-art developments in the field and classical methods.

Reflecting the wide range of current research in statistics, the series encompasses applied, methodological and theoretical statistics, ranging from applications and new techniques made possible by advances in computerized practice to rigorous treatment of theoretical approaches.

This series provides essential and invaluable reading for all statisticians, whether in academia, industry, government, or research.

† ABRAHAM and LEDOLTER · Statistical Methods for Forecasting
  AGRESTI · Analysis of Ordinal Categorical Data, *Second Edition*
  AGRESTI · An Introduction to Categorical Data Analysis, *Second Edition*
  AGRESTI · Categorical Data Analysis, *Second Edition*
  ALTMAN, GILL, and McDONALD · Numerical Issues in Statistical Computing for the
    Social Scientist
  AMARATUNGA and CABRERA · Exploration and Analysis of DNA Microarray and
    Protein Array Data
  ANDĚL · Mathematics of Chance
  ANDERSON · An Introduction to Multivariate Statistical Analysis, *Third Edition*
\* ANDERSON · The Statistical Analysis of Time Series
  ANDERSON, AUQUIER, HAUCK, OAKES, VANDAELE, and WEISBERG ·
    Statistical Methods for Comparative Studies
  ANDERSON and LOYNES · The Teaching of Practical Statistics
  ARMITAGE and DAVID (editors) · Advances in Biometry
  ARNOLD, BALAKRISHNAN, and NAGARAJA · Records
\* ARTHANARI and DODGE · Mathematical Programming in Statistics
\* BAILEY · The Elements of Stochastic Processes with Applications to the Natural
    Sciences
  BAJORSKI · Statistics for Imaging, Optics, and Photonics
  BALAKRISHNAN and KOUTRAS · Runs and Scans with Applications
  BALAKRISHNAN and NG · Precedence-Type Tests and Applications
  BARNETT · Comparative Statistical Inference, *Third Edition*
  BARNETT · Environmental Statistics
  BARNETT and LEWIS · Outliers in Statistical Data, *Third Edition*
  BARTOSZYNSKI and NIEWIADOMSKA-BUGAJ · Probability and Statistical Inference
  BASILEVSKY · Statistical Factor Analysis and Related Methods: Theory and
    Applications
  BASU and RIGDON · Statistical Methods for the Reliability of Repairable Systems
  BATES and WATTS · Nonlinear Regression Analysis and Its Applications
  BECHHOFER, SANTNER, and GOLDSMAN · Design and Analysis of Experiments for
    Statistical Selection, Screening, and Multiple Comparisons
  BEIRLANT, GOEGEBEUR, SEGERS, TEUGELS, and DE WAAL · Statistics of
    Extremes: Theory and Applications

\*Now available in a lower priced paperback edition in the Wiley Classics Library.
†Now available in a lower priced paperback edition in the Wiley–Interscience Paperback Series.

BELSLEY · Conditioning Diagnostics: Collinearity and Weak Data in Regression
† BELSLEY, KUH, and WELSCH · Regression Diagnostics: Identifying Influential
    Data and Sources of Collinearity
BENDAT and PIERSOL · Random Data: Analysis and Measurement Procedures,
    *Fourth Edition*
BERNARDO and SMITH · Bayesian Theory
BERRY, CHALONER, and GEWEKE · Bayesian Analysis in Statistics and
    Econometrics: Essays in Honor of Arnold Zellner
BHAT and MILLER · Elements of Applied Stochastic Processes, *Third Edition*
BHATTACHARYA and WAYMIRE · Stochastic Processes with Applications
BIEMER, GROVES, LYBERG, MATHIOWETZ, and SUDMAN · Measurement Errors
    in Surveys
BILLINGSLEY · Convergence of Probability Measures, *Second Edition*
BILLINGSLEY · Probability and Measure, *Third Edition*
BIRKES and DODGE · Alternative Methods of Regression
BISGAARD and KULAHCI · Time Series Analysis and Forecasting by Example
BISWAS, DATTA, FINE, and SEGAL · Statistical Advances in the Biomedical Sciences:
    Clinical Trials, Epidemiology, Survival Analysis, and Bioinformatics
BLISCHKE AND MURTHY (editors) · Case Studies in Reliability and Maintenance
BLISCHKE AND MURTHY · Reliability: Modeling, Prediction, and Optimization
BLOOMFIELD · Fourier Analysis of Time Series: An Introduction, *Second Edition*
BOLLEN · Structural Equations with Latent Variables
BOLLEN and CURRAN · Latent Curve Models: A Structural Equation Perspective
BOROVKOV · Ergodicity and Stability of Stochastic Processes
BOSQ and BLANKE · Inference and Prediction in Large Dimensions
BOULEAU · Numerical Methods for Stochastic Processes
BOX · Bayesian Inference in Statistical Analysis
BOX · Improving Almost Anything, *Revised Edition*
BOX · R. A. Fisher, the Life of a Scientist
BOX and DRAPER · Empirical Model-Building and Response Surfaces
\* BOX and DRAPER · Evolutionary Operation: A Statistical Method for Process
    Improvement
BOX and DRAPER · Response Surfaces, Mixtures, and Ridge Analyses, *Second Edition*
BOX, HUNTER, and HUNTER · Statistics for Experimenters: Design, Innovation,
    and Discovery, *Second Editon*
BOX, JENKINS, and REINSEL · Time Series Analysis: Forcasting and Control, *Fourth*
    *Edition*
BOX, LUCEÑO, and PANIAGUA-QUIÑONES · Statistical Control by Monitoring
    and Adjustment, *Second Edition*
BRANDIMARTE · Numerical Methods in Finance: A MATLAB-Based Introduction
† BROWN and HOLLANDER · Statistics: A Biomedical Introduction
BRUNNER, DOMHOF, and LANGER · Nonparametric Analysis of Longitudinal Data in
    Factorial Experiments
BUCKLEW · Large Deviation Techniques in Decision, Simulation, and Estimation
CAIROLI and DALANG · Sequential Stochastic Optimization
CASTILLO, HADI, BALAKRISHNAN, and SARABIA · Extreme Value and Related
    Models with Applications in Engineering and Science
CHAN · Time Series: Applications to Finance with R and S-Plus®, *Second Edition*
CHARALAMBIDES · Combinatorial Methods in Discrete Distributions
CHATTERJEE and HADI · Regression Analysis by Example, *Fourth Edition*
CHATTERJEE and HADI · Sensitivity Analysis in Linear Regression
CHERNICK · Bootstrap Methods: A Guide for Practitioners and Researchers,
    *Second Edition*
CHERNICK and FRIIS · Introductory Biostatistics for the Health Sciences

\*Now available in a lower priced paperback edition in the Wiley Classics Library.
†Now available in a lower priced paperback edition in the Wiley–Interscience Paperback Series.

\*Now available in a lower priced paperback edition in the Wiley Classics Library.

†Now available in a lower priced paperback edition in the Wiley–Interscience Paperback Series.

EDLER and KITSOS · Recent Advances in Quantitative Methods in Cancer and Human
  Health Risk Assessment
\* ELANDT-JOHNSON and JOHNSON · Survival Models and Data Analysis
ENDERS · Applied Econometric Time Series
† ETHIER and KURTZ · Markov Processes: Characterization and Convergence
EVANS, HASTINGS, and PEACOCK · Statistical Distributions, *Third Edition*
EVERITT · Cluster Analysis, *Fifth Edition*
FELLER · An Introduction to Probability Theory and Its Applications, Volume I,
  *Third Edition,* Revised; Volume II, *Second Edition*
FISHER and VAN BELLE · Biostatistics: A Methodology for the Health Sciences
FITZMAURICE, LAIRD, and WARE · Applied Longitudinal Analysis, *Second Edition*
\* FLEISS · The Design and Analysis of Clinical Experiments
FLEISS · Statistical Methods for Rates and Proportions, *Third Edition*
† FLEMING and HARRINGTON · Counting Processes and Survival Analysis
FUJIKOSHI, ULYANOV, and SHIMIZU · Multivariate Statistics: High-Dimensional and
  Large-Sample Approximations
FULLER · Introduction to Statistical Time Series, *Second Edition*
† FULLER · Measurement Error Models
GALLANT · Nonlinear Statistical Models
GEISSER · Modes of Parametric Statistical Inference
GELMAN and MENG · Applied Bayesian Modeling and Causal Inference from
  Incomplete-Data Perspectives
GEWEKE · Contemporary Bayesian Econometrics and Statistics
GHOSH, MUKHOPADHYAY, and SEN · Sequential Estimation
GIESBRECHT and GUMPERTZ · Planning, Construction, and Statistical Analysis of
  Comparative Experiments
GIFI · Nonlinear Multivariate Analysis
GIVENS and HOETING · Computational Statistics
GLASSERMAN and YAO · Monotone Structure in Discrete-Event Systems
GNANADESIKAN · Methods for Statistical Data Analysis of Multivariate Observations,
  *Second Edition*
GOLDSTEIN · Multilevel Statistical Models, *Fourth Edition*
GOLDSTEIN and LEWIS · Assessment: Problems, Development, and Statistical Issues
GOLDSTEIN and WOOFF · Bayes Linear Statistics
GREENWOOD and NIKULIN · A Guide to Chi-Squared Testing
GROSS, SHORTLE, THOMPSON, and HARRIS · Fundamentals of Queueing Theory,
  *Fourth Edition*
GROSS, SHORTLE, THOMPSON, and HARRIS · Solutions Manual to Accompany
  Fundamentals of Queueing Theory, *Fourth Edition*
\* HAHN and SHAPIRO · Statistical Models in Engineering
HAHN and MEEKER · Statistical Intervals: A Guide for Practitioners
HALD · A History of Probability and Statistics and their Applications Before 1750
HALD · A History of Mathematical Statistics from 1750 to 1930
† HAMPEL · Robust Statistics: The Approach Based on Influence Functions
HANNAN and DEISTLER · The Statistical Theory of Linear Systems
HARMAN and KULKARNI · An Elementary Introduction to Statistical Learning Theory
HARTUNG, KNAPP, and SINHA · Statistical Meta-Analysis with Applications
HEIBERGER · Computation for the Analysis of Designed Experiments
HEDAYAT and SINHA · Design and Inference in Finite Population Sampling
HEDEKER and GIBBONS · Longitudinal Data Analysis
HELLER · MACSYMA for Statisticians
HERITIER, CANTONI, COPT, and VICTORIA-FESER · Robust Methods in
  Biostatistics

HINKELMANN and KEMPTHORNE · Design and Analysis of Experiments, Volume 1: Introduction to Experimental Design, *Second Edition*

HINKELMANN and KEMPTHORNE · Design and Analysis of Experiments, Volume 2: Advanced Experimental Design

HINKELMANN (editor) · Design and Analysis of Experiments, Volume 3: Special Designs and Applications

HOAGLIN, MOSTELLER, and TUKEY · Fundamentals of Exploratory Analysis of Variance

\* HOAGLIN, MOSTELLER, and TUKEY · Exploring Data Tables, Trends and Shapes

\* HOAGLIN, MOSTELLER, and TUKEY · Understanding Robust and Exploratory Data Analysis

HOCHBERG and TAMHANE · Multiple Comparison Procedures

HOCKING · Methods and Applications of Linear Models: Regression and the Analysis of Variance, *Second Edition*

HOEL · Introduction to Mathematical Statistics, *Fifth Edition*

HOGG and KLUGMAN · Loss Distributions

HOLLANDER and WOLFE · Nonparametric Statistical Methods, *Second Edition*

HOSMER and LEMESHOW · Applied Logistic Regression, *Second Edition*

HOSMER, LEMESHOW, and MAY · Applied Survival Analysis: Regression Modeling of Time-to-Event Data, *Second Edition*

HUBER · Data Analysis: What Can Be Learned From the Past 50 Years

HUBER · Robust Statistics

† HUBER and RONCHETTI · Robust Statistics, *Second Edition*

HUBERTY · Applied Discriminant Analysis, *Second Edition*

HUBERTY and OLEJNIK · Applied MANOVA and Discriminant Analysis, *Second Edition*

HUITEMA · The Analysis of Covariance and Alternatives: Statistical Methods for Experiments, Quasi-Experiments, and Single-Case Studies, *Second Edition*

HUNT and KENNEDY · Financial Derivatives in Theory and Practice, *Revised Edition*

HURD and MIAMEE · Periodically Correlated Random Sequences: Spectral Theory and Practice

HUSKOVA, BERAN, and DUPAC · Collected Works of Jaroslav Hajek— with Commentary

HUZURBAZAR · Flowgraph Models for Multistate Time-to-Event Data

IMAN and CONOVER · A Modern Approach to Statistics

† JACKMAN · Bayesian Analysis for the Social Sciences

† JACKSON · A User's Guide to Principle Components

JOHN · Statistical Methods in Engineering and Quality Assurance

JOHNSON · Multivariate Statistical Simulation

JOHNSON and BALAKRISHNAN · Advances in the Theory and Practice of Statistics: A Volume in Honor of Samuel Kotz

JOHNSON and BHATTACHARYYA · Statistics: Principles and Methods, *Fifth Edition*

JOHNSON, KEMP, and KOTZ · Univariate Discrete Distributions, *Third Edition*

JOHNSON and KOTZ · Distributions in Statistics

JOHNSON and KOTZ (editors) · Leading Personalities in Statistical Sciences: From the Seventeenth Century to the Present

JOHNSON, KOTZ, and BALAKRISHNAN · Continuous Univariate Distributions, Volume 1, *Second Edition*

JOHNSON, KOTZ, and BALAKRISHNAN · Continuous Univariate Distributions, Volume 2, *Second Edition*

JOHNSON, KOTZ, and BALAKRISHNAN · Discrete Multivariate Distributions

JUDGE, GRIFFITHS, HILL, LÜTKEPOHL, and LEE · The Theory and Practice of Econometrics, *Second Edition*

JUREČKOVÁ and SEN · Robust Statistical Procedures: Aymptotics and Interrelations

*Now available in a lower priced paperback edition in the Wiley Classics Library.

†Now available in a lower priced paperback edition in the Wiley–Interscience Paperback Series.

*Now available in a lower priced paperback edition in the Wiley Classics Library.

†Now available in a lower priced paperback edition in the Wiley–Interscience Paperback Series.

*Now available in a lower priced paperback edition in the Wiley Classics Library.

†Now available in a lower priced paperback edition in the Wiley–Interscience Paperback Series.

    * RUBIN · Multiple Imputation for Nonresponse in Surveys

    RUBINSTEIN and KROESE · Simulation and the Monte Carlo Method, *Second Edition*

    RUBINSTEIN and MELAMED · Modern Simulation and Modeling

    RYAN · Modern Engineering Statistics

    RYAN · Modern Experimental Design

    RYAN · Modern Regression Methods, *Second Edition*

    RYAN · Statistical Methods for Quality Improvement, *Third Edition*

    SALEH · Theory of Preliminary Test and Stein-Type Estimation with Applications

    SALTELLI, CHAN, and SCOTT (editors) · Sensitivity Analysis

    * SCHEFFE · The Analysis of Variance

    SCHIMEK · Smoothing and Regression: Approaches, Computation, and Application

    SCHOTT · Matrix Analysis for Statistics, *Second Edition*

    SCHOUTENS · Levy Processes in Finance: Pricing Financial Derivatives

    SCHUSS · Theory and Applications of Stochastic Differential Equations

    SCOTT · Multivariate Density Estimation: Theory, Practice, and Visualization

    * SEARLE · Linear Models

    † SEARLE · Linear Models for Unbalanced Data

    † SEARLE · Matrix Algebra Useful for Statistics

    † SEARLE, CASELLA, and McCULLOCH · Variance Components

    SEARLE and WILLETT · Matrix Algebra for Applied Economics

    SEBER · A Matrix Handbook For Statisticians

    † SEBER · Multivariate Observations

    SEBER and LEE · Linear Regression Analysis, *Second Edition*

    † SEBER and WILD · Nonlinear Regression

    SENNOTT · Stochastic Dynamic Programming and the Control of Queueing Systems

    * SERFLING · Approximation Theorems of Mathematical Statistics

    SHAFER and VOVK · Probability and Finance: It's Only a Game!

    SHERMAN · Spatial Statistics and Spatio-Temporal Data: Covariance Functions and Directional Properties

    SILVAPULLE and SEN · Constrained Statistical Inference: Inequality, Order, and Shape Restrictions

    SINGPURWALLA · Reliability and Risk: A Bayesian Perspective

    SMALL and McLEISH · Hilbert Space Methods in Probability and Statistical Inference

    SRIVASTAVA · Methods of Multivariate Statistics

    STAPLETON · Linear Statistical Models, *Second Edition*

    STAPLETON · Models for Probability and Statistical Inference: Theory and Applications

    STAUDTE and SHEATHER · Robust Estimation and Testing

    STOYAN, KENDALL, and MECKE · Stochastic Geometry and Its Applications, *Second Edition*

    STOYAN and STOYAN · Fractals, Random Shapes and Point Fields: Methods of Geometrical Statistics

    STREET and BURGESS · The Construction of Optimal Stated Choice Experiments: Theory and Methods

    STYAN · The Collected Papers of T. W. Anderson: 1943–1985

    SUTTON, ABRAMS, JONES, SHELDON, and SONG · Methods for Meta-Analysis in Medical Research

    TAKEZAWA · Introduction to Nonparametric Regression

    TAMHANE · Statistical Analysis of Designed Experiments: Theory and Applications

    TANAKA · Time Series Analysis: Nonstationary and Noninvertible Distribution Theory

    THOMPSON · Empirical Model Building: Data, Models, and Reality, *Second Edition*

    THOMPSON · Sampling, *Third Edition*

    THOMPSON · Simulation: A Modeler's Approach

    THOMPSON and SEBER · Adaptive Sampling

    THOMPSON, WILLIAMS, and FINDLAY · Models for Investors in Real World Markets

*Now available in a lower priced paperback edition in the Wiley Classics Library.

†Now available in a lower priced paperback edition in the Wiley–Interscience Paperback Series.

Printed and bound by CPI Group (UK) Ltd, Croydon, CR0 4YY

16/04/2025

14658535-0004